Finnie's Handling the Young Child with Cerebral Palsy at Home

Commissioning Editor: *Rita Demetriou-Swanwick*
Associate Editor: *Siobhan Campbell*
Development Editor: *Veronika Watkins*
Project Manager: *Sukanthi Sukumar*
Designer: *Charles Gray*
Illustration Manager: *Kirsteen Wright*
Illustrator: *Annabel Milne*

Finnie's Handling the Young Child with Cerebral Palsy at Home

Fourth Edition

Edited by

Eva Bower
PhD FCSP
Honorary Senior Lecturer, School of Health
Professions and Rehabilitation Sciences,
University of Southampton, Southampton, UK

Illustrated by

Annabel Milne

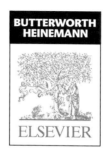

BUTTERWORTH
HEINEMANN

ELSEVIER

EDINBURGH LONDON NEW YORK OXFORD PHILADELPHIA ST LOUIS SYDNEY TORONTO 2009

BUTTERWORTH
HEINEMANN
ELSEVIER

An imprint of Elsevier Ltd.

First edition 1968
Second edition 1974
Third edition 1997
Fourth edition 2009

ISBN: 978-0-7506-8810-9

British Library Cataloguing in Publication Data
A catalogue record for this book is available from the British Library

Library of Congress Cataloging in Publication Data
A catalog record for this book is available from the Library of Congress

Notice
Knowledge and best practice in this field are constantly changing. As new research and experience broaden our knowledge, changes in practice, treatment and drug therapy may become necessary or appropriate. Readers are advised to check the most current information provided (i) on procedures featured or (ii) by the manufacturer of each product to be administered, to verify the recommended dose or formula, the method and duration of administration, and contraindications. It is the responsibility of the practitioner, relying on their own experience and knowledge of the patient, to make diagnoses, to determine dosages and the best treatment for each individual patient, and to take all appropriate safety precautions. To the fullest extent of the law, neither the Publisher nor the Editor or Contributors assume any liability for any injury and/or damage to persons or property arising out or related to any use of the material contained in this book. It is the responsibility of the treating practitioner, relying on independent expertise and knowledge of the patient, to determine the best treatment and method of application for the patient.

The Publisher

 ELSEVIER   your source for books, journals and multimedia in the health sciences
www.elsevierhealth.com

Working together to grow
libraries in developing countries

www.elsevier.com | www.bookaid.org | www.sabre.org

ELSEVIER   BOOK AID International   Sabre Foundation

The Publisher's policy is to use **paper manufactured from sustainable forests**

Printed in the United States of America

Transferred to Digital Printing, 2012

Contents

Contents

DEDICATION

Nancie Finnie was one of the first therapists to consider the problems of CP from a largely practical and functional point of view. The publication of the first edition of this book in 1968 was a landmark in the history of the management of young children with CP. Nancie understood the needs of young children at home, in their own environments, together with those of their parents and families. It is a great tribute to her that the book has stood the test of time, is still widely read today and has been translated into many different languages.

I feel privileged to have been entrusted with the job of editing this fourth edition and hope that I have done justice to it.

I dedicate this edition to the late Nancie Finnie.

The Nancie Finnie Charitable Trust (Registered Charity number 1082707)

The Trustees of the Nancie Finnie Charitable Trust invite applications from suitably qualified therapists wishing to undertake research in the area of rehabilitation of the child with cerebral palsy. Multidisciplinary projects are encouraged, but only research to be carried out in the United Kingdom can be supported.

Application forms can be obtained from 18 Nassau Road, Barnes, London SW13 9QE

List of contributors

J Bavin MB BS BSc FRC Psych DPM
Former Consultant Psychiatrist to Leavesden Hospital, Charing Cross Hospital, Hammersmith Hospital and Gloucestershire Area Health Authority

Jasia Beaumont RGN HVcert
Specialist Nurse, Southampton Children's Sleep Disorder Service, Southampton, UK

Eva Bower PhD FCSP
Honorary Senior Lecturer, School of Health Professions and Rehabilitation Sciences, University of Southampton, Southampton, UK

Mark Bower PhD FRCP FRCPath
Professor of Medical Oncology, Chelsea and Westminster Hospital, London, UK

Helen Cockerill BSc(Hons) MRCSLT
Consultant Speech and Language Therapist, Guy's and St Thomas', NHS Foundation Trust, London, UK

Caroline Fitzgerald RGN RSCN BSs(Hons)
Children's Community Nurse, Team Leader, Kensington and Chelsea Primary Care Trust, London, UK

Mary Gardner BSc (Econ) DipEd DipPsych
Honorary Child Psychologist, Charing Cross Hospital, London

Julia Graham MCSP MSc
Paediatric Therapy Services Manager, The Basingstoke and North Hampshire Hospital, Basingstoke, UK

Dido Green PhD MSc DipCOT
Research Training Fellow, NIHR GSTFT/KCL Biomedical Research Centre and Clinical Expert Paediatric Occupational Therapist, Newcomen Centre, Guy's Hospital, London, UK

Renzo Guerrini MD
Professor, Division of Child Neurology and Psychiatry, Director, Paediatric Neurology Unit and Laboratories, Children's Hospital A. Meyer-University of Florence, Italy

Rosie Kelly RSCN MSc Nursing
Paediatric Outreach Nurse, Evelina Children's Hospital, London, UK

Tara Kerr Elliott RN(Child) BSc(Hons) PGDip
Children's Palliative Care Nurse Specialist, Kensington and Chelsea Primary Care Trust, London

Ingeborg Krägeloh-Mann MD
Professor of Paediatrics, Director, University Children's Hospital, Director, Department of Paediatric Neurology and Developmental Medicine, Tübingen, Germany

Cathy Laver-Bradbury
SRN RSCN HV cert MSc Nursing
Consultant Nurse, Module Leader CAMHS, School of Nursing and Midwifery, University of Southampton, Southampton, UK

John F McLaughlin MD
Professor of Pediatrics, University of Washington and Children's Hospital and Regional Medical Center, Seattle, Washington, USA

Christopher Morris MSc DPhil
Principal Orthotist, Madigan Army Medical Center; MRC Training Fellow in Health Services Research, Department of Public Health and Junior Research Fellow, Wolfson College, University of Oxford

Simona Pellacani MD
Associated Researcher, Children's Hospital A. Meyer, Florence, Italy

Dinah Reddihough MD BSc FRACP FAFRM
Director of Developmental Medicine, Royal Children's Hospital, Victoria, Australia

Peter Rosenbaum MD FRCP(C)

Professor of Paediatrics, McMaster University, Canada Research Chair in Childhood Disability, CanChild Centre for Childhood Disability Research, Director, McMaster Child Health Research Institute, Hamilton, Ontario, Canada

Daniel S Roy MD

Fellow, Developmental and Behavioural Pediatrics, Madigan Army Medical Centre, Fort Lewis, Washington, USA

David Scrutton MSc MCSP

Former Honorary Senior Lecturer, Department of Neurosciences, The Institute of Child Health, University College London and Department of Paediatrics, Guy's, King's College & St. Thomas' Hospitals' Schools of Medicine, Dentistry & Biomedical Sciences, King's College, London, UK

Marko Wilke MD

Research Associate, University Children's Hospital, Tübingen, Germany

Anne J Wright

MBBCh MRCPCH MSc Community Paediatrics

Consultant Paediatrician, Evelina Children's Hospital, St Thomas Hospital, London, UK

Foreword

As the parent of a young disabled child, I first read and treasured Nancy Finnie's *Handling the Young Child with Cerebral Palsy at Home* in the early 1970s. The birth and diagnosis of a disabled child challenges the whole family. We, like Philip Larkin in his poem to a new goddaughter, just wanted our child to be '*ordinary, nothing special*'. But life was anything but ordinary and, living at the time in Central Africa, Nancy's book became our family bible! Suddenly our child was understandable; we had something with which to help the multiple and often confused professionals who wanted to help us and we had a sense of the future.

Life has changed in the past three decades since Simon's birth. Partnership with parents, '*the equivalent expertise of families and professionals*' as the late Professor Sheila Wolfendale described it, is seen as key to all children's futures. In England we have an *Early Support Programme*, with a strong focus on the active, welcome and supported engagement of parents as key players in their disabled child's growth and development. Disabled children are seen in public policy as having potential, and services and support for disabled people in general now focus on '*life chances*' and *outcomes* rather than the crisis intervention which characterised much of my son's early childhood.

But partnership with parents can be challenging. In the British Parliamentary Hearings which informed the DfES/Treasury's publication of *Aiming High*[1], parents talked of fragmented services; of multiple assessments and, as one mother put it, '*a feeling that if you have a disabled child, that child becomes a jigsaw, multiple pieces that don't always fit, and is no longer Lily or John, whole children belonging to a family with expectations for the future*'. Therefore, I warmly welcome this new edition. It not only emphasises the crucial importance of parent participation in the care and development of their child with cerebral palsy, but it also provides invaluable information for the multiple professionals and staff working in the voluntary sector who will become engaged in those families' lives.

As a former Director of the Council for Disabled Children, as a Disability Rights Commissioner and now as Chair of the British Prime Minister's Standing Commission on Carers, I acknowledge and welcome the thrust in public policy towards family support that acknowledges both practical and emotional needs. We now expect that disabled children could and should achieve the '*Every Child Matters*' five key outcomes but we are also all aware that the rhetoric is sometimes very different from the reality for the families who are coming to terms with diagnosis and what one parent described as '*the child we love but didn't expect!*'

Launching '*Aiming High*, the British Government emphasised the importance of ensuring that all children have the best start in life and the ongoing support that they and their families need to fulfil their potential. But it also acknowledged that '*disabled children and their families face a unique and often challenging set of circumstances that demand a unique and sometimes specialised response from both the universal and targeted services that support them*'. This new edition is particularly timely, for, as early years services expand; parents themselves are anxious to play proactive roles in improving outcomes for their disabled children but at the same time, families may have personal and emotional barriers which hinder their participation without high quality support.

---

[1] Aiming High for Disabled Children: Better Support for Families (May 2007), HM Treasury and DfES (available at hm-treasury.gov.uk)

In this edition, we have a new *'bible'*, which will help to transform the lives of many families and professionals as the earlier edition did for many others and myself. I am delighted to have been invited to write the foreword for a publication which I know will help us move towards the National Service Framework's Standard 8 ambition of *'an ordinary life'* for some very extraordinary children, parents and those who support them.

Philippa Russell,
July 2008

Acknowledgements

Firstly I wish to thank all the people who kindly gave both their expertise and time to write new chapters for this book.

Secondly I wish to thank Heidi Allen, Siobhan Campbell, Veronika Watkins, Glenys Norquay and Sukanthi Sukumar of Elsevier for their help and patience during the production of this book and Annabel Milne for undertaking the illustrations. Lastly, but not least, I wish to thank my grand-daughter Jessica for all her help with the typing and formatting and my husband John for his constant support.

Introduction

This book has been written to help the parents of a child with cerebral palsy (CP) assist their child towards achieving the most comfortable independence in all activities. It is hoped to show how, by using typical parenting skills, which involve guiding and exposing a child to develop through challenging experiences, the child with CP will also develop. The book is also intended to help professionals and other carers new to this field understand, support and encourage young children with CP and their families.

The book is not prescriptive, nor is it intended to supplant or substitute the interventions of the various professionals who will almost certainly be involved with your child.

Throughout the text the emphasis is not on diagnostic categories, although the terms are explained; rather the emphasis is on how children present to their parents and on the difficulties most commonly encountered. There are wide variations in the pressures found within a family and between families. I have tried to address the needs of the child while at the same time taking into account those of the family.

A good analogy during the early years (0–5 years of age are covered in this book) is that of a kaleidoscope, an ever-changing panorama of emotional, social, intellectual, communication and motor performance by the child. A time when lots of nice things are happening, sometimes clouded by the child's difficulties. A time for parents when the hours at home without the benefit of a professional's support can sometimes seem to make even simple tasks daunting.

For most parents the knowledge that their child has suffered some degree of brain damage and has been diagnosed as having CP is not only a grievous shock but also induces a sense of panic. They ask themselves questions such as 'What is CP?', 'How can I help my child?', 'I don't know anything about it, what can we expect?' Visits to the hospital to see the various staff responsible for the diagnosis, assessment, treatment and management of their child can be both reassuring and at the same time somewhat terrifying. I hope that readers will be reassured firstly, that they are not alone in these feelings and secondly, that all the members of the team responsible for the management of their child's care expect to respond to their questions.

The treatment and management of a child with CP involve tackling a wide range of problems due to the variability of the disorder. All children with CP have difficulty in moving purposefully and efficiently but no two children experience exactly the same difficulties, for example:

1. A child with stiffness (increased postural tone) will have a paucity of movements which are stereotyped.

2. A child who is sometimes stiff and sometimes floppy (fluctuations in postural tone), although able to move, does so in a disorganized manner, lacking both postural control and stability.

3. A child with floppiness (decreased postural tone) will have excessive incoordination of voluntary movements and difficulty in timing and grading movements.

Some children have a mixture of the above problems. In some children these abnormalities may lead to the later development of muscular skeletal deformities. There may also be associated disabilities of vision, hearing, speech, epilepsy, learning and behaviour.

A wide spectrum of intellect is found in children with CP, ranging from the typical to the more severely subnormal. In a number of children their chronological age may not correspond to their developmental age, which in some children may be lower in all aspects, whereas in other children there may be a scatter of achievement in the child's development. For example: a child of 4 years may not progress in all areas of development beyond that of a 9-month-old whereas another child may be within typical limits as regards fine motor skills but have difficulty using the legs for walking and have a problem with vision.

However, not all the difficulties described will apply to any one child.

All children need similar daily care: to be fed, carried, bathed, dressed and toileted. These tasks are often demanding when a first-time mother is developing her own mothering skills. She is rewarded by the warm bond that gradually develops between herself and her child and both parents take pleasure in each new skill their child achieves. The same joy is there for the mother of a child with CP but the presence of abnormalities may make the daily tasks mentioned above more difficult for her to undertake and create barriers to learning together.

Repetition and overlap between the content of the various chapters are at times unavoidable, firstly because different aspects of the same problem will be seen from a different perspective by different contributors and secondly, because there is naturally occurring overlap in activity as development proceeds. For example, Chapter 9 discusses the early interaction between a mother and her child and the important role she plays in helping the development of vision and hearing; these aspects are also discussed in the chapters on fine motor movement (Chapter 19) and communication (Chapter 18). I have deliberately not edited out repetition as readers will not necessarily read the chapters in the order in which they are presented and it may serve to remind the reader that there is carry-over of learning from one situation to another.

Over the years since the first edition of this book was written, ideas on appropriate therapies have changed and developed. Similarly, opinion on early intervention has changed and the method of delivery of service has in some places moved from centralization to home-based or community provision. The emphasis however remains on a holistic approach to the child's needs, seeing the difficulties in relation to the overall development of the child as a unique person from childhood to adulthood. Although the text is only intended to cover the early years, that is, from birth to 5 years of age, the tasks and activities described are those that are fundamental to eventual independence in adulthood.

Suggestions on how to use this book

Readers who have taken this book off the shelf have their own motivation for doing so, but it is probably because they have recently been confronted with the difficulties of a child with cerebral palsy (CP). A parent, carer or professional new to the field may initially find most helpful the earlier chapters on the need for two-way communication between parents and professionals, information regarding hospital appointments and admissions, the various medical aspects and problems experienced by parents.

Soon the chapters on how children learn and behave, suggestions to help with emotional problems and early learning strategies may also be helpful. As time goes on the more practical chapters on understanding movement, specific techniques on holding and moving your child, or 'handling', as Nancie called it, and the different care routines may come into their own as problems are encountered.

When she wrote the first edition of this book, Nancie Finnie included a number of strategies for the handling of children with CP which, however effective, are no longer socially acceptable. For example, when bathing a child who cannot sit, a parent may get in the bath with the child and support the child in sitting by placing the child between his or her legs. I have endeavoured to take all the current (2008) thinking into account in view of the higher profile of the question of physical and sexual abuse of children. Nevertheless, over the years some of the strategies I am advocating may suffer a similar fate and this must always be borne in mind.

Depending upon the individual's previous knowledge and experience the book may be read in its entirety but it is likely to be more useful if dipped into for relevant information and returned to at different times for further information as needed.

The chapters on communication, fine and gross motor movement, chairs, mobility aids, play and leisure and fitness may be found helpful as those topics become important to the care of the child.

The chapters on deformities, orthoses and spasticity may become useful to parents as the child grows. However it is suggested that forewarned is forearmed and it may be helpful for any parent whose child has stiffness (increased postural tone) to read these chapters, and especially Chapter 25 on deformity.

The final chapter on complementary and alternative medicine may help parents if they are considering using therapies outside the general remit of conventional medical practice.

In Appendices 1 and 2 you will find a brief outline of the early stages of the general development of a typical child, followed by a very brief synopsis of the early gross motor development of a typical child. Appendix 3 describes some of the more commonly used gross motor and functional measures used by physicians and therapists. Appendix 4 suggests some ideas on intervention planning using the Gross Motor Function Classification System (see Chapter 20). Appendix 5 describes some of the terminology used by physicians and therapists although most are described within the context of the chapters in which they are used.

In conclusion, please remember that if your child is to achieve a degree of independence, however limited that may be, he or she should be given opportunities and encouragement to communicate, use the hands and move about throughout the day.

Chapter One

Communication between parents and professionals

Revised by Eva Bower

I feel that any programme of intervention for the child with cerebral palsy (CP) may only be successful if, right from the start, it is based on a sound foundation of communication between parents and professionals. Only in this way will the needs and changing priorities of both the child and the family be addressed.

What is meant by communication? At the least, communication has two parts: speaking and listening. This does not necessarily bring understanding. The participants need to use the same code to decipher the idea or message being transmitted. This is of importance in the relationship between parents and professionals, where incorrect assumptions about understanding are sometimes made. The reality is that both parents and professionals have much to contribute to the caring programme for the child with CP. When there is a communication gap it is to the detriment of the child's total intervention programme and that is why it is important to work towards establishing a partnership of mutual understanding and respect for what each can bring to the child's care.

Some years ago I attended a seminar where the mother of a child with CP was speaking to an audience of medical students about her experience of attending doctors' clinics and hospital departments with her child for routine tests and appointments. At the end of the presentation, the chairman asked if she would give her audience of future doctors a final message. She replied: 'Please listen to us, the parents.' It was a message we should all try to remember.

Exchange of information

Parents' reactions when they receive their child's initial diagnosis of CP varies, and these reactions go through many phases during the ensuing days, weeks, months and years. Most parents soon reach a stage where they want more information and clarification and have countless questions. The questions often relate to the diagnosis, the meaning of some clinical tests and, possibly more importantly, a desire to know their child's prognosis.

I urge all parents to ask their paediatrician, therapist or other professionals their questions, and to go on asking their questions until they receive and understand the answers, rather than keeping anxieties and worries to themselves or within the family group or trying to find out the answers by asking family and friends. To make sure that you do not forget to ask the right questions at the clinic appointment, I suggest you write down the questions and take the list with you. It is likely that the answers to some of the questions will have an impact on the whole family; for example, you may like a clearer picture of your child's prognosis and what demands an intervention programme may make on your time, so that you can plan to integrate this with other commitments that you may have, such as work or activities with other members of the family. The answers may also affect later decisions in relation to employment opportunities or choice of house, its type and location.

I would also caution you about the well-meaning advice which may be offered to you by friends and other family members who have heard of a new therapy programme that claims to offer great benefit, if not a miracle cure. It is wise to note these and discuss them with your paediatrician at the next follow-up appointment before embarking on a new programme. Professionals will usually be willing to discuss the advantages and disadvantages of a new approach with you. This is really more satisfactory than 'shopping around' on your own.

Therapists have skills which help them to analyse your child's problems and identify the potential for future development. They do this by successive assessments, in which the parents should be active and full participants. This process should identify and continually monitor the child's changing needs. One of the therapist's roles may be to help parents to modify their caregiving activities so that each daily task, whether it is feeding, bathing or dressing, may be made easier for the child and the carer. With the older child this may mean identifying specific skills and self-help tasks which the child finds difficult and then breaking them down into small steps, hopefully

making it easier for the child. The role of professionals is to give guidance and support, not to make you – the parents – professional experts or to supplant your role as parents.

It is important that you, the parents, are involved from the beginning in any decision-making regarding your child's management, which underlines once more the importance of the two-way flow of communication between you, the parents, and us, the professionals.

Both during the early sessions with your therapist and later on, it is helpful if you share with the therapist the wealth of knowledge that you have about your child. The type of information needed will come in response to some of the following questions.

1. What is it about your child's development that makes you think the child is 'behind' or 'different'?

2. What do you feel are the main problems?

3. Has your child ever done something that you had previously thought was beyond your child's ability?

4. Has it occurred to you that if you did less for your child, the child might achieve more on his or her own?

Assessing the ability of a child with CP

For intervention programmes to be helpful, the criteria for using them must first be clearly understood. During the assessment process you will be aware that the therapist is documenting different aspects of your child's behaviour. An important part of the assessment process is learning about the child's behaviour by the simple, unsophisticated method of observation. The way the child moves spontaneously and interacts with you while you talk and play together speaks volumes about the child's level of competence. Through the eyes of your therapist you may learn to recognize and understand that, although your child may have little difficulty in moving, the movements may not be purposeful and efficient. You may observe that the movements are poorly coordinated and therefore abnormally executed and the abnormal postures and movements may be affecting other aspects of development and preventing the child from functioning effectively.

A typical day in the life of the child

Any programme of intervention will inevitably make additional demands of time and effort on parents. For this reason, before putting any plan into action it is useful for professionals involved in the care of the child to know how you previously organized your time as a family, and how you would now like to plan your day. The programme can then be structured around your day, so that working with your child does not become intrusive. I have found that the best way of doing this is to ask parents to describe 'a typical day in the life of the family'. Then together we can structure a programme that puts minimal strain on the parents while at the same time addressing the needs of the child and the family.

This is invaluable information that tells the therapist something about the family's routine, the child's routine, the child's method of self-expression, likes and dislikes, and the time when the child is most susceptible to being worked with.

Following are some examples to illustrate this approach.

How the day starts

For many families, especially when there are other children, the start to the day is usually described as a 'mad rush', a time when mother, having fed the child and got herself dressed, is then busy seeing to the needs of the rest of the family, perhaps preparing breakfast, getting the other children ready for school and seeing her partner off to work. This is a time when their needs come first, certainly not one when she, or other members of the family, can be expected to give their undivided attention to the child with CP.

During the early months, the majority of children sleep after a feed, and it is only when this pattern starts to change that some children with

CP, unable to play and amuse themselves because of their immature development, become bored and frustrated and demand attention. We need to ask ourselves why the child is distressed, and then find ways of organizing this part of the day so that we make sure that the child has every opportunity to look, react, explore, practise and use those abilities of which we know the child to be capable without our participation or supervision. We need to be sure that the activities we expect of the child, and the toys that we select, are at the child's developmental or functional level and not necessarily the child's chronological age, so that every effort made on the child's part is rewarded by success, in this way stimulating and sustaining interest.

For example, the child who with your help enjoys the experience of getting the hands together, feeling, looking and taking them to the mouth may be able to practise doing this independently of you if supported on the side or in a cut-out wedge. Alternatively the child may enjoy the visual stimulus of focusing and following a moving object so that, if you provide a favourite mobile whose colour, movement and changing shape attract the attention, the child will not only become more visually alert, but happy and contented while alone. The child who can reach out and grasp will need toys to play with that stimulate interest while at the same time offering the opportunity to practise these skills. It is worth remembering that even when a child becomes skilful at using the hands, the child will continue for quite a time to take toys to the mouth to explore them further. It is therefore worthwhile having a couple of toys nearby or attached to the cot so that the child can pull them closer, to suck, bite and explore further.

It is vital to ensure that any toy or play material given to a child is safe and not harmful for that child at his or her current developmental/ functional age.

The child's routine

We have seen that parents' description of a typical day provides us with invaluable information about their child's daily routine and the child's methods of self-expression, likes and dislikes. It is helpful to know:

1. When the child is most alert and responsive.
2. Whether the child is one who is contented during the day but becomes unsettled during the evening or vice versa.
3. Whether the child has a prolonged period of responsiveness following a bath or a feed, or perhaps is a child who immediately likes to doze.

We can then channel input on to those activities the child enjoys and avoid those the child actively dislikes. This is particularly important in the beginning, as many children do not welcome the extra demands made on them by intervention.

Fortunately most routine activities, such as nappy changing, are repeated throughout the day, which means that we can choose the time when the child is most responsive to intervene. For example, if a mother describes her child as being niggling and unsettled towards the evening and that the child is most active during times when the nappy is being changed, we would know that:

1. Nappy-changing times offer an opportunity for intervention.
2. The morning period is when the child is most receptive.

Similarly, if a child had reached the stage of starting to feed independently with a spoon, and if lunchtime is the only meal when food is really enjoyed, rather than having a battle, it would be sensible for the mother to concentrate on the one meal where she would be sure that the child would be responsive, only gradually introducing self-feeding at other mealtimes later on.

It is helpful to remember that the same fundamental skills used in one particular activity are often also used in other tasks, and these should also be practised in order to encourage carry-over.

Setting priorities and communicating goals

There is always the danger when discussing short- and long-term goals and the immediate priorities

in intervention for your child that by concentrating on one aspect of a child's development we forget to explain that at the same time the child should be given opportunities to accomplish other activities and skills. It is of importance to emphasize that all aspects of the child's development, and not only one aspect, should be considered.

Turning now to the responsibilities of the professional, you must continue discussing with parents, from time to time, how their child spends the day. It is an excellent way of finding out whether you have been successful in communicating with parents. You might find, for example, that because the goal had been to help the child use the hands in sitting, the child has been sitting most of the day, as the importance of also being on the floor and being encouraged to move about while playing had not been explained. There is a danger that if the child spends too much time in sitting, the muscles at the front of the hips and behind the knees become tight and deformities develop. The child who is limited in the ability to move around is likely to become what I call a 'container baby', spending the day sitting in a highchair, corner seat or specially adapted chair, and in some cases in a baby swing and, when taken out, sitting in a pushchair or car seat. On occasion I have found that the only time the child is not sitting is when having a nappy changed or when in the cot. Again, activities with a child while being dressed might not have been undertaken because the holding and moving techniques shown to the mother were not clear. Going through how the child spends the day may also help to clarify how often and in which situations a piece of equipment is being used.

The use of video recording as a means of communication

Observation and analysis of problems

Observing how a child performs is never easy and this is where video recording is a useful tool for recording the initial and sequential evaluations, enabling the child's progress to be monitored. Video recording offers another way of facilitating communication between parents and professionals and between professionals. Furthermore, the recording may allow the parents to distance themselves from the child, allowing them to see that their child is much more independent than they had given the child credit for or to appreciate where the difficulties arise.

Learning new techniques

When it is impossible for both parents to attend a therapy session, I find a video recording may be valuable in providing parents with an opportunity to review the child's performance at home and observe any modifications that have been made to the intervention programme. Through discussion together they can decide on any points they do not understand, disagree with or want clarified.

A short sequence of film can also act as a back-up for parents, for example, as a reminder of any special techniques they have been shown or to help them identify the different stages necessary for the acquisition of a particular skill.

The use of video recording may also help parents to master particular holding and moving skills. For example, I have filmed a parent holding and moving her child when a new technique has been demonstrated. Then, together, we have been able to look at the sequence and make any further changes that were necessary.

Similarly a short sequence filmed at home by the parents of their child moving spontaneously in the home environment, or using a new piece of equipment, may offer a new insight to a doctor or therapist who only sees the child in the foreign environment of the clinic.

Two-way communication in the intervention programme

Various professionals will evaluate your child's physical and social development, language and communication and response to learning. Based on these assessments, the total intervention programme embracing all these aspects is planned. The programme will require changing over time to reflect the changing needs and priorities of the child and family. I cannot overemphasize that programmes should be developed in partnership. The professionals contribute their base knowledge of development, understanding of the child's problems and intervention skills, while the parents bring to the partnership their expert knowledge of their child, knowledge of the needs and abilities of other members of the family and knowledge of their own needs and priorities. Partnership does not mean that there will always be total agreement, but effective communication should mean that there is an open door to resolving differences and reaching an understanding, whether this be on setting priorities, use of a particular technique or even accepting that long-term estimates of your child's potential for development are not possible at an early stage.

In summary, effective communication between parents and professionals, and between professionals of different disciplines, is essential in the assessment of the child's needs and in planning and implementing intervention programmes.

I hope that the foregoing has made clear the need for a two-way flow of communication and emphasized the importance of the parents' contribution in this process.

Chapter Two

Preparing for and coping with hospital appointments, assessments and admissions

Caroline Fitzgerald • Tara Kerr Elliott

CHAPTER CONTENTS

The purpose of this chapter is to offer advice and ideas to help you and your child to prepare for and cope with visiting hospital. Although hospital admissions are referred to in the greatest detail, much of the advice may also be applicable to hospital assessments and appointments and also to those occasions when your child may be visited at home by a health care, educational or social services professional.

Appointments and assessments

It is likely that a number of different professionals want to see your child, and the number of appointments and assessments may seem daunting. A calendar or diary may be a very useful way of keeping track of the many appointments, and you may also want to use it to record the names and contact numbers of everyone who is involved with your child. Although it may not be possible, it is always worth asking if appointments at the same hospital can be arranged on the same day.

There is a range of doctors with whom your child may have appointments (Box 2.1). The appointments may be at your local hospital, child development centre, school or nursery, or at a specialist regional hospital. It is a good idea to make sure you understand what each appointment is for, but it may be confusing, so do not be afraid to ask someone such as your general practitioner (GP), health visitor or community children's nurse.

Box 2.1

Range of medical specialists (doctors)

- General paediatrician (hospital children's doctor)
- Community paediatrician (community children's doctor)
- Neurologist (brain)
- Ear, nose and throat (ENT) consultant
- Gastroenterologist (digestion)
- Ophthalmologist (vision)
- Audiologist (hearing)
- Orthopaedic consultant (bones, muscles and joints)
- Respiratory consultant (breathing)

Professionals who may be involved in the assessment, treatment and management of your child

- Health visitor
- Special needs health visitor
- Community children's nurse
- Nurse specialists (e.g. neuro-nurse, continence nurse)
- Speech and language therapist (communication)
- Speech and language therapist (feeding)
- Dietician
- Physiotherapist (movement)
- Occupational therapist in England (health, function)
- Occupational therapist in England (social services, equipment)
- Clinical psychologist (behaviour)
- Educational psychologist (cognition)
- Peripatetic teacher (e.g. for the visually impaired)
- Portage/home learning worker
- Respite coordinator
- Respite carer
- Social worker (general)
- Social worker (children with disabilities team)

It may be useful to write down any questions or issues you want to discuss before you go to the appointment, as it is very easy to forget on the day. You may also find it helpful to take a friend or relative to the appointment with you, as the amount of information you are expected to remember may sometimes feel overwhelming. You could ask this person to make notes for you during the appointment for you to review later at home.

It is helpful to take a list of people to whom you would like reports and clinic letters sent, otherwise correspondence may only be circulated to a few contacts, such as the GP.

Many hospitals or community trusts in England have a multidisciplinary team of therapists and other professionals who assess, treat, manage and review children with disabilities. Members of the team may include physiotherapists, occupational therapists, speech and language therapists, psychologists and specialist nurses or health visitors (Box 2.2).

Although assessments may seem time-consuming, repetitive and sometimes intrusive, they are a necessary way of establishing your child's abilities and needs, and then a means of planning treatment or management strategies to help your child. However, if you do not understand the purpose of any particular assessment that is planned for your child it is important to ask for an explanation.

You may find that you are offered a multidisciplinary assessment for your child where several therapists will be present. The advantage of this is that the therapists can assess a number of different areas of function, and should work together to develop a treatment or management programme for your child. Although the assessment can be lengthy, it reduces the number of assessments or appointments that you have to attend.

Home visits

Professionals may visit you at home to continue to offer treatment and therapy, to review and amend treatment or management programmes, and to offer advice and support to you and your child. Once your child starts nursery or school, therapists are likely to visit him or her there, again to offer support and advice to staff, and also to teach staff specific positioning or therapy techniques helpful to your child.

Home visits are considered beneficial for several reasons. Your child is in a familiar environment and likely to feel more relaxed and better able to attempt the tasks asked. For you it may be more comfortable, because you have not needed to rush to an appointment and in your own environment you may feel better able to ask questions of the therapist. However, having a lot of professionals visiting your home can be stressful. Many parents report that they prefer home visits, but the sheer number of visits can be overwhelming, especially in the early stages. Keeping free time for you, your child and other family members is vital in order to maintain some normality, and to allow you the freedom, time and space to be your child's parent, friend and nurturer. Some parents have suggested that they have needed to block out a day or two each week to ensure that, on these days at least, they have both their child and their home to themselves.

As illustrated in Box 2.2, the list of professionals who may be involved with your child can appear endless. It can be very confusing understanding who does what and why, where they are from, and, most importantly, what is the benefit to your child and your family. Do not be afraid to ask why somebody needs to see your child, and what he or she may be offering. Some professionals may be from the National Health Service (NHS) (they may be members of the child development centre multidisciplinary team, mentioned previously), whereas others may be from social services, education or voluntary agencies working in your area. It would be highly unlikely that a professional would arrive at your home without an appointment; even so, make sure you ask to see identification. Ask what the purpose of this visit is so that you can have realistic expectations or ask for a referral to someone more appropriate if you feel that other needs of your child are not going to be met. Some professionals have very similar job titles but offer different services. For example, in England an occupational therapist from the NHS will be concerned with function, perception and cognition, whereas the occupational therapist from social services is likely to be the person who provides or recommends the pieces of equipment to aid with function and activities of daily living, such as toileting or bath aids, and house adaptations.

Each time your child is seen by a professional, remember to ask him or her to write in your *personal child health record* (PCHR – the red book given to you by your health visitor) as this will aid communication between professionals and help you to keep track of events. The PCHR is issued by the health visitor to every child in England when the child is about 10 days old, and contains pages to record growth, development and immunizations, contacts with professionals, and useful advice and essential health information. If you do not live in England, it may be a good idea to provide such a book yourself and keep similar records.

Hospital admissions

The team of professionals working with you and your child should, whenever possible, try to avoid the need for hospital admissions, as there has been much research demonstrating the negative effects on children of having to stay in hospital (Ministry of Health 1959; Department of Health 1991, 2003). Being separated from their parents and fear about what is going to happen to them can cause great anxiety. Fifty per cent of all children will have to stay in hospital at some stage and this figure is even higher for disabled children (Audit Commission Fact Sheet for Disabled Children). In recent years health care professionals have realized what parents and children have known for much longer, which is that a child's life is turned completely upside down when the child is admitted to hospital.

There may be a wide range of reasons why admission to hospital is suggested to you. These may include investigations, treatment for illness, surgery or respite. Always try to establish if there are any alternatives to staying in hospital. For example, could your child visit the hospital as an outpatient for investigations or could a community nurse give the necessary treatment at home?

Respite care is a supportive mechanism for families and individuals who are caring for a dependent child or adult. Caring for a child with disabilities can take up an immense amount of time and energy. Respite care allows time for the child to socialize away from the parents, and for parents to have a break together, or to spend time with their other children. At its best, respite care will be tailored to meet the needs of the affected child, and family members, and can be provided in a number of ways (Department of Health 2004). Provision varies greatly from area to area, but services may include carers coming to the home or short breaks away from home, to stay with either another family or at dedicated respite units. Respite care homes or units may be provided by the voluntary sector, charitable services or social services. Historically, and where services are very limited, admission to hospital has been used as a form of respite. A children's ward is not the best place for you and your child to receive respite care, due to hospital-acquired infections and lack of suitable play and opportunities for socializing. Talk to your social worker, health visitor or community children's nurse and ask for help in investigating the best services available in your area.

Preparing for hospital admission

Obviously, there are occasions when admission to hospital is unavoidable, but there are many ways you can help your child to prepare for, and cope with, the experience. There are many books, for children of all ages and levels of understanding, explaining and describing hospital routines, staff and procedures. Find out whether the hospital offers tours to familiarize your child with the unit to which he or she will be admitted and ask to meet with the play specialist who can work with your child to help allay fears and anxieties. The play specialist may be able to loan you books or play equipment prior to your child's admission. Alternatively your local library is likely to have a range of books available (see Box 2.3 for examples). If your child is unable to understand such explanations due to age or disability, it is still worth talking to the play specialist as he or she may be able to help your child to feel more relaxed during the stay or during certain procedures. Examples of suitable techniques include using massage; distraction techniques, such as singing to your child or blowing bubbles during a procedure; music; and multisensory toys, such as sound and light toys.

Box 2.4

Items you may wish to take into hospital

- Communication aids
- Favourite comforter/toys
- Nappies
- Day and night clothes
- Specialized feeding equipment – spoons, cups
- Any special milk or dietary additives
- Medicines
- Sleeping aids – special pillows, wedges, splints
- Bathing aids
- Toileting aids
- Slings (if your child uses a hoist)
- A book/magazine for yourself
- Money for the telephone (you may not be able to use a mobile phone on the ward)

If your child is more able, he or she may like to be involved in preparing for hospital. For example, your child may be able to help with packing, such as preparing a small bag with favourite items from home (Box 2.4).

You can also help to prepare your child by communicating honestly before hospital visits, admissions and procedures. Never use doctors or nurses, or hospital admissions or treatment, as a threat when your child is misbehaving. When these are required it is vital that your child does not perceive them as punishment.

During the hospital stay

On the day of hospital admission both a doctor and a nurse will probably assess your child. At this point you will be able to inform the nursing staff about your child's individual likes, dislikes, needs and routines. It is important for you to take the time to describe your child's method of communicating; for example, the use of gesture or eye pointing to indicate discomfort, hunger and thirst. If your child uses symbols or pictures to communicate you may need to prepare a new range appropriate to the hospital stay, such as 'nurse',

Box 2.3

Books which may be helpful to you and your child before admission to hospital

Adamson J, Adamson G. Topsy and Tim go to hospital. London: Ladybird/Penguin, UK, 2003
Barbour J. People who help us in hospital. East Sussex: Wayland, UK, 1998
Church D. Operation fix-it. London: British Heart Foundation, UK, 2003
Hunter R. My first visit to hospital. London: Evans Brothers, UK, 2000

'medicine' or 'sore'. It may take a while for information to filter through to other departments and staff, so you may find you need to explain things several times.

Although it can be difficult, it is important to be honest with your child. For example, if you know a procedure is going to be painful, it is better that your child is warned of this, rather than being told it will not hurt. If you have not been entirely truthful, your child may find it hard to trust and be comforted by future reassurances. Your child should be reassured that if he or she feels sore or uncomfortable he or she will be given medicines to make it feel better. If your child is unable to communicate through speech, gestures or signing, the nursing staff should welcome your help with identifying occasions when your child is uncomfortable. Children can respond very differently to pain, so do not assume you are wrong if no one else has noticed signs which you feel suggest your child is uncomfortable. Some children may cry or appear very restless whereas others become very still or withdrawn. Notice changes in your child's facial expression, breathing pattern, muscle tone and pallor or colour and ask for pain relief or other help if you are concerned.

It is important that, wherever possible, your child is given the chance to understand the reason for a procedure and what it involves. An example of this would be prior to orthopaedic surgery, after which your child may be in a plaster cast. If your child has been told that the surgery will help walking and then wakes up to find that he or she is unable to get up as one or both legs are in plaster, your child will have every reason to feel let down and frustrated. Encourage your child to ask questions, make choices and express feelings or needs whenever possible.

If your child is attending school, ask the teacher to liaise with staff from the hospital school prior to, and during, the admission. By sharing information about your child's abilities, likes and dislikes, the teachers within the hospital will be able to provide activities which are appropriate for your child to enjoy during this hospital stay.

Children in England have the right to have their parents stay with them in hospital (Department of Health 2003). This is government policy, so check

facilities and accommodation for parents before your child is admitted. It is recognized that family circumstances mean it will not always be possible for parents to stay with their child. However, if you are planning to stay, it is at this stage that you will also need to prepare for and make arrangements for your other children. There is much evidence that siblings of disabled or sick children can feel jealous of their sibling or excluded from their care (Miller 1996). It is a good idea to try to arrange for them to visit your child in hospital. This should promote your family well-being and identity and is likely to benefit your child as well.

Frequent hospital appointments or admissions can prove costly (Department of Health 2003). If you are working it can mean losing pay. You may also find that the extra expense on transport or paying for food in the hospital is causing problems for you financially. If this is the case, ask to speak either to your own social worker or to the social worker attached to the unit where your child is staying, as help may be available.

There may be occasions when you are unable to plan or prepare for admission to hospital, because your child requires treatment suddenly or unexpectedly. In this situation, once your child is admitted and more settled you could request that someone brings in particular items such as a comforter or favourite toy, and any necessary equipment. If your child's condition is such that hospital admissions are likely to be frequent and unpredictable, try to negotiate an open admissions policy with your hospital, rather than using the Accident and Emergency Department, as your child may then benefit from being treated by staff who are familiar.

Coming home from hospital

As your child begins to recover from illness, surgery or treatment, the hospital staff should start to help you plan for going home. This should be done as soon as possible and it should involve professionals involved with caring for your child at home, such as your GP, community children's nurse and therapists. Do not be afraid to remind them of this, and if you can provide names and contact telephone numbers this will be very helpful.

It is Government policy in England that children should be discharged from hospital as soon as they are clinically well, but not before their needs can be safely met at home. Prior to discharge, ensure you fully understand and feel confident with any new treatments or medicines that need to be continued once home. Also make sure you are aware of what the follow-up arrangements are. For example, when is your child's next outpatient appointment? Alternatively, if the next appointment is a home visit, ensure that you know who to expect and when.

Despite preparation and careful consideration, children's experiences of hospital admission or treatment may sometimes still be traumatic, for example during an unexpected or particularly prolonged admission or if the child has been very unwell. Children may show signs of distress in different ways and this can be especially true for young or disabled children, who may be unable to express their anxieties or concerns in words. It may help you to be aware of these behaviours, as they may continue for a short while even after your child has come home. It may be particularly upsetting to see your child appear to lose skills previously acquired, or if the child seems to return to earlier stages of development. This will usually be temporary. Other signs may include nightmares, tantrums or becoming withdrawn. They may have problems with sleeping, with bed-wetting or refusal to eat. Remember that these behaviours are just your child's way of expressing unhappiness about the experience and, as the child settles again at home, the behaviours should disappear. However, if you are worried, you can discuss this with your GP, health visitor, community children's nurse or psychologist.

If you are unhappy with any aspect of your child's care or treatment in hospital, or by staff visiting your child at home, you can contact the Patient Advocacy and Liaison Service (PALS) for advice. In England every hospital and Primary Care Trust (which employs many of the community-based staff who will visit your child at home) will have such a service, which can help you to investigate and deal with any problems you may have experienced. Box 2.5 lists some useful websites.

Box 2.5

Useful websites for further reference

- www.goshkids.nhs.uk (a website for children about illness and hospitals; includes sections for under-5s, children and teenagers)
- www.dh.gov.uk (from which can be downloaded *Standards for Children in Hospital: a Guide for Parents and Carers*)
- www.healthcarecommission.org.uk (details of a current review of children's hospital services; the opportunity to feed back your experiences)
- www.audit-commission.gov.uk/ disabledchildren/factsheet6.asp (parents' fact sheet entitled *Disabled Children: Making the best of an admission to hospital*)
- www.familyfund.org.uk
- www.cafamily.org.uk/hospitals.html
- www.ccaa.org.uk/disability_benefits.htm (offers practical advice regarding hospital treatment and admission, including possible financial assistance)

References

Audit Commission Fact Sheets. Available online at: www.audit-commission.gov.uk/disabledchildren/factsheet6.asp

Department of Health. Getting the right start: the National Service Framework for children, young people and maternity services – standard for hospital services. Department of Health, London, 2003.

Department of Health. Disabled child standard, National Service Framework for children, young people and maternity services – disabled children and young people and those with complex health needs. Department of Health, London, 2004.

Miller S. Living with a disabled sibling: a review of the literature. Paediatric Nursing 1996; 8:21–24.

Ministry of Health. The welfare of children in hospital – report of the committee, chaired by Sir H Platt. HMSO, London, 1959.

Further reading

Conners C, Stalker K. The experiences and views of disabled children and their siblings: implications for practice and policy. Jessica Kingsley, London, 2003.

Department of Health. The welfare of children and young people in hospital. HMSO, London, 1991.

Department of Health. What should a really good hospital look like? [A booklet for children.] Department of Health, London, 2003.

Department of Health. Disabled child standard, National Service Framework for children, young people and maternity services – disabled children and young people and those with complex health needs. Department of Health, London, 2004.

Chapter Three

Medical aspects of cerebral palsy: causes, associated problems and management

Dinah Reddihough

CHAPTER CONTENTS

Movement is a complex process. Getting up from a chair, riding a bicycle, turning a page, switching on the stove and even turning around to watch the cat all involve pathways that begin in the brain (Figure 3.1). The brain controls all that we do. Messages travel from the brain down the spinal cord, then out from the spinal cord via nerves to muscles in various parts of the body. The muscles are responsible for carrying out the movement. Some movements are automatic, for example, we withdraw

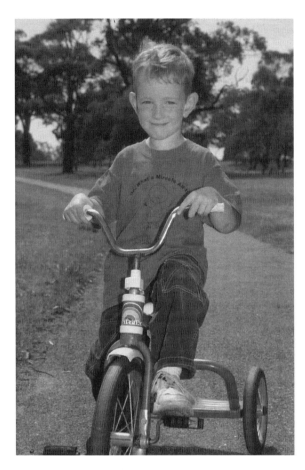

Figure 3.1 • The process of riding a tricycle involves pathways that begin in the brain.

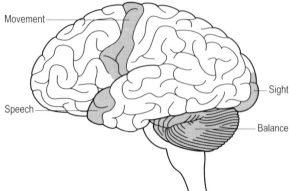

Figure 3.2 • Schematic drawing of brain with various areas marked.

However, the term 'cerebral palsy' is used when the problem has occurred before birth, around the time of birth or early in life (up to the age of about 5 years), whilst the brain is still undergoing rapid development. Every child with CP is different and some people say that we should use the term 'cerebral palsies', as the term is like an umbrella term that describes a whole range of different problems. The movement problems are sometimes also called motor problems. They can range from mild to severe. In mild CP, the child may be slightly clumsy in one arm or leg, and the problem may be barely noticeable. In more severe CP, the child may have a lot of difficulties in performing everyday tasks and movements. Children with CP can have weak, stiff, awkward, slow or shaky movements and they can also have difficulties with balance.

our hands quickly from a hot surface, whereas other movements may require a lot of thought, for example, getting out of bed on a cold wet morning.

Many different diseases or conditions can affect this pathway, for example, there can be problems with the brain, the spinal cord, the nerves themselves or the muscles. In cerebral palsy (CP) there is damage to, or lack of development in, one or more areas of the brain.

So what does the term 'cerebral palsy' mean? 'Cerebral' refers to the brain and 'palsy' means weakness or paralysis or lack of muscle control. CP is therefore a disorder of movement that results from damage to part of the brain (Figure 3.2). People can acquire damage to the brain at any time of life from accidents such as motor vehicle accidents and from other problems such as strokes.

What are the different types of CP?

The descriptions used for children with CP can be quite confusing. It is also possible for the movement problems to change, particularly during the first 2 years of life.

There are three different ways in which the movement problems are classified.

1. The type of movement disorder.

2. The parts of the body affected.

3. The severity of the movement problems.

The type of movement disorder

Spastic CP is the most common type of CP. Spasticity means stiffness or tightness of muscles. The muscles are stiff because the messages to the muscles are relayed incorrectly from the damaged parts of the brain. When people without CP perform a movement, groups of muscles contract whilst the opposite groups of muscles relax in order to perform the movement. In children with spastic CP, both groups of muscles may contract together, making the movement difficult.

Dyskinetic CP refers to a group of cerebral palsies with involuntary movements and is characterized by abnormalities of muscle tone involving the whole body. Several terms are used within this group.

1. *Dystonia* is a term used for involuntary muscle contractions. Children with dystonia are often quite 'floppy' or have low muscle tone but then suddenly develop stiffness or spasms.

2. *Athetosis* (or athetoid CP) is the word used for the uncontrolled movements that occur in this type of CP. This lack of control is often most noticeable when the child starts to move, for example, when the child attempts to grasp a toy or a spoon. In addition, children with athetoid CP often have very weak muscles or feel floppy when carried.

Ataxic CP is the least common type of CP. Ataxic (or ataxia) is the word used for unsteady shaky movements or tremor. Children with ataxia also have problems with balance.

Many children have not just one type, but a mixture of several of these movement problems.

The parts of the body affected

This varies from one child to another. Different words are used to describe the parts affected (Figure 3.3).

1. *Hemiplegia* – the leg and arm on one side of the body are affected (also described as hemiparesis). Children with hemiplegia usually walk independently. The upper limb can be slightly, moderately or severely impaired.

2. *Diplegia* – both legs are predominantly affected. Children with diplegia usually also have some involvement with their arm and hand movements and may walk independently or with

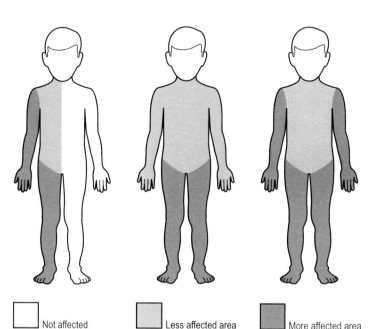

Figure 3.3 • Schematic drawing of body parts involved in the various types of cerebral palsy: (a) hemiplegia; (b) diplegia; (c) quadriplegia. Note that children with quadriplegia may also have some involvement of the head and neck.

☐ Not affected   ▨ Less affected area   ▧ More affected area

(a)   (b)   (c)

a frame or walking sticks. A few children with diplegia are wheelchair-dependent.

3. *Quadriplegia* – both arms and both legs are affected (also described as quadriparesis). The muscles of the face, mouth and throat may also be involved. Many children with quadriplegic CP require a wheelchair for mobility.

Other terms used are *triplegia* (three limbs involved) and, rarely, *monoplegia* (one limb involved).

The severity of the movement problems

A classification system, called the Gross Motor Function Classification System, provides information about the movement problems of children with CP based on their functional ability and their need for walking frames, wheelchairs and other mobility devices (Palisano et al. 1997). There are five levels: children in levels 1 and 2 walk independently, children in level 3 generally need walking frames or elbow crutches and children in levels 4 and 5 use wheelchairs. For more information, see Chapter 20.

How often does CP occur?

CP registers have been established in many parts of the world, including all of the states of Australia, parts of the UK and North America and in Scandinavia. Registers are very useful as they help us to understand trends in the occurrence of CP and how the causes are varying over the years. In all of these parts of the world, CP occurs in about 2.0–2.5 per 1000 live births (Stanley et al. 2000).

What are the causes of CP?

There are many different causes, resulting from problems during the pregnancy, around the time of birth or in the days or weeks following birth, and up to the age of about 5 years when there is still rapid brain development.

Before birth

1. If the brain does not grow or form properly during the early part of pregnancy, brain malformations may result. These malformations usually occur between about the 12th and 20th week of pregnancy and different types are identified with brain scans. Magnetic resonance imaging (MRI) is the preferred scan. Most of these malformations have unusual names such as lissencephaly, holoprosencephaly and cerebellar hypoplasia, and some have a genetic basis (Figure 3.4).

2. If mothers are exposed to certain infections during the early months of pregnancy, such as rubella (German measles) or cytomegalovirus, there may be an abnormality in early brain development. Both rubella and cytomegalovirus infections may be quite mild in the mother and may be passed off as a cold or flu-like illness. An immunization is now available for rubella but not for cytomegalovirus.

3. Some children appear to have had a 'stroke' during pregnancy. This is evident on brain scans done after birth (Figure 3.5).

4. Rarely, metabolic problems may cause brain damage.

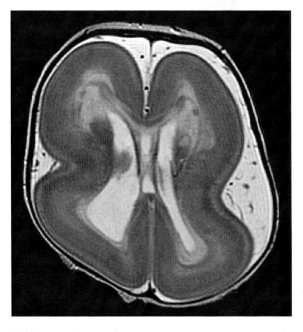

Figure 3.4 • Brain scan of a child with a brain malformation. The surface of the brain is much smoother than normal and it lacks the many folds normally present.

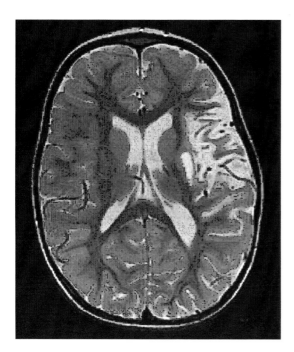

Figure 3.5 • Brain scan of a child with a middle cerebral infarct. The dark space represents fluid which has replaced the normal brain tissue.

During and shortly after birth

1. The baby may not receive enough oxygen during labour or birth. There are many reasons for this. For example, the mother may have a haemorrhage, the cord may prolapse out of the uterus, or there may be some difficulties with the delivery. If there is lack of oxygen, the baby will usually have an illness after birth called hypoxic–ischemic encephalopathy or neonatal encephalopathy. This is a condition associated with irritability, impaired alertness, difficulty with feeding and seizures.

2. Brain damage may result when an infant develops a severe infection, such as meningitis, in the first few days or weeks of life.

In the early months and years of life

1. If children have accidents, for example, motor vehicle accidents or near-drowning episodes, in the early years of life, permanent brain injury may result.

2. Severe brain infections such as meningitis and encephalitis can cause brain damage during this period.

In some children, despite a careful review and various tests, the cause of CP remains unknown (Nelson 2003). With new technologies such as MRI brain scans and sophisticated blood tests, more causes are slowly being identified. It has been suggested that most children with CP should now have these specialized radiological investigations (Ashwal et al. 2004). For more information, see Chapter 4.

Current research suggests that approximately 75% of all CP is caused by problems that occur during pregnancy, 10–15% by difficulties at birth or in the newborn period and a further 10% by illnesses or accidents in the early weeks, months or years of life. Problems that lead to permanent neurological deficits up to the age of 5–6 years are included in the CP group (Stanley et al. 2000).

Many risk factors for CP have been identified. Children particularly at risk are those infants who have been born extremely prematurely (Figure 3.6). It is sometimes difficult to be sure whether the neurological problem predated the premature delivery or whether the problems that occurred due to prematurity are responsible for the child's CP. The particular brain lesion often found in premature children is called periventricular leukomalacia. This term describes the changes that are seen in the white matter of the brain close to the ventricles (inner cavities).

Often parents worry about the cause of the CP and spend a lot of time wondering why it happened. This is understandable and a natural response. They may blame themselves for something they may or may not have done during the pregnancy or birth. Usually the event for which the family blame themselves is either not the cause or could not have been prevented. It is helpful if families can discuss the problem and share their concerns with each other and with the people involved in the care of their child.

Diagnosis

The diagnosis of CP is not always easy, particularly in children born prematurely. Neurological signs may develop over the first year of life, for example, spasticity is not usually present in the

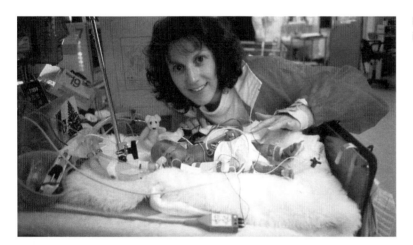

Figure 3.6 • Mother with premature infant.

early weeks of life. By contrast, abnormal neurological signs may disappear during this time. This is a difficult period for families who are anxious to know whether their child has CP. CP usually comes to attention in the following ways:

1. Follow-up of 'at-risk' infants, such as those born prematurely or those with a history of neonatal encephalopathy.

2. Delayed motor milestones, particularly delay in learning to sit, stand and walk.

3. Development of uneven movement patterns, for example, strong preference for one hand in the early months of life.

4. Abnormal muscle tone, particularly spasticity (stiffness) or hypotonia (floppiness).

The doctor takes a careful history of the pregnancy, birth and newborn period, and observes the child: such observation often provides more information than a 'hands-on' examination. This observation provides information about the presence or absence of age-appropriate motor skills and their quality. The examination involves a search for abnormalities in muscle tone and reflexes. There is no single test for CP. The diagnosis is made from the history, observing the child and conducting a physical examination. Tests such as a brain scan may assist in determining the cause.

What other problems may the child have?

Some children may have disabilities associated with CP, others may have specific health issues and, in addition, there are some consequences of the motor disorder. No one child has all these problems, and the list can seem quite frightening. However, there are specific treatments for many of the problems.

Hearing problems

Children hear from a very young age, even before they are born. The young baby will quieten, blink, startle or cry to sounds, more particularly to those sounds that are within the general range of the pitch and loudness of the human voice. As development proceeds, children may turn their eyes, and later move their heads, in the direction of various noises. They will learn to differentiate human speech from other sounds.

Hearing is vitally important for the development of speech and communication. Difficulties with hearing are uncommon but all children with CP should have their hearing checked by an audiologist (specialist in hearing) before commencing preschool, or sooner if there are any concerns. The audiologist uses a soundproof room and introduces various sounds, watching to see if the young child turns appropriately to the various noises that are made. More sophisticated testing with headphones is possible later.

There are various types of hearing loss. Surgery to drain middle-ear fluid along with placement of drainage tubes is sometimes helpful. Hearing aids can be used in certain types of hearing loss. An increasing number of children with severe or profound hearing loss are being offered cochlear implants. For children with severe physical disabilities who may not be able to develop oral speech, cochlear implantation may enable them to become more aware of their environment and more settled in their behaviour, hence improving their quality of life.

Problems with vision

The development of vision takes place rapidly in the first few months of life. At birth, infants can react to light. The ability to focus on near objects, particularly the mother's face, gradually develops in the early weeks of life so that infants are able to focus on near objects just as well as adults can by about 3 months of age.

Concerns about vision should be taken seriously and investigated promptly. Children with CP can have a variety of problems with their eyesight. Testing the vision of young children can be quite difficult. All children with CP should be checked by an eye specialist (ophthalmologist) within weeks or months if there are concerns, and in the early years of life routinely.

Visual problems include squints (turned eye or strabismus) that may require patching, eye drops or surgery. Refractive errors, such as being long-sighted or short-sighted, may be improved by the use of glasses (spectacles). In addition some children do not see well because of problems arising in the part of the brain that controls vision. This is called cortical visual impairment.

Epilepsy

Epilepsy may develop in about one in three of all children with CP. There are various types of epilepsy and medication is prescribed following a careful diagnosis of the seizure type. Doctors attempt to prescribe medications with the fewest side-effects whilst providing good seizure control. Some children may only have very occasional seizures whereas in others the problem may be more persistent, and may require the advice of a paediatric neurologist. For more information, see Chapter 5.

Intellectual or learning disability

There is a wide range of intellectual ability in children with CP. Although it is often difficult to assess learning ability in the early years of life, a psychologist can be helpful in providing some information about intellectual ability. Children with severe physical disabilities may have normal intelligence.

Speech and language problems

Receptive and expressive language delays and articulation problems frequently occur. For more information, see Chapter 18.

Perceptual difficulties

Problems such as judging the size and shape of objects are termed perceptual difficulties, and may not be apparent until school age.

Health problems

Children with CP have the same health problems as other children of a similar age. They are just as likely to develop coughs and colds and other common childhood illnesses such as chickenpox. Routine immunizations are very important. There are some specific health issues for children with CP.

Failure to thrive (undernutrition)

Some children with severe CP have difficulties with chewing and coordinating their swallowing, causing prolonged or difficult meal times. This in turn may lead to inadequate food intake and failure to thrive. Other children with CP seem to have poor weight gains despite adequate calorie

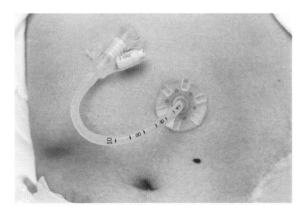

Figure 3.7 • Gastrostomy tube in place.

intake. A dietician can provide useful advice about adequate nutrition and may also provide advice about nutritional supplements. For children with major eating difficulties or at risk of aspiration, alternative methods of feeding, such as the use of nasogastric or gastrostomy tubes, need to be considered (Figure 3.7). Placement of a gastrostomy tube involves a small operation and insertion of a tube directly from the abdominal wall into the stomach. Unless there is a high risk of aspiration (see below), children may still have some food and fluids by mouth.

Obesity

Some children with normal eating abilities have a tendency to put on weight. This may be due to reduced physical activity. Excessive weight gain can be particularly disadvantageous for children learning to walk.

Constipation

This is common in children with CP. The cause is not always clear, but lack of normal mobility, difficulties with eating a high-fibre diet and poor fluid intake play a major part. It is important that constipation is managed with dietary modification (more fibre and increased fluids). If dietary manipulation is inadequate, then careful use of laxatives is generally helpful. Suppositories and enemas are also used on occasions. For more information, see Chapter 15.

Gastro-oesophageal reflux

Food comes back up the oesophagus (gullet) more commonly in children with CP. Symptoms may include vomiting and discomfort during feeds. A complication of gastro-oesophageal reflux is inflammation of the lower oesophagus (called oesophagitis). Children with this problem may be unsettled or irritable and have a poor appetite. Conservative measures, such as ensuring that the infant or child is propped upright after a meal and thickening liquids, may be helpful. Sometimes medication is used to reduce the acid content of the stomach. Occasionally surgery for reflux (called a fundoplication) is necessary when other measures have failed to control the problem. For further information, see Chapter 13.

Recurrent chest infections

This is a problem in only a very small group of children with CP. It is most likely to occur in children who have difficulties with chewing and swallowing. Some of the food and drink may inadvertently pass into the lungs. This is called aspiration. The child may cough and wheeze during or after meals and these symptoms may mimic asthma. Aspiration can sometimes occur without any signs. Children can also develop pneumonia and asthma like other children.

Chronic lung disease

If aspiration episodes are persistent the child may develop recurrent attacks of pneumonia, and chronic lung disease. There is no 'gold standard' test for aspiration but barium videofluoroscopy may be helpful. Alternative feeding regimes such as the use of a gastrostomy should be considered if aspiration is present.

Dental health

Children are at risk for dental problems and should be regularly monitored.

Osteoporosis

Many children with CP are relatively immobile and have some degree of osteoporosis. Fractures can occur with very minor injuries and sometimes during normal activities such as napkin change or putting an arm through a sleeve. Some children need special medication to promote bone mineralization.

Emotional problems

Emotional problems are frequent. They may be responsible for suboptimal performance either with academic tasks or in the self-care area. Children with CP need the same love, care and acceptance as all other children, and are more like other children than unlike them. It is important to remain optimistic about children's progress, yet realistic when the problems are severe. This is often a difficult balance to achieve. Despite all the difficulties faced by children and families, it is important to remember that the greatest achievement is the development of the child into a mature person able to adjust to life. For more information, see Chapters 6–8.

Consequences of the motor disorder

Poor saliva control (dribbling or drooling)

Children often dribble in the early years of life and this can persist in children with CP, due to problems with control of the muscles around the mouth. Dribbling results in damage to clothing and books and impedes successful integration to preschool, school and to home and community life. It is often associated with eating and drinking difficulties and with delayed or absent oral speech.

There are a number of treatments available (Johnson and Scott 2004). The speech pathologist has an important role and can provide strategies to improve dribbling problems, such as encouraging lip seal and helping the child to learn to recognize the damp secretions on the chin and to wipe them away.

For children where these strategies are not effective, medication to dry oral secretions is occasionally used, particularly in children over the age of 6 years. For older children with persistent dribbling problems, surgical treatment can be offered, which involves redirecting salivary ducts and removing some salivary glands. There are a number of different operations. One of the commonly used approaches is an operation whereby the submandibular ducts are redirected and the sublingual glands are removed. Operations usually reduce drooling but do not lead to an unduly dry mouth. It is important that children undergoing this procedure have regular dental follow-up as there is an increased risk of dental cavities.

Less common interventions occasionally tried for dribbling include the use of various orthodontic appliances and the injection of botulinum toxin A into the salivary glands.

Incontinence

Children may be late in achieving bowel and bladder control due to learning problems or lack of opportunity to access toileting facilities because of physical disability and/or inability to communicate. Sometimes children have overactivity of the bladder muscles causing urgency, frequency and incontinence. If continence is not achieved, a continence nurse may be helpful in suggesting various pads and protectors. See Chapter 15 for more information.

Undescended testes is a common but often unrecognized problem in boys with CP. The testes may be in the scrotum at birth but gradually retract upwards into the abdomen. A surgical opinion should be sought.

Spasticity

Stiffness or tightness of muscles may increase as the child grows and develops. Spasticity management is aimed at improving function, comfort and care and requires a team approach. Some of the interventions are useful for spasticity involving parts of the body (localized spasticity), for example, the use of splints, plaster casts and botulinum toxin injections. Other interventions are aimed at reducing spasticity throughout the body (generalized spasticity) and include oral medications, intrathecal baclofen and selective dorsal rhizotomy. Paediatric physiotherapists and occupational therapists play a key role in the management of spasticity in addition to encouraging optimal movement patterns and function. For more information, see Chapter 27.

Treatment for localized spasticity

Orthoses/splints

Many children use orthoses (sometimes known as braces) for the lower limbs at some stage in their development. They are made of a light-weight material and are individually fitted for each child. They fulfil a number of functions, including control of spasticity in the calf. In the upper limb, splints are sometimes made to maintain range of movement, facilitate better grasp and improve overall function of the arm and hand. These splints are usually of plastic material.

Plaster casts

Plaster casts are sometimes applied to lower limbs to stretch the calf muscles and to improve the position of the foot during walking. The casts are changed every 1–2 weeks, the child walks in the plasters, and generally the plasters remain in use for about 6 weeks. These plasters are sometimes called 'inhibitory casts'.

Botulinum toxin A

Botulinum toxin A has become very useful in the management of children with CP (Boyd and Graham 1997). It is injected into tight or spastic muscles and acts as a nerve blocker, preventing the transmission of messages from the nerves to the tight muscles. As a result, the muscles relax and spasticity is reduced, usually for a period of about 3–6 months. This provides a period of more normal muscle growth, which may be accompanied by progress in the child's movement abilities. It is most commonly injected into the lower limb when calf or hamstring spasticity is interfering with progress in learning to move. Disadvantages include

the fact that the administration of botulinum toxin A requires multiple injections, the effects of the drug are not completely predictable (sometimes it works well and at other times it is less effective) and are of short duration and the toxin is costly. For more information, see Chapter 27.

Treatments for generalized spasticity

Oral medications

Oral medications may be used for generalized spasticity but are often not effective or may cause too many unwanted effects.

Intrathecal baclofen

Intrathecal baclofen involves the administration of a medication called baclofen. The medication is given via a pump that is implanted underneath the skin of the abdominal wall (Figure 3.8). The pump

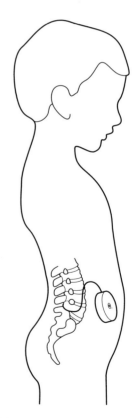

Figure 3.8 • Schematic drawing of baclofen pump in place.

is connected to a tube which delivers the drug into the space around the spinal cord. Dose adjustments are made by an external computer. The pumps remain in the body for an extended period, up to about 7 years. This treatment is suitable for a small number of children with severe spasticity that is interfering with comfort and quality of life.

Selective dorsal rhizotomy

Selective dorsal rhizotomy is a major operation on the spine. Nerve roots are cut to reduce spasticity. The operation is most successful in young children (aged about 4–6 years) who have spastic diplegia. Following the procedure a very extensive rehabilitation period, of at least 1–2 years, is required.

Orthopaedic problems

As children grow and develop, muscles with spasticity or stiffness may become shortened, causing muscle or joint deformity. This is most likely to occur at the ankle, knee, hip, elbow and wrist. Surgery is mainly undertaken on the lower limb, but is occasionally helpful in the upper limb. Gait laboratories are useful in planning the surgical programme for children who are able to walk independently or with sticks or walking frames. Physiotherapists are essential in the postoperative rehabilitation phase.

The hip

Children with CP are at risk for developing hip subluxation, that is, movement of the head of the thigh bone out of the hip socket, and dislocation (Figure 3.9). This is most likely to occur in children who are not walking independently. Regular monitoring with hip X-rays is important. If there is evidence that the hip is at risk of dislocation, children are referred for an orthopaedic opinion. Soft-tissue surgery, that is, release of muscles, is often effective for children when the hip problems are detected at an early stage, hence the importance of regular X-rays. If subluxation progresses towards dislocation, more extensive surgery to the hip bones is required. A dislocated hip can result in pain and difficulty with hygiene (Dobson et al. 2002).

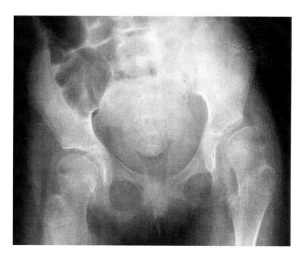

Figure 3.9 • Hip X-ray. The left hip is normally positioned but the right hip is subluxed (partially displaced out of the hip socket).

The knee

Lengthening of the hamstrings can help the knee straighten and so improve the walking pattern. Sometimes transferring a muscle from the front to the back of the knee can also help by reducing stiffness around the knee.

The ankle

Equinus deformity at the ankle, standing on the toes, is the commonest orthopaedic problem in children with CP. It is treated conservatively in young children with orthoses, inhibitory casts and botulinum toxin A therapy. Older children benefit from surgery for a definitive correction of the deformity.

Multilevel surgery

Sometimes children require surgery at several different levels (for example, hip, knee and ankle). This involves a single hospitalization and is called 'single-event multilevel surgery'. It is of most benefit to children who walk independently or with the assistance of walking frames or sticks. The usual age is 8–12 years. The aims of surgery are to correct deformities and to improve both the appearance and efficiency of walking. An accurate

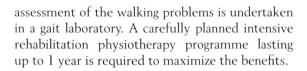

assessment of the walking problems is undertaken in a gait laboratory. A carefully planned intensive rehabilitation physiotherapy programme lasting up to 1 year is required to maximize the benefits.

Upper limb

A number of procedures are available for the upper limb, aimed at improving function or cosmesis. An intensive occupational therapy programme is essential following most procedures.

Spine

Children with CP may develop scoliosis, and spinal surgery to correct the curve may sometimes be necessary. For more information, see Chapters 25–27.

Questions commonly asked by parents

Will my child get better?

'Cerebral palsy' refers to a permanent condition, and the problems associated with this condition, such as muscle weakness or stiffness and unwanted movements, remain throughout the lifetime of a person with CP. However, children can learn to cope with the condition as they grow. Treatment often brings about improvement, though not a cure.

Will my child's condition deteriorate?

The answer is 'no'. The damage done to the brain early in life does not worsen. But sometimes it does seem that the child's condition becomes worse. This may be because of tightening of muscles, other illnesses, poorly controlled epilepsy, side-effects of medication or emotional stress. If the child appears to be losing previous skills, parents should consult their doctor.

Will my child learn to walk?

Parents generally want to know the answer to this question shortly after CP is diagnosed.

Unfortunately, it is often not possible to be sure until after the child has been observed by the paediatrician and therapist for a period of time. Knowledge about how children's motor function develops has progressed with the work that has been done to create growth motor curves (Rosenbaum et al. 2002). This is discussed in Chapter 20.

Will my child learn to talk?

The development of speech involves a number of factors, including learning to control the movements around the mouth and attaining the necessary learning skills. Some children with CP will not have any difficulties in learning to talk; others will need help from a speech pathologist to develop speech or alternative methods of communication.

Will my child be able to look after him- or herself?

The aim of intervention is to encourage the child to learn to be as independent as possible. Some children with mild CP will not have any problems in achieving independence. For others, it will be a slow process. In some with severe difficulties, considerable assistance from others will always be needed. It is important for parents to encourage children to do as much as possible for themselves.

Will my child have a normal life expectancy?

Most children with CP are healthy, and can expect a normal lifespan. A very small group of children with extremely severe CP and associated conditions such as epilepsy may be at risk of reduced life expectancy. For example, they may develop recurrent chest infections or have a prolonged seizure.

Will my next child have CP?

This is extremely unlikely, but you should discuss this with your doctor. Parents should feel free to seek advice from their doctor about genetic counselling and obstetric care of future pregnancies.

Who is available to help my child?

A number of professionals work with children with CP and their families. Depending on needs, some children may be seen by all of these people, others only by one or two. Different professionals will be helpful at various stages of the child's development. Some of the people involved are the family doctor (general practitioner), the paediatrician, nurses, therapists, social workers, psychologists, special education teachers, orthotists and orthopaedic surgeons.

Is there any research being carried out?

In many areas of the world there is research going on into the causes of CP. Research is also being carried out to help find the best methods of management and treatment or intervention. For more information about research, you should speak to your paediatrician or therapist. You may also find the websites of the following organizations helpful: United CP (USA) (www.UCP.org), Scope (UK) (www.scope.org.uk), American Academy of CP and Developmental Medicine (www.aacpdm.org), Canchild (www.canchild.ca) and CP Australia (www.cpaustralia.com.au).

References

Ashwal S, Russman B, Blasco P et al. Practice parameter: diagnostic assessment of the child with CP. Neurology 2004; 62:851–863.

Boyd R, Graham HK. Botulinum toxin A in the management of children with cerebral palsy: indications and outcome. Eur J Neurol 1997; 4:15–S22.

Dobson F, Boyd RN, Parrott J et al. Hip surveillance in children with cerebral palsy: impact on the surgical management of spastic hip disease. J Bone Joint Surg (Br) 2002; 84-B:720–726.

Johnson H, Scott A. A practical approach to the management of saliva, 2nd edn. Pro-ed, Arizona, 2004.

Nelson KB. Can we prevent cerebral palsy? N Engl J Med 2003; 18:1765–1769.

Palisano R, Rosenbaum P, Walter S et al. Development and reliability of a system to classify gross motor function in children with CP. Dev Med Child Neurol 1997; 39:214–223.

Rosenbaum P, Walter S, Hanna S et al. Prognosis for gross motor function in CP – creation of gross motor curves. JAMA 2002; 288:1357–1363.

Stanley FJ, Blair E, Alberman E. Cerebral palsies: epidemiology and causal pathways. Clinics in Developmental Medicine no. 151. MacKeith Press, London, 2000.

Chapter Four

4

The role of different brain-imaging techniques in the diagnosis of cerebral palsy

Ingeborg Krägeloh-Mann • Marko Wilke

With the development of advanced neuroimaging methods it has become possible to obtain information about the brain in a living person during his or her lifetime (in vivo). Brain imaging can be undertaken consecutively, and thus show the development of a harmful process occurring in the brain. This chapter aims to present some of the different brain-imaging techniques used routinely in clinical practice and to discuss them with respect to the diagnosis of CP, considering:

1. What they can show and what they are not able to show.

2. When they should be performed and when they should not or no longer be performed.

Brain imaging has significantly helped to enhance our understanding of cerebral palsy (CP), especially when it comes to unravelling the mechanisms leading to brain changes responsible for the neurological abnormalities characteristic of children with CP, such as spastic, dyskinetic or ataxic movement disorders. Brain imaging may also help us to understand the additional problems, such as learning difficulties, epilepsy and visual deficits, present in many children with CP. Before imaging techniques were available, the main source of knowledge on the brain disorder behind CP was the study of the brain after death (postmortem neuropathology). However, this was only available in a few cases, and the insights gained from such studies are limited.

Neuroimaging methods

There are three main approaches to investigating brain structure: (1) ultrasound (US); (2) computed tomography (CT); and (3) magnetic resonance imaging (MRI). Over the following paragraphs, we will give a very brief overview of each approach and discuss their respective advantages and disadvantages. This chapter will not discuss neuroimaging techniques such as positron emission tomography (PET) and single-photon emission computed tomography (SPECT) which are currently not routinely used in children with CP.

Ultrasound

Principle

Ultrasound, as the name implies, relies on generating high-frequency sound waves inaudible to the human ear which are transmitted from and received by a small hand-held probe. The signals are analysed in an attached computer and visualized on a screen in real time. The basic principle behind these images is that different tissue types reflect the ultrasound waves in different ways. This means that, for example, brain tissue (grey matter, the neurons, and white matter, the neuronal fibres) can clearly be distinguished from cerebrospinal fluid (CSF), for example, in the CSF chambers within the brain ventricles.

Procedure

The examiner places the ultrasound probe directly on the open fontanelles of the head, with the child usually lying in a supine position. The examination can be performed in a child who is either asleep or awake, and takes around 10 minutes. Contrast agent is not used.

Advantages

Ultrasound is not harmful. It is fast and shows images in real time. It is widely available. In skilled hands, it is a valuable method as it allows repeated, fast examinations at the bedside, and is especially useful for very small infants in the neonatal intensive care unit.

Disadvantages

Image quality and interpretation are very dependent on the experience of the operator, and image sections are harder to standardize than with other imaging modalities, making it a much more subjective method. It is therefore often necessary to confirm ultrasound-based diagnoses with other imaging modalities, such as CT or MRI. Structures in the middle of the brain can be visualized better than the cortex (the outer sections of the brain, consisting of grey matter). An open fontanelle is a prerequisite for high resolution ultrasound brain imaging. It is thus unusable after the fusion of skull bones at the age of about 1½–2 years. Figure 4.1 shows a normal infant's brain as seen by ultrasound.

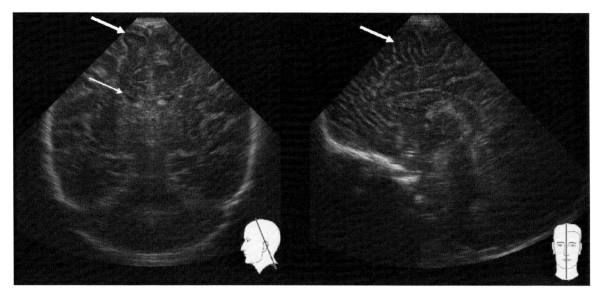

Figure 4.1 • Ultrasound of a normal child's brain at the age of 5 months. The orientation of the slice is shown in the drawing of a head (lower, right). The thick arrow indicates the cortex, and the thin arrow the lateral ventricle.

Computed tomography

Principle

CT is an X-ray-based technique. It involves a rotating X-ray emitter/detector which circles around the head to take numerous independent images from different angles. Computerized postprocessing then constructs three-dimensional images that delineate bone in detail and provide good soft-tissue visualization.

Procedure

The child lies supine on a moving table which is used to position the head in the centre of the circular detector. The investigation may take up to 20 minutes, depending on the extent of images necessary, but a fast snapshot can be obtained in only a few minutes. Imaging is silent, and contrast agent may be used, depending on the investigation needed.

Advantages

CT is still the gold standard when it comes to assessing bone structures and for detecting blood and calcifications within soft tissue. It is also faster and more widely available than MRI and therefore more likely to be available in the case of an emergency or with children less able to lie still for prolonged periods of time. It may also be the only advanced imaging option in the presence of sensitive metallic implants.

Disadvantages

As CT relies on X-ray absorption, it invariably involves radiation exposure, especially so if non-adapted protocols from adult patients are used with children. Soft-tissue delineation is not as good as with MRI, and artefacts from bone may make interpretation difficult, especially in the lower parts of the brain.

Magnetic resonance imaging

Principle

Magnetic resonance describes a phenomenon that occurs when certain atoms are exposed to a strong magnetic field and are then excited by means of a radiofrequency pulse. In the clinical situation, magnets with field strength between 0.5 and 1.5 Tesla (T) are used. The resulting signal is detected by so-called coils and, by means of computerized processing, is turned into an image that basically reflects the distribution of water in the brain, as hydrogen, yielding the bulk of the obtained signal, is most abundant in water. Numerous modifications of the original approach allow the assessment not only of structure but also nowadays of function and biochemical information. Structural images are acquired with different sequences, which lead to different signals – hyperintense and hypointense, which means bright or dark in the image. The basic sequences are:

1. The so-called T1-weighted sequence (T1w), where water appears dark and lipids bright. Thus CSF is dark, compounds of neurons are grey and myelinated white matter is white.

2. The T2w sequence, where water appears bright and lipids dark. Thus CSF is bright, compounds of neurons are grey and myelinated white matter is dark. Examples are shown in Figures 4.2–4.7: Figure 4.3 illustrates a lesion seen on T2w images only.

Procedure

The child is brought into the centre of the magnet for examination. Due to the constrained space within the large machine, claustrophobia may be a problem with adults, but is much less so with children. Parents can usually stay in the room as no harmful radiation is generated. When the brain is investigated, a special coil like an astronaut's helmet surrounds the head. The investigation usually takes 30–45 minutes. Imaging is noisy so ear protection should be provided. Contrast media may be necessary.

Advantages

MRI yields good soft-tissue contrast and very high resolution without harmful radiation exposure and without interference from surrounding bone structures, making it the method of choice for brain tissue assessment. It is especially advantageous when inflammatory or malignant processes are suspected.

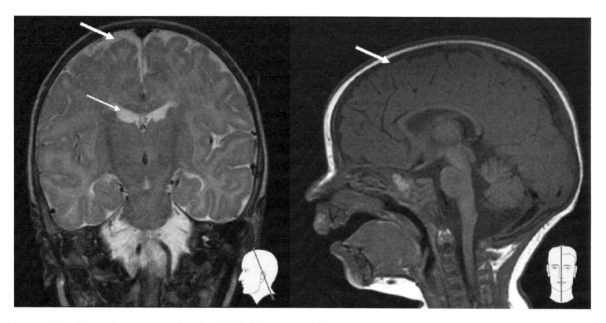

Figure 4.2 • Magnetic resonance imaging (MRI) of the same child as in Figure 4.1, illustrating the superior spatial resolution and contrast that MRI offers over ultrasound. On the left is a T2w image, on the right a T1w image, both showing a slice corresponding to the ultrasound in Figure 4.1.

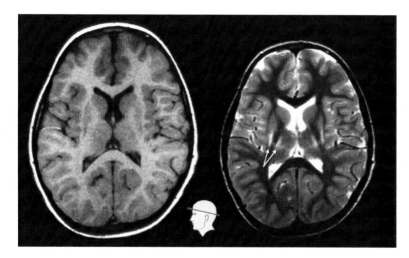

Figure 4.3 • This figure illustrates how the different magnetic resonance imaging sequences have different sensitivities to show lesions. The T1w image on the left does not show a clear abnormality, whereas the T2w image on the right shows clear lesions of the basal ganglia and thalamus (arrows), which give rise to a very disabling movement disorder, dyskinetic cerebral palsy.

A special advantage that has revolutionized the clinical care for patients with a stroke is the much earlier detection of tissue damage due to insufficient blood supply. In contrast to the other imaging modalities, MRI can show the process of myelination. Myelination, the insulation around nerve fibres, starts during late pregnancy and has its main spurt during the first 24 months of life (see Figure 4.4).

Disadvantages

The magnetic field necessary to achieve the effect needs to be very strong, which requires quite an amount of infrastructure and technical effort. This explains some of the higher costs of an MRI. Availability therefore may be less than for CT scans. The presence of the strong magnetic field prevents the scanning of patients with certain metallic implants, such as cardiac pacemakers. Bone and blood cannot be detected with a high degree of reliability. The large machine may intimidate younger children, and scanning times tend to be longer than for a CT scan, which makes it more

vulnerable to motion artefacts. Consequently, in younger children, it often needs to be performed under sedation or general anaesthesia.

Figure 4.2 shows a normal infant's brain seen by MRI (similar to Figure 4.1).

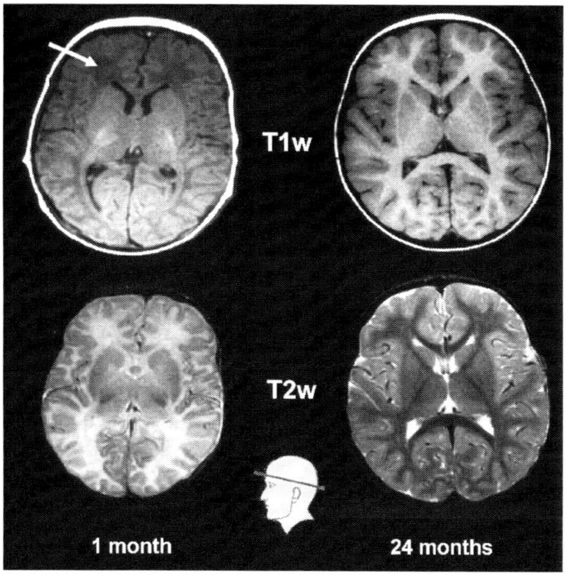

Neuroimaging techniques in the diagnosis of CP

To understand what neuroimaging can show in children with CP it is helpful to have some basic knowledge of normal and abnormal brain development.

Normal and abnormal brain development

The child's brain undergoes complex changes during its development which are not complete at birth. When something harmful happens to the brain, the result in the brain may depend more on the timing than on the nature of the event. For example, different mechanisms such as a lack of oxygen, an infection or a poison can cause a malformation when occurring during early brain development and a defect when occurring later. The reason is that in the first case the brain was disturbed in its gross architecture, which went wrong and a 'different and wrong form' was established, whereas in the second case, the gross architecture

Figure 4.4 • Magnetic resonance images at 1 and 24 months to illustrate different periods of myelination: top, T1w images; bottom, corresponding T2w images. At 1 month, when myelination is just starting, the entire white matter (arrow) is dark on the T1w and bright on T2w image; at 24 months myelination is nearly complete and white matter appears uniformly bright on the T1w and dark on the T2w image.

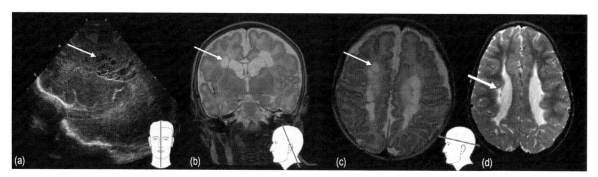

Figure 4.5 • These images illustrate different stages of a severe form of lesion: cystic periventricular leukomalacia, seen with ultrasound and magnetic resonance imaging (MRI) in a child born at 31 weeks, who developed severe bilateral spastic cerebral palsy. (a) Ultrasound at 5 months, showing cysts in the depth of the brain, next to the ventricles (arrow). MRI at the same time in coronal (b) and axial (c) orientation showing these cysts (thin arrows). (d) MRI at a later age (6 years) in axial orientation showing the end-stage of periventricular leukomalacia with tissue loss and scars (arrow).

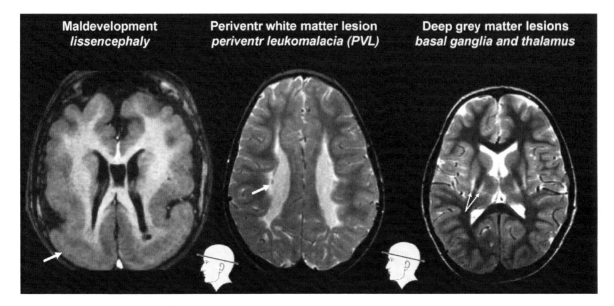

Figure 4.6 • Examples for the three major groups of brain abnormalities which are mainly found in cerebral palsy. Children are all older than 5 years at the time of imaging. Left: lissencephaly with a thick and non-gyrated cortex (arrow; T1-weighted image). Middle: periventricular leukomalacia with periventricular tissue loss and scarring (arrow). Right: the same basal ganglia and thalamus lesions as in Figure 4.3 (T2-weighted image).

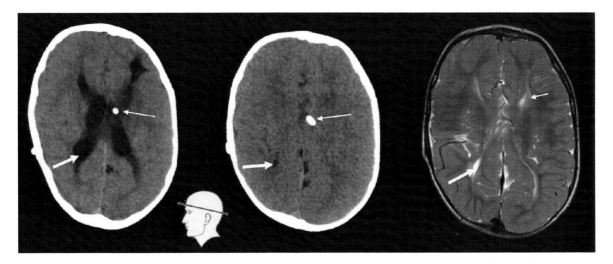

Figure 4.7 • Computed tomography (CT: left) acutely done in a 3-year-old child because of suspected shunt dysfunction (and consequently increased intracranial pressure, leading to vomiting and headache). Indeed, the inner chambers (ventricles) were enlarged (thick arrow), in comparison to the CT done 6 months earlier (middle), when the ventricles were very small (thick arrow). The child is a former preterm who developed hydrocephalus after severe intraventricular bleeding. Magnetic resonance imaging (right) at the time of the middle CT shows much better the cortex/white-matter differentiation and the gliosis (small, thin arrow), which indicate that the child also has periventricular leukomalacia. The shunt, however, is only clearly seen on the CT scans (long thin arrow).

was already finished and the harmful event led to destruction of part of the brain, which left a defect.

Gross architecture of the normal brain is established during the first approximately 24 weeks of gestation (also called the first and second trimester: a trimester covers 3 months). This period is mainly characterized by the production of brain cells, that is neurons, and their precursors and is called the period of proliferation. These cells, neuronal precursors, then wander to their future places in the brain, called the period of migration. The migration is mainly to the cortex, where they then organize themselves in the cell layers of the cortex. This is called the period of organization. Harmful events, as discussed above, cause malformations or maldevelopments of the brain. These maldevelopments are classified according to the periods when they occurred, that is: (1) disorders of proliferation; (2) disorders of migration; and (3) disorders of organization. Typical examples are: (1) severe microcephaly (the brain is far too small) due to too little proliferation; (2) lissencephaly, in which the brain is smooth, and without gyri due to abnormal migration; and (3) polymicrogyria, in which the cortex consists of too many small gyri due to abnormal organization. It is important to appreciate that these early changes in brain development can be genetic or acquired, whereas disturbances of brain development later on are usually acquired. Causes can include infections and lack of oxygen.

Once the basic formation of the brain has been established before the last approximately 15 weeks of pregnancy (called the third trimester), the finer, more subtle processes of the brain develop and the brain grows. This goes on long after birth. The finer, more subtle processes of brain development consist of the formation of axons, dendrites and synapses, that is the sprouting of cell processes and their connections. Myelination occurs, which entails the formation of insulating sheaths around axons. Disturbances of brain development during this later period predominantly result in so-called lesions or defects. Causes may be infections, lack of oxygen and insufficient blood supply to the brain. Early during the third trimester, when the infant is around 24–36 weeks of age, periventricular white matter, the nerve fibres next to the CSF

chambers within the brain, is especially sensitive to insults, whereas towards the end of the third trimester and around birth, grey matter appears to be more vulnerable. Grey matter consists primarily of neurons, which form the cortex and are also assembled in the deep brain structures called basal ganglia and thalamus. These are connecting stations between the outer parts of the brain and the spinal cord conveying the brain's commands to the body and vice versa. The deep brain structures are also a relay station of the cerebral networks.

Abnormalities of brain development and CP

CP is defined as being due to a lesion/abnormality/disturbance of the brain occurring during its development. As discussed above, harmful events during brain development lead to different kinds of damage depending on timing, that is, maldevelopments during the first and second trimester of pregnancy and lesions during the third trimester and at birth. We shall now address the question of whether brain-imaging techniques can identify these problems and how often they are found in CP.

Maldevelopments are found in less than 10% of children with CP. They can best be identified by MRI, irrespective of the age of the child. It is possible to undertake MRI soon after birth and also later on. Ultrasound may detect important maldevelopments, especially those located in the middle of the brain, but depicts the cortex less well. In CP, however, cortical maldevelopments are the most important, which is why ultrasound alone is of limited help. Ultrasound may raise suspicion which should then be followed up with an MRI. CT also has a very limited potential to depict cortical maldevelopments, but, in contrast to ultrasound, it can be undertaken later on, when brain ultrasound is no longer feasible.

Lesions are responsible for around 75% of CP; around 55% are periventricular white-matter lesions and around 20% are cortical or deep grey-matter lesions. From what we have explained it follows that these lesions arise near birth, somewhat before, around or even thereafter. Imaging, thus, may show the development of a lesion. It takes some time between cell swelling, cell death and the cell's decomposition, the end-stage of a lesion.

Periventricular white-matter lesions are mainly seen in children born preterm. Two main forms may be distinguished: (1) periventricular leukomalacia (PVL), that is, tissue destruction along the inner CSF chambers of the brain which results in scars; and (2) defects after intraventricular haemorrhage (IVH) or bleeding. Ultrasound is good for detecting IVH itself, but less sensitive in showing the extent of tissue destruction IVH may cause; here CT and, even better, MRI can show the long-term effects of such haemorrhage. None of the three neuroimaging techniques is very sensitive in detecting the early development of a PVL; only the so-called cystic PVL, a severe form with lacunar degeneration of periventricular tissue, can be depicted early using all three techniques. The end-stage of PVL and IVH can be best seen on MRI. It is important to note that the full extent of PVL can only be seen in the already myelinated brain, that is, in the older child. As ultrasound is available in the neonatal unit and can be performed repeatedly, it is the method of choice for the early diagnosis of periventricular white-matter lesions, whereas MRI is the method of choice for definite diagnosis, that is, after the age of 1½ years or, even better, 2 years, when the brain is myelinated. Figure 4.5 illustrates cystic PVL in ultrasound and in MRI at the same time and later on.

Cortical or deep grey-matter lesions mainly arise around birth in the term-born child. They are the typical consequences of severe birth asphyxia. Early identification is difficult in cortical lesions, but overall brain swelling (oedema) may be an indicator of extensive brain damage with cortical lesions, and can be seen by ultrasound, CT or MRI. At this early stage, the definite extent of the lesions cannot yet be seen. Deep grey-matter lesions are also best seen by MRI, but it is important to note that this may not be before 8–10 days after the acute event. The definite extent of grey-matter lesions, whether cortical or deep, is again best seen on MRI, and again it is very important to note that the best point in time is after myelination.

Figure 4.6 gives examples for these three groups.

Conclusion

Neuroimaging is of great importance in the diagnosis of CP. MRI is clearly the method of choice in a child where, due to abnormal neurological signs, CP is suspected or clearly diagnosed. In such a situation, MRI has an 85% chance of showing the underlying brain damage.

Our knowledge from systematic imaging studies in children with CP suggests that this will be a brain maldevelopment in about 10% of children. It is important to recognize this entity as it may be genetically determined.

However, in the majority of affected children (around 75%) a lesion is found, that is, a defect following an insult in the third trimester or around birth. Recognizing this can have some implications: (1) it confirms that the condition is permanent, but non-progressive and non-genetic; and (2) it usually helps to explain the degree of the motor disability and the additional problems, such as epilepsy, visual deficits or severe learning difficulties.

In some children with CP (around 15%), MRI does not reveal a clear pathology. It is either normal or shows unspecific findings. In such a situation two main considerations are important:

1. Are the images obtained sufficient? If it was done before the age of 2 years it should be repeated as a lesion may not yet be clearly delineated due to ongoing myelination.

2. Is the clinical diagnosis of CP certain? A child with normal or unspecific MRI undertaken at 2 years or later should always be carefully followed with respect to other diagnoses, for example progressive genetic disease, which may require different treatment and genetic counselling.

Ultrasound continues to be the method of choice in the neonatal period to depict an evolving lesion. It allows repeated examinations without being too stressful for the child. However, findings may need to be confirmed and extended by a follow-up MRI.

CT has a limited role to play in the diagnosis of CP. It may be used in specific situations when it is important to detect calcifications, for example

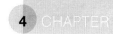

as a late consequence of a prenatal infection. It is an essential modality for imaging in the acute setting, for example in the diagnosis and follow-up of high-pressure hydrocephalus, which is often seen as a consequence and complication of IVH in preterm children (Figure 4.7).

Further reading

Ashwal S, Russman BS, Blasco BA et al. Practice parameter: diagnostic assessment of the child with cerebral palsy. Neurology 2004; 62:851–863.

Barkovich AJ, Kuzniecky RI, Jackson GD et al. Classification system for malformations of cortical development. Neurology 2001; 57:2168–2178.

Krägeloh-Mann I. Imaging of early brain injury and cortical plasticity. Exp Neurol 2004; 190:84–90.

Krägeloh-Mann I, Horber V. The role of MR imaging in elucidating pathogenesis of cerebral palsy – a systematic review. Dev Med Child Neurol 2007; 47:144–151.

Chapter Five

5

Epilepsy in cerebral palsy

Renzo Guerrini • Simona Pellacani

CHAPTER CONTENTS

Definitions and terminology

Epilepsy is characterized by the repetition of seizures (fits). The causes and the clinical spectrum of epilepsy are extremely wide in children. Seizures are descriptively characterized with standard terminology (Blume et al. 2001, Fisher et al. 2005) and, where possible, classified into specific epilepsy types or syndromes (Commission 1989, Engel 2001), as described in Box 5.1. A syndrome is a complex of signs and symptoms defining a unique epileptic condition. Syndrome classification is described on the basis of seizure types, clinical context, neurophysiology and neuroimaging (Commission 1989, Engel 2001). Epilepsy can be: (1) focal (partial) if clinical and electroencephalogram (EEG) manifestations suggest focal onset (Engel 2001); or (2) generalized, if all seizures and EEG abnormalities are generalized. Symptomatic epilepsies result from a brain lesion, which is not necessarily detected by neuroimaging. Cerebral palsy (CP) is one of the major causes of symptomatic epilepsy.

Epidemiology of epilepsy in cerebral palsy

Epileptologists know that CP is the most common neurological disorder associated with epilepsy.

Box 5.1

Definitions of key terms (modified from Engel 2001, Fisher et al. 2005)

Epilepsy

A disorder of the brain characterized by an enduring predisposition to generate epileptic seizures and by the neurobiological, cognitive, psychological and social consequences of this condition. The definition of epilepsy requires the occurrence of at least one epileptic seizure

Epileptic seizure

A transient occurrence of signs and symptoms, or both, as a result of abnormal excessive or synchronous neuronal activity in the brain

Epileptic seizure type

An ictal event believed to represent a unique pathophysiological mechanism and anatomic substrate. This is a diagnostic entity with aetiologic, therapeutic and prognostic implications

Epilepsy syndrome

A complex of signs and symptoms that define a unique epilepsy condition. Epilepsy syndrome must involve more than just the seizure type: thus, frontal-lobe seizures per se, for instance, do not constitute a syndrome

Epileptic disease

A pathological condition with a single specific, well-defined cause. Thus, progressive myoclonus epilepsy is a syndrome, but Unverricht–Lundborg is a disease

Epileptic encephalopathy

A condition in which the epileptiform abnormalities themselves are believed to contribute to the progressive disturbance in cerebral function

Benign epilepsy syndrome

A syndrome characterized by epileptic seizures that are easily treated, or need no treatment, and remit without sequelae

Reflex epilepsy syndrome

A syndrome in which all epileptic seizures are precipitated by sensory stimuli. Reflex seizures that occur in focal and generalized epilepsy syndromes that are also associated with spontaneous seizures are listed as seizure types. Isolated reflex seizures can also occur in situations that do not necessarily need a diagnosis of epilepsy. Seizures precipitated by other special circumstances, such as fever or alcohol withdrawal, are not reflex seizures

Focal seizures and syndromes

Replaces the terms 'partial seizures' and 'localization-related syndromes'

Simple and complex partial epileptic seizures

These terms are no longer recommended, nor will they be replaced. Ictal impairment of consciousness will be described when appropriate for individual seizures, but will not be used to classify specific seizure types

Idiopathic epilepsy syndrome

A syndrome that is only epilepsy, with no underlying structural brain lesion or other neurological signs or symptoms. These are presumed to be genetic and are usually age-dependent

Symptomatic epilepsy syndrome

A syndrome in which the epileptic seizures are the result of one or more identifiable structural lesions of the brain

Probably symptomatic epilepsy syndrome

Synonymous with, but preferred to, the term 'cryptogenic', used to define syndromes that are believed to be symptomatic, but for which no cause has been identified

However, from the perspective of the carer of children with CP it is more helpful to know that the frequency of epilepsy in CP varies between 15% and 60% (Aksu 1990, Hadjipanayis et al. 1997, Stephenson 1997), with rates differing according to the type of CP. In the series of Hadjipanayis et al. (1997), epilepsy was present in 50% of children with quadriplegia, in 47% of those with hemiplegia but in only 27% of those with spastic diplegia. A different category is represented by children with acquired postconvulsive hemiplegia (the hemiconvulsion hemiplegia (HH) syndrome) in whom the frequency of epilepsy is highest (80%) (Aicardi et al. 1969). Only about 25% of people with dyskinetic CP have seizures; these are more common in dystonic types than in athetoid or other dyskinetic forms, respectively 32% and 11% (Kyllerman 1981). The incidence of epilepsy in ex-preterm infants with diplegia was as low as 11% in one series (Amess et al. 1998), probably a result of the predominance of deep white-matter lesions in such cases.

Epileptic seizures and main epilepsy syndromes

All types of seizures may occur in children with CP. Seizures may include a single symptom or have complex symptomatology.

Partial motor seizures

Partial motor seizures are the most common in children with hemiplegia (73%) but can be observed in any child with CP. Clinical manifestations may be either simple (a jerk) or complex (complex organized movements: Box 5.2). The epileptic discharges responsible for partial motor seizures may remain localized to a relatively small cortical area or they may spread to involve neighbouring areas that may be relatively distant from the site of origin. Simple clonic (repetitive and rhythmic) and tonic (stiffening of one body segment) phenomena are often present from the start or may become clonic after an initial brief tonic contraction.

Clonic seizure activity is characterized by rhythmic jerking or twitching of usually contiguous body segments, due to short (50–200 ms) muscle contractions alternating with silent periods. Purely tonic focal motor seizures may also occur. Any part of one side of the body can be affected. Resulting from the respective sizes of the cortical representation of movement, the seizures tend to involve preferentially the thumb, fingers, lips, eyelids and big toe. In children, involvement of the muscles of the face, tongue, pharynx and larynx, with consequent salivation and speech difficulties, is especially common. In some seizures, the convulsions remain narrowly localized, e.g. to one segment or limb.

Partial motor seizures may vary in duration from a few seconds to several hours. When they are prolonged, they are usually clonic. Postictal hemiplegia or a more restricted motor deficit is common following long seizures and may last from minutes to several days.

Unilateral clonic seizures are frequent in childhood. They are characterized by synchronous rhythmic jerking of most or all muscles of one-half of the body. Jerks may sometimes be very mild and only affect the eyeballs or the labial muscles.

Box 5.2

Features of partial motor seizures

Definition

Partial seizures are those in which the first clinical and electroencephalographic changes indicate activation of a system of neurons limited to part of one cerebral hemisphere. In children with cerebral palsy the cortical areas of the brain where movement is represented are often damaged and are involved in the epileptogenic zone. Therefore, focal seizures in which motor manifestations are the initial or the only symptom are frequent. When consciousness (responsiveness or awareness) is not impaired, the seizure is classified as a *simple partial motor seizure*; if the child becomes unresponsive (unconscious or unresponsive), the seizure is usually classified as a *complex partial motor seizure*

Who gets them?

Most commonly children with hemiplegia, but partial motor seizures may be observed in any child with cerebral palsy

Main features

Clinical manifestations may be either simple (repetitive jerking) or complex (complex patterned movements). The focal motor symptoms may be with or without a march (Jacksonian march, i.e. beginning with localized twitching of a body segment – usually distal – and progressively spreading to contiguous segments). There may also be versive, postural and phonatory (vocalization or arrest of speech) manifestations

Duration

Variable, from a few seconds to hours (focal status epilepticus)

Possible complications

Postictal hemiplegia or hemiparesis or a more restricted motor deficit is common following prolonged seizures and may last from minutes to hours or days if the seizure has been very prolonged

Unresponsiveness is often, but not always, observed and can be either initial or gradual. Autonomic phenomena, including pallor, perspiration or hypersalivation, are frequent. Consciousness may recover quickly, as seizure activity ceases, while postictal hemiparesis is still present (Dravet 1992).

Some motor seizures are characterized by asymmetric tonic motor phenomena. The term *versive* seizures designates the ictal turning of the head and eyes to one side (Wyllie et al. 1986). Repetitive vocalization or loud moaning may be heard and some people may try to speak during attacks or are able to respond as soon as tonic contraction relaxes (Bleasel and Lüders 2000). However, speech arrest is more common. As a result of the predominantly axial involvement

and preserved consciousness, children may still have spontaneous activity which, together with modifications in intensity and distribution of muscle contraction, may lead to slow writhing, dystonic movements (Bleasel and Lüders 2000). Consciousness is usually preserved during attacks, but the person may become unresponsive or a secondary generalization with stiffening and subsequent clonic jerks of the whole body may follow. Seizure duration is brief, usually between 10 and 40 seconds, and postictal confusion is rarely observed (Bleasel and Lüders 2000).

Some focal seizures feature prominent bilateral postural movements involving primarily the trunk, pelvis and proximal extremities resembling natural movements and therefore different from the tonic, clonic or dystonic movements occurring during bilateral asymmetric motor phenomena. Characteristic patterns of repetitive movements and automatic activities include kicking, cycling, thrashing, crossing and uncrossing the legs, rocking, genital manipulations and a peculiar repetitive vocalization. The term 'hypermotor seizures' was introduced to describe the whole phenomenology (Lüders et al. 1998).

Alteration of consciousness has classically been considered the hallmark of complex partial seizures, as opposed to simple partial seizures in which awareness is preserved. However, alteration of consciousness indicates extensive seizure spread but no origin or distribution (Munari et al. 1980).

Typical complex partial seizures include an initial rising epigastric sensation with fear, oroalimentary automatisms (chewing, swallowing, lip smacking), alteration of consciousness with staring and postictal confusion (Mohamed et al. 2001).

In verbal children, aphasia is often observed when the dominant hemisphere is involved.

In infants and small children, reduction of motor activity may be the prominent feature, without automatisms (hypomotor seizures) (Hamer et al. 1999).

Postictal sleepiness is frequent in children and has major relevance for differential diagnosis with respect to nonepileptic attacks.

Infantile spasms

Infantile spasms are a unique seizure type, typical of the first year of life but often observed beyond that age. They are usually resistant to conventional antiepileptic drugs and are associated with developmental delay or deterioration, and a hypsarrhythmic EEG pattern, which expresses a chaotic disorganization of electrogenesis (Box 5.3). In West syndrome, all these elements occur together. However, infantile spasms may occur without the typical EEG or developmental features.

Infantile spasms are manifested as clusters of increasing plateau–decreasing intensity brisk (0.5–2.0 seconds) flexions or extensions of the neck, with abduction or adduction of the upper limbs. Sometimes spasms are simply manifested as repetitive upward eye deviation, especially at the beginning of a cluster. A crescendo is often

Box 5.3

Features of infantile spasms

Definition

A distinctive seizure disorder with sudden, generally bilateral flexor or flexoextensor contraction of muscles of the neck, trunk and extremities. Developmental delay, stagnation or deterioration and a characteristic electroencephalogram (EEG) pattern (hypsarrhythmia) co-occur in West syndrome

Who gets them?

Usually, although not exclusively, children in the first year of life

Main features

Symmetric or asymmetric spasms, often in clusters, which recur frequently during the day, especially upon awakening. Flexion or extension of the neck, with abduction or adduction of the upper limbs and/or rising of the lower limbs in a large brisk flexor movement, may occur. Sometimes spasms are simply manifested as repetitive upward eye deviation, especially at the beginning of a cluster

Duration

Clusters may include a few spasms rising to several dozens of spasms and may be repeated many times per day

Possible complications

In the more severe cases clusters of spasms may recur many times per day and in prolonged series so that a sort of status epilepticus occurs. This condition is usually accompanied by a regression in the child's psychomotor skills and ability to interact

observed within the same cluster, with initial upward eye deviation and subsequent progressive involvement of the neck, trunk and upper limbs. Clusters include a few units to several dozens of spasms and are repeated many times per day. After a series, the child is usually exhausted. Asymmetric spasms are often associated with a lateralized or asymmetric brain lesion (Kramer et al. 1997), although unilateral lesions may cause symmetric spasms. Other seizure types can coexist. Developmental delay predates the onset of spasms in about 70% of children (Arzimanoglou et al. 2004). Disappearance of social smile, loss of visual attention (Kramer et al. 1997) or autistic withdrawal is often observed with the onset of spasms. Misdiagnosis of colic, startles, Moro response or shoulder shrugs still happens frequently. Duration of spasms is variable, depending both on treatment and on their tendency to remit or evolve into other seizure types. Rapid spontaneous remission is rare. In about 50% of children, spasms disappear before the age of 3 years and in 90% before the age of 5 years (Cowan and Hudson 1991).

Prognosis depends more on the cause than on treatment (Guerrini 2006).

Unfavourable prognostic factors for children with CP include early onset (before 3 months), pre-existing seizures other than spasms, asymmetric EEG (Saltik et al. 2002) and relapse after initial response to treatment.

Good prognostic indicators include typical hypsarrhythmia, rapid response to treatment and no regression after onset of spasms or its short duration (Kivity et al. 2004).

About 80% of patients have residual cognitive or behavioural impairment (Kivity et al. 2004), which will worsen the overall prognosis of a child with CP.

About 50% of children will have other epilepsy types.

Infantile spasms must be differentiated from rarer, earlier-onset conditions with ominous prognosis, such as the early infantile epileptic encephalopathy and the early myoclonic encephalopathy (Arzimanoglou et al. 2004).

Generalized motor seizures

Generalized motor seizures, whose manifestations involve the whole body, predominate in dystonic or quadriplegic CP, in which they represent 75% of seizure types. The main generalized seizure types that are usually observed in children with CP include tonic seizures, clonic seizures, tonic-clonic seizures and atypical absence seizures (Box 5.4). They can be observed as the only seizure type or

occur in various combinations in the same child with CP.

The association of brief tonic and atonic seizures, atypical absences and a generalized interictal EEG pattern of spike and slow wave discharges is typical of the Lennox–Gastaut syndrome. Its incidence peaks between 3 and 5 years of age. Cognitive and psychiatric impairment are frequent. About 40% of children have previous infantile spasms. Tonic seizures are particularly frequent during sleep and are characterized by stiffening of the whole body, eye opening and upward eye deviation, with transient apnoea, lasting from a few seconds to about 15 seconds. Tonic seizures occurring while the child is awake can cause the child to collapse heavily. Sudden loss of postural control may also cause the child to fall down when atonic seizures occur. Atonic seizures are a rare phenomenon and tend to occur in the Lennox–Gastaut syndrome. They are characterized by sudden inhibition of muscle activity. The consequences of falling due to an atonic seizure can be severe, as the child falls without any postural reaction that would prevent head injury. Differentiating between seizures causing drop attacks due to tonic or atonic mechanisms is particularly difficult based on clinical observation only and video-EEG recording with simultaneous sampling of EEG and muscle (EMG) activity is often needed. Proper characterization is important since the choice of drug treatment may vary according to the pathophysiological mechanisms underlying such more severe seizure types.

Myoclonic seizures are characterized by brief (usually one-tenth of a second), isolated or repetitive jerks, involving the whole body or predominating in the axial muscles (shoulders and neck) that cause the child to startle, stagger or fall, determined by the position of the body at the time of the occurrence and the intensity of the jerk. Myoclonic jerks in children with CP are also caused by an exaggerated startle reaction, which is related to spasticity. Differentiating myoclonic jerks of epileptic origin from an exaggerated startle reaction often requires video-EEG and EMG recording.

Generalized clonic seizures are characterized by rhythmic jerking of the whole body at about

Box 5.4

Features of generalized seizures

Definition

Generalized seizures are those in which the first clinical and electroencephalographic changes indicate initial involvement of both hemispheres. Consciousness (responsiveness or awareness) may be impaired and this impairment may be the initial manifestation. Motor manifestations, if any, are bilateral

Who gets them?

Generalized motor seizures predominate in dystonic or quadriplegic cerebral palsy in which they represent 75% of seizure types

Main features

Myoclonic seizures

Brief, isolated or repetitive jerks, involving the whole body or predominating in the axial muscles (shoulders and neck)

Generalized clonic seizures

Rhythmic jerking of the whole body at about one jerk per second and with loss of consciousness. The intensity of clonic muscle contractions is variable and in some cases may be limited to simple eyeball jerking or localized twitching of the distal limbs

Generalized tonic-clonic seizures

Sudden, abruptly maximal stiffening of the whole body, usually protracted for several seconds, followed by a clonic phase. In children, the tonic phase of a convulsive seizure tends to be rather 'vibratory', resembling a clonic seizure with high-frequency rhythmic jerking

Atypical absences

Impaired awareness with an 'empty' expression, slow nodding of the head and, sometimes, drooling

Duration

Myoclonic seizures are brief, usually one-tenth of a second, though may be repeated in small bouts of two to several jerks
Generalized clonic seizures have a variable duration

Possible complications

Massive myoclonic and atonic seizures may both cause sudden falls
After generalized clonic seizures postictal impairment of consciousness, with drowsiness or sleep, is often observed, especially after prolonged attacks
Repeated absences may translate into non-convulsive status, in which the child becomes unresponsive or severely apathetic

---

one jerk per second and by loss of consciousness. Their duration is variable and the rate of jerking may progressively slow down. The intensity of clonic muscle contractions is extremely variable and in some cases may be limited to simple eyeball jerking or seemingly localized twitching of the distal limbs. Postictal deficit of consciousness and

sleep is often observed, especially after prolonged attacks.

Generalized tonic-clonic seizures are characterized by a sudden, initial maximal stiffening of the whole body, which is usually protracted for several seconds, followed by a clonic phase. In children, the tonic phase of a convulsive seizure tends to be rather 'vibratory', resembling a clonic seizure with high-frequency rhythmic contractions.

Atypical absences are characterized by impaired awareness with an 'empty' expression, slow nodding of the head and drooling. When an atonic component is present, the child tends to lose postural control slowly and collapse. Repeated absences may translate into non-convulsive status, in which the afore-mentioned manifestations tend to be quasicontinuous and the child becomes unresponsive or severely apathetic.

Status epilepticus

Status epilepticus is defined as recurrent seizures, lasting for more than 30 minutes, without interictal resumption of baseline central nervous system function (Blume et al. 2001). About 70% of episodes of status epilepticus are the initial seizure.

Status epilepticus can occur with motor manifestations (convulsive status) or without (non-convulsive status) (Box 5.5). However, this distinction is not necessarily sharp. Convulsive status can sometimes be simply manifested as localized twitching or eyeball jerking occurring in a drowsy, unresponsive child.

Non-convulsive status can be manifested as reduced motor activity and unsteady postural control or full-blown unresponsiveness. Subtle forms often escape recognition, especially in children with developmental delay. Prompt recognition is crucial, as serious consequences can sometimes derive from prolonged status.

Febrile status epilepticus (20–30% of all cases) occurs in infants or small children with no history of seizures or acute central nervous system infection. Its occurrence in children with CP is possible but is unrelated to pre-existing brain pathology. Most often, status epilepticus occurring in the brain-injured child is defined as remote symptomatic (14–23% of all cases). CP is not, however, a major etiological factor of status epilepticus. Acute symptomatic status epilepticus (23–50% of all cases) complicates an acute illness affecting the central nervous system, and represents 75% of status epilepticus in children younger than 1 year and 28% in those older than 3 years. Antiepileptic drugs can sometimes precipitate status epilepticus if

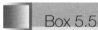

Box 5.5

Features of status epilepticus

Definition

The term is used whenever seizure activity lasts for a sufficient length of time or is repeated frequently enough that recovery between attacks does not occur

Who gets them?

In theory any child with known epilepsy is at risk. However, withdrawal of drugs and non-compliance are the most frequent precipitants in children with known epilepsy. De novo cases are rarely observed

Main features

Status epilepticus can occur with motor manifestations (convulsive status) or without them (non-convulsive status)

Duration

More than 30 minutes

Possible complications

Status epilepticus, especially convulsive status, is a medical emergency and should be recognized and treated promptly

inappropriately chosen or as a result of paradoxical reaction (Guerrini et al. 1998, Wong and Lhatoo 2000).

A chain of metabolic and excitotoxic events accompanying convulsive status epilepticus has been causally related to neuronal damage. Seizure clusters might evolve into status epilepticus.

Benzodiazepines administered by paramedics out of hospital are effective in terminating prolonged seizures and seizure clusters (Alldredge et al. 1995).

Prehospital treatment with rectal diazepam, buccal-nasal midazolam or sublingual lorazepam has been advised (Alldredge et al. 2001, Livingston 2004). However, acute parenteral treatment should be carefully supervised as it causes drowsiness or sleep and, occasionally, cardiorespiratory collapse (Shorvon 2000).

Convulsive status epilepticus that is resistant to initial benzodiazepine administration should always be approached according to a management protocol (Working Group on Status Epilepticus 1993).

EEG recording is essential for diagnosis of non-convulsive status epilepticus. Non-convulsive status epilepticus is not immediately life-threatening; it should nonetheless be treated promptly.

Diagnosis

1. History-taking is the main diagnostic instrument. It should assemble a coherent sequence of manifestations that is made likely by the functional characteristics of the brain, according to age and neurological status. It is often overlooked that children with CP have particular motor patterns, such as spasticity and dyskinesia, that represent the way their motor system functions. As a consequence, seizure activity involving the motor system will often be manifested through the same pathways and patterns, not as would be expected from classical observations obtained in individuals with normal motor patterns. In older children, direct questioning can clarify subjective symptoms. Description of seizures should be focused on the very initial ictal manifestations and include the whole sequence and postictal symptoms, circumstances of occurrence and precipitating factors. Parents can be asked to emulate attacks and use home videotape recordings.

2. Clinical examination should include neurological, skin and ocular assessment, and the measurement of head circumference.

3. EEG may reveal paroxysmal abnormalities. However, with few exceptions, diagnosis does not depend primarily on EEG, as interictal abnormalities are observed in 5–8% of healthy children (Arzimanoglou et al. 2004) and in a much higher proportion of children with CP, even if they have never had seizures. Sleep EEG enhances the positivity rate of routine EEG from 60% to 90%. Video-EEG recordings, with simultaneous sampling of EEG, electromyogram, electrocardiogram, respirogram and electro-oculogram, are invaluable for characterizing complex clinical manifestations. Long-term cable telemetry is essential to capture and quantify seizures.

A normal interictal EEG does not exclude epilepsy when there is a convincing clinical history. Surface EEG can sample electrical activity only originating from the scalp convexity, leaving the mesiobasal brain surface and the inner cortex virtually unexplored.

The International League Against Epilepsy has proposed a diagnostic scheme (Engel 2001) that is divided into five parts, or axes. The diagnostic axes include: descriptive terminology for ictal semiology (axis 1); detailed descriptions of epileptic seizure types (axis 2); epileptic syndromes (axis 3); diseases frequently associated with epileptic seizures or syndromes (axis 4); and the impairment classification derived from the World Health Organization *International Classification of Functioning, Disability and Health* (axis 5). Their most recent versions can be found at the International League Against Epilepsy website (http://www.epilepsy.org).

Differential diagnosis between epilepsy and non-epileptic paroxysmal manifestations in children with cerebral palsy

Children with CP are at risk of exhibiting a number of motor manifestations that are misdiagnosed as epilepsy as they are often presumed to have epilepsy (Stephenson 1997).

Misdiagnosis is frequent and is an important cause of pseudorefractory epilepsy (Metrick et al. 1991).

The interictal EEG is often of little help since it may show epileptiform activity which is related to the underlying structural brain lesion, even in children with CP who have no epileptic seizures (Perlstein et al. 1953). Exaggerated startle phenomena are common in children with spasticity and they closely resemble massive myoclonic jerks or tonic seizures. Although the relationship with sudden stimulations and the absence of a postictal phase are usually sufficient to differentiate a startle from a seizure, some children may require video-EEG monitoring to be accurately assessed. A correct diagnosis may be even more difficult in children who exhibit startle-induced epileptic seizures in which tonic attacks are closely related to a preceding exaggerated startle reaction.

A manifestation which may closely mimic infantile spasms is the so-called repetitive sleep start, sometimes observed in children with spasticity, with or without epilepsy (Fusco et al. 1999). These starts might represent a pathological enhancement of hypnagogic jerks, which are cyclically repeated while the infants are falling asleep. Video-EEG monitoring is often necessary.

Reflex anoxic seizures (Stephenson 1997) are often misdiagnosed as tonic or tonic-clonic seizures. Roving eye movements that are sometimes observed in children with severe dystonia may closely resemble upward eye deviation that may accompany myoclonic or absence seizures, but they do not exhibit the episodic character they have when they are an expression of epileptic brain activity.

Gastro-oesophageal reflux is manifested in small children as episodes of change in colour, respiratory rate disturbances or bradycardia. Dystonic posturing and opisthotonos may occur (Pranzatelli and Pedley 1991). Night terrors or pavor nocturnus typically appear after sleeping for a few hours. The child screams while sitting terrified in bed for several minutes. Attempts to establish a reassuring contact are unsuccessful until the child falls asleep again, having no recollection of the event. Such episodes can occur regularly for a period of time but disappear by school age (Di Mario and Emery 1987). Differential diagnosis of epilepsy and sleep-related seizures of frontal or frontotemporal origin may need ictal recordings.

Course of epilepsy

Figure 5.1 shows a simple flow diagram of the course of epilepsy in children with CP.

Onset of epilepsy in children with CP is usually early. Fifty per cent of children in one series had an onset before the age of 2 years, although onset was usually later in children with hemiplegia (3–5 years). The course of epilepsy in these children was variable. Delgado et al. (1996) found that only 69 of 531 patients (12.9%) with both CP and epilepsy achieved a remission of 2 years or more. In other series, a higher remission rate of 30–40% was observed but in some cases was only reached after many years. However, relatively benign epilepsies may be seen in children with CP, especially with hemiparesis (Goutières et al. 1972). Both neurological difficulties and cognitive problems tend to be more severe when more severe seizures are also present. Some studies seem to indicate that epilepsy associated with CP considerably aggravates the total disability of children as a result of the inconvenience of the seizures and increasing social rejection. In children with hemiplegic CP, the presence of epilepsy is clearly associated with more severe and increasing cognitive problems. Vargha-Khadem et al. (1992) have suggested that such children function at lower levels than children

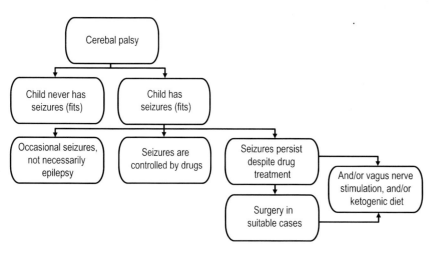

Figure 5.1 • Flow diagram of the course of epilepsy in children with cerebral palsy.

with the same form of CP without seizures in both intelligence and memory. The decrease in achievement seems to be directly correlated to the occurrence of epilepsy rather than to the extent of brain damage as children with small lesions and epilepsy do less well as a group than those with larger lesions without epilepsy. Uvebrandt (1988) found epilepsy to be five times more frequent in hemiplegic children with cognitive impairment than in those with normal intellect, and Goutières et al. (1972) reported that 71.4% of the hemiplegic children with epilepsy were cognitively impaired as against 28.6% of those without epilepsy.

However, epilepsy associated with CP is not always refractory to drug treatment. Most studies have been conducted in centres where only the more difficult cases are seen and studies that have assessed the rate of seizure freedom may thus provide a biased view of the problem. Reaching seizure freedom is difficult in any child who has a brain lesion but minimizing seizure frequency using a simple antiepileptic drug treatment with limited side-effects is a reasonable target.

What to do if a convulsive seizure occurs

1. When a child has a convulsive seizure it is inappropriate to make any attempt at stopping the movements made by the child using physical restraint.

2. No attempt should be made either to open the mouth of the child or to try to introduce anything into the mouth of the child. Such attempts are likely to increase the risk of the child vomiting and may in addition cause injury to the child's teeth and soft palate.

3. The child's head and body should be protected from hard or sharp objects which might cause the child injury.

4. In the postictal period the child should be put into a semiprone position to prevent aspiration and blockage of the nasopharynx.

5. It is unnecessary to take a child to hospital in the postictal period following an uncomplicated seizure.

6. If seizures recur within a short interval and the child does not seem to have regained habitual level of alertness, medical advice should be sought.

When to start treatment with antiepileptic drugs

The decision to begin treatment should be individually tailored for each child. Treatment can be withheld without major risk in many children with single unprovoked seizures. Likewise, children with profound developmental impairment and mild epilepsy that does not affect the overall picture should probably not be treated if the drug administration involves additional practical difficulties and side-effects without any positive outcome. Convulsive status epilepticus should be treated promptly if further episodes pose an immediate danger. The risk of accidental death related to severe seizures must also be considered, particularly in the neurologically impaired (Camfield et al. 2002). Delaying treatment may have devastating effects when clinically subtle or epileptic activity sustains cognitive impairment (Binnie 2003).

Setting the targets of drug treatment

The targets of treatment differ considerably according to the type of epilepsy and the severity of the seizures.

Seizure control without adverse effects, with possibly one drug and in the most convenient and least expensive form, is a reasonable target in most children with CP. Drug choices for such purposes vary little.

For complex and severe epilepsies the main goal should not necessarily be complete seizure control at all costs. Such an attitude may lead to drug escalation and to increased polytherapies with more severe cognitive side-effects, the consequences of which may be even worse than those of the seizures. There is an increased risk of seizures becoming worse with heavy polytherapies (Beghi et al. 1987, Guerrini et al. 2002, Guerrini 2006).

Therefore, the aim should be to reduce seizure frequency, ensuring the best possible quality of life, which should result from a balance between the cognitive side-effects of the drugs and the intrinsic severity and frequency of the seizures. Table 5.1 lists the more commonly used drugs.

Monitoring of antiepileptic drug treatment

Regular clinical supervision, paying special attention to sedative side-effects, is essential. Monitoring the concentration in the blood is not routinely indicated (Aicardi 1998). However, some epileptologists recommend this practice when using certain drugs or in some specific circumstances. Monitoring is also required to assess compliance, especially in cases of breakthrough seizures, clinically suspected toxicity and drug interactions.

In children who are seizure-free with monotherapy and a concentration in the blood of the drug that is below the therapeutic range, no dosage adjustment is needed. Conversely, the dose should be raised to the limit of clinical tolerance in resistant cases without considering blood concentrations. Blood concentrations are not helpful with some drugs and are difficult to interpret with others. When a dose of a medication is missed, it should be added to the next dose.

Cognitive and behavioural effects of antiepileptic drugs

Cognitive impairment, which often occurs in children with epilepsy, is in part attributed to antiepileptic drugs. Although a detrimental dose-dependent effect of some antiepileptic drugs on cognition is self-evident, only a few controlled studies have addressed this factor in children (Loring and Meador 2004).

Clear evidence has only been obtained concerning reduction of IQ scores in children treated with phenobarbital (Farwell et al. 1990, Sulzbacher et al. 1999). It appears that such effects are reversible with drug withdrawal, but the enduring consequences in academic achievement suggest that prolonged decrease in cognitive processing may not be compensated in prospect (Sulzbacher et al. 1999).

Carbamazepine does not affect IQ (Riva and Devoti 1999), but might slightly impair children's memory, without affecting academic achievement (Seidel and Mitchell 1999, Bailet and Turk 2000).

Phenytoin may slightly affect IQ, but its effects on academic achievement are unknown (Loring and Meador 2004).

Effects of valproate on memory were found to be less pronounced than those of phenytoin and carbamazepine (Forsythe et al. 1991), but may not have been adequately studied (Loring and Meador 2004).

There are no studies that have scientifically addressed the neuropsychological effects of the new antiepileptic drugs in children (see Table 5.1).

Discontinuation of drug treatment

The optimum time for discontinuing antiepileptic drugs in children in remission is difficult to establish. Evidence from randomized trials suggests that after seizure remission at least 2 years should elapse (Sirven et al. 2001). However, specific syndromes have different relapsing rates (Baruzzi et al. 1998).

A ketogenic diet

The ketogenic diet has been shown to have some efficacy in the treatment of children with drug-resistant epilepsies (Freeman et al. 1998, Vining et al. 1998), but no comparative trials have been undertaken. No specific syndrome responds more effectively than others, and an assessment of the risks and benefits needs further study. The mechanisms of action are unknown, but the predominantly fatty nutrition maintains ketosis in the long term and high concentrations of ketone bodies have been correlated with better seizure control (Huttenlocher 1976). The diet may be too restrictive, resulting in diarrhoea, vitamin

Table 5.1 Antiepileptic drugs in children (modified from Guerrini 2006)

Antiepileptic drugs	Usual dose (oral) in mg/kg per day	No of daily doses	Side-effects	Serious toxicity
Carbamazepine	10–20	2–3	Ataxia, diplopia, rashes	Aplastic anaemia (rare)
Clobazam	0.5–1.0 (maximum 30 mg/day)	1–3	Sedation	
Clonazepam	Slow titration: 0.1–0.2	2–3	Fatigue, drowsiness, hypotonia; behaviour disturbances, salivary and bronchial hypersecretion	Respiratory depression (only IV route)
Ethosuximide	20–30	1–2	Gastric discomfort, hiccups, rash, blurred vision, headache	Aplastic anaemia (rare)
Felbamate	15–45	2	Somnolence, anorexia, gastric discomfort, nervousness	Aplastic anaemia (300 per million adult patients treated); hepatotoxicity (164 per million adult patients treated)
Gabapentin	23–35	2–3	Fatigue, weight gain	Rarely, behavioural problems: hostility
Lamotrigine	Slow titration: 5–15 (add-on enzyme inducers); 1–3 (add-on valproate); 1–5 (add-on valproate + inducer)	2	Dizziness, diplopia, ataxia, somnolence, rash	Stevens–Johnson syndrome, Lyell's syndrome
Levetiracetam	20–40	2	Somnolence, asthenia, headache, anorexia	Psychotic events (rare)
Nitrazepam	0.25–2.50	2	Hypotonia, drowsiness, drooling	Drooling and aspiration causing pneumonia
Oxcarbazepine	30–45	2	Somnolence, headache, ataxia, vomiting, hyponatraemia, rash	
Phenobarbital	15–20 IV in newborns; 3–5 < 5 years; 2–3 > 5 years	2 or 1 at bedtime	Behaviour disturbances, drowsiness, rash, might affect cognitive function. Systemic toxicity	Hypersensitivity reactions (rare)
Phenytoin	15–20 IV in newborns; 8–10 < 3 years; 4–7 > 3 years	2	Ataxia, diplopia, nystagmus, acne, gum hypertrophy, hirsutism, cognitive and sedative effects, peripheral neuropathy	Megaloblastic anaemia, lymphoma, encephalopathy, choreoathetosis

(Continued)

Table 5.1 Continued

Antiepileptic drugs	Usual dose (oral) in mg/kg per day	No of daily doses	Side-effects	Serious toxicity
Primidone	10–20	2–3	Behaviour distubances, drowsiness, rash, might affect cognitive function	Anaemia (rare)
Sodium valproate	15–40	2–3	Nausea and epigastric pain, tremor, alopecia, weight gain, hyperammonaemia	Encephalopathy, hepatitis, and pancreatitis (rare)
Sulthiame	5–15	2	Ataxia, paraesthesia	
Tiagabine	0.5–2.0	2	Dizziness, abdominal pain, nervousness, difficulty with concentration	Non-convulsive status epilepticus
Topiramate	Slow titration: 4–6	2	Weight loss, paraesthesias, emotional lability, difficulty concentrating and word-finding, hypohidrosis	Kidney stones
Vigabatrin	20–80; 100–150 for infantile spasms	2	Excitation, drowsiness, weight gain	Psychosis (rare). Visual field defects (40%; not always clinically detectable)
Zonisamide	4–12	2	Somnolence, dizziness, ataxia, abdominal discomfort, decreased spontaneity, rash, hypohidrosis	Psychiatric disorders

IV, intravenous.

deficiency, renal stones and potentially lethal cardiomyopathy (Kang et al. 2004).

Homeopathy

This treatment involves the ingestion of herbs. Its use is not recommended in epilepsy as there have been no scientifically controlled trials to determine either its efficacy or its potential for seizure aggravation.

Vagus nerve stimulation

Vagus nerve stimulation may be used as an adjunct to treat drug-resistant epilepsy. A stimulator is placed under the skin and emanates adjustable pulsed stimuli to an electrode that is wrapped around the left vagus nerve (Crumrine 2000). Interesting results have been obtained in children with severe epilepsies that are untreatable by surgery, but which epilepsy syndromes are likely to benefit is still undetermined. Adverse effects of hoarseness, cough and pain are usually tolerated (Privitera et al. 2002).

Surgical treatment

Some children who are refractory to antiepileptic drugs can benefit from surgical treatment.

1. Resective surgery implies removal of the neuronal aggregate that is responsible for the seizure generation.

2. Palliative or functional surgery aims at preventing or limiting propagation of seizure activity without targeting seizure control.

Several factors need to be considered when identifying a child who may benefit from surgery. Medical intractability should be ascertained, perhaps limited to the more appropriate drugs and not exceeding 2 years (Berg et al. 2003). The level of seizure-related disability should be established on the basis of each child's clinical presentation. In children with CP, the surgical treatment of epilepsy is only indicated in a very small number of well-selected cases.

General care and risks in daily life

Children with epilepsy are at increased risk of accidents, but only some epilepsies have a high risk, relating to seizure types and the time of seizure occurrence. In children with severe epilepsy, special precautions are needed. At home, the kitchen and bathroom are the most dangerous places: (1) burning accidents should be prevented with shields for sources of heat; and (2) the child should never be left alone when bathing (Sonnen 1991). Beyond these specific precautions, reasonable restrictions should be adapted to the individual child.

General anaesthesia can be used for children with epilepsy. Anaesthetic drugs which lower seizure threshold (such as meperidine, halothane and isoflurane) should however be avoided. Only some antiepileptic drugs are available for intravenous administration in the sedated child. When epilepsy is particularly active, and anaesthesia is scheduled for a relatively long procedure, a drug load corresponding to the 24 hours total intake should be given. Drug monitoring is advised following the surgical procedure in children who are difficult to treat.

References

Aicardi J. Diseases of the nervous system in children, 2nd edn. Cambridge University Press, Cambridge, 1988.

Aicardi J, Amsli J, Chevrie JJ. Acute hemiplegia in infancy and childhood. Dev Med Child Neurol 1969; 11:162–173.

Aksu F. Nature and prognosis of seizures in patients with CP. Dev Med Child Neurol 1990; 32:661–668.

Alldredge BK, Wall DB, Ferriero DM. Effect of prehospital treatment on the outcome of status epilepticus in children. Pediatr Neurol 1995; 12:213–216.

Alldredge BK, Gelb AM, Isaacs SM et al. A comparison of lorazepam, diazepam, and placebo for the treatment of out-of-hospital status epilepticus. N Engl J Med 2001; 345:631–637.

Amess PN, Baudin J, Townsend J et al. Epilepsy in very preterm infants: neonatal cranial ultrasound reveals a high-risk subcategory. Dev Med Child Neurol 1998; 40:724–730.

Arzimanoglou A, Guerrini R, Aicardi J. Epilepsy in children, 3rd edn. Lippincott/Williams and Wilkins, Philadelphia, 2004.

Bailet LL, Turk WR. The impact of childhood epilepsy on neurocognitive and behavioral performance: a prospective longitudinal study. Epilepsia 2000; 41:426–431.

Baruzzi A, Procaccianti G, Tinuper P et al. Antiepileptic drug withdrawal in childhood epilepsies: preliminary results of a prospective study. In: Faienza C, Prati GL (eds) Diagnostic and therapeutic problems in pediatric epileptology. Elsevier Science, Amsterdam, 1998, pp. 117–123.

Beghi E, Bollini P, Di Mascio R et al. Effects of rationalizing drug treatment of patients with epilepsy and mental retardation. Dev Med Child Neurol 1987; 29:363–369.

Berg AT, Langfitt J, Shinnar S et al. How long does it take for partial epilepsy to become intractable? Neurology 2003; 60:186–190.

Binnie CD. Cognitive impairment during epileptiform discharges: is it ever justifiable to treat the EEG? Lancet Neurol 2003; 2:725–730.

Bleasel AF, Lüders HF. Tonic seizures. In: Lüders HO, Noachtar S (eds) Epileptic seizures: pathophysiology and clinical semiology. Churchill Livingstone, Philadelphia, 2000, pp. 389–411.

Blume WT, Lüders HO, Mizrahi E et al. Glossary of descriptive terminology for ictal semiology: report of the ILAE task force on classification and terminology. Epilepsia 2001; 42:1212–1218.

Camfield CS, Camfield PR, Veugelers PJ. Death in children with epilepsy: a population-based study. Lancet 2002; 359:1891–1895.

Commission on Classification and Terminology of the International League Against Epilepsy. Proposal for revised classification of epilepsy and epileptic syndromes. Epilepsia 1989; 30:389–399.

Cowan LD, Hudson LS. The epidemiology and natural history of infantile spasms. J Child Neurol 1991; 6:355–364.

Crumrine PK. Vagal nerve stimulation in children. Semin Pediatr Neurol 2000; 7:216–223.

Delgado MR, Riela AR, Mills J et al. Discontinuation of antiepileptic drug treatment after two seizure-free years in children with CP. Pediatrics 1996; 97:192–197.

Di Mario FJ Jr., Emery ES. The natural history of night terrors. Clin Pediatr 1987; 26:505–511.

Dravet C et al. Comments on an epileptic syndrome with unilateral seizures. In: Roger J, Dravet C, Bureau M et al (eds) Epileptic syndromes in infancy, childhood and adolescence, 2nd ed. John Libbey Eurotext, London, 1992, pp. 273–277.

Engel J, International League Against Epilepsy (ILAE). A proposed diagnostic scheme for people with epileptic seizures and with epilepsy: report of the ILAE Task Force on Classification and Terminology. Epilepsia 2001; 42:796–803.

Farwell JR, Lee YJ, Hirtz DG et al. Phenobarbital for febrile seizures – effects on intelligence and on seizure recurrence. N Engl J Med 1990; 322:364–369.

Fisher RS, van Emde Boas W, Blume W et al. Epileptic seizures and epilepsy: definitions proposed by the International League Against Epilepsy (ILAE) and the International Bureau for Epilepsy (IBE). Epilepsia 2005; 46:470–472.

Forsythe I, Butler R, Berg I et al. Cognitive impairment in new cases of epilepsy randomly assigned to carbamazepine, phenytoin and sodium valproate. Dev Med Child Neurol 1991; 33:524–534.

Freeman JM, Vining EP, Pillas DJ et al. The efficacy of the ketogenic diet – 1998: a prospective evaluation of intervention in 150 children. Pediatrics 1998; 102:1358–1363.

Fusco L, Pachatz C, Cusmai R et al. Repetitive sleep starts in neurologically impaired children: an unusual non-epileptic manifestation in otherwise epileptic subjects. Epileptic Disord 1999; 1:63–67.

Goutières F, Challamel MJ, Aicardi J et al. Les Hémiplégies congénitales: sémiologie, étiologie et pronostic. Arch Fr Pédiatr 1972; 29:839–851.

Guerrini R. Epilepsy in children. Lancet 2006; 367:449–524.

Guerrini R, Belmonte A, Genton P. Antiepileptic drug-induced worsening of seizures in children. Epilepsia 1998; 39(suppl 3):2–10.

Guerrini R, Arzimanoglou A, Brouwer O. Rationale for treating epilepsy in children. Epileptic Disord 2002; 4(suppl 2):9–21.

Hadjipanayis A, Hadjichristodoulou C, Youroukos S. Epilepsy in patients with CP. Dev Med Child Neurol 1997; 39:659–663.

Hamer HM, Wyllie E, Lüders HO et al. Symptomatology of epileptic seizures in the first three years of life. Epilepsia 1999; 40:837–844.

Huttenlocher PR. Ketonemia and seizures: metabolic and anticonvulsant effects of two ketogenic diets in childhood epilepsy. Pediatr Res 1976; 10:536–540.

Kang HC, Chung da E, Kim DW et al. Early- and late-onset complications of the ketogenic diet for intractable epilepsy. Epilepsia 2004; 45:1116–1123.

Kivity S, Lerman P, Ariel R et al. Long-term cognitive outcomes of a cohort of children with cryptogenic infantile spasms treated with high-dose adrenocorticotropic hormone. Epilepsia 2004; 45:255–262.

Kramer U, Sue W-C, Mikati M. Focal features in West syndrome indicating candidacy for surgery. Pediatr Neurol 1997; 16:213–217.

Kyllerman M. Dyskinetic CP. Ph D thesis. Department of Pediatrics, University of Göteborg, Gothenburg, Sweden, 1981.

Livingston JH. Status epilepticus. In: Wallace SJ, Farrell K (eds) Epilepsy in children, 2nd edn. Arnold, London, 2004, pp. 290–303.

Loring DW, Meador KJ. Cognitive side-effects of antiepileptic drugs in children. Neurology 2004; 62:872–877.

Lüders H, Acharya J, Baumgartner C et al. Semiological seizure classification. Epilepsia 1998; 39:1006–1013.

Metrick ME, Ritter FS, Gates JR et al. Nonepileptic events in childhood. Epilepsia 1991; 32:322–328.

Mohamed A, Wyllie E, Ruggieri P et al. Temporal lobe epilepsy due to hippocampal sclerosis in pediatric candidates for epilepsy surgery. Neurology 2001; 56:1643–1649.

Munari C, Bancaud J, Bonis A et al. Impairment of consciousness in temporal lobe seizures: a stereoelectroencephalographic study. In: Canger R, Angeleri F, Penry JK (eds) Advances in epileptology: XIth Epilepsy International Symposium. Raven Press, New York, 1980, pp. 111–114.

Perlstein MA, Gibbs EL, Gibbs FA. The electroencephalogram in infantile CP. Am J Phys Med 1953; 34:477–496.

Pranzatelli MR, Pedley TA. Differential diagnosis in children. In: Dam M, Gram L (eds) Comprehensive epileptology. Raven Press, New York, 1991, pp. 423–447.

Privitera MD, Welty TE, Ficker DM et al. Vagus nerve stimulation for partial seizures. Cochrane Database Systemat Rev 2002; 1:CD002896.

Riva D, Devoti M. Carbamazepine withdrawal in children with previous symptomatic partial epilepsy: effects on neuropsychologic function. J Child Neurol 1999; 14:357–362.

Saltik S, Kocer N, Dervent A. Informative value of magnetic resonance imaging and EEG in the prognosis of infantile spasms. Epilepsia 2002; 43:246–252.

Seidel WT, Mitchell WG. Cognitive and behavioral effects of carbamazepine in children: data from benign rolandic epilepsy. J Child Neurol 1999; 14:716–723.

Shorvon SS. The treatment of epilepsy. Blackwell Science, London, 2000.

Sirven JI, Sperling M, Wingerchuk DM. Early versus late antiepileptic drug withdrawal for people with epilepsy in remission. Cochrane Database Systemat Rev 2001; 3:CD001902.

Sonnen AEH. How to live with epilepsy. In: Dam M, Gram L (eds) Comprehensive epileptology. Raven Press, New York, 1991, pp. 753–767.

Stephenson JBP. CP. In: Engel J Jr, Pedley TA (eds) Epilepsy. A comprehensive textbook, vol. 3. Lippincott-Raven, Philadelphia, 1997, pp. 2571–2577.

Sulzbacher S, Farwell JR, Temkin N et al. Late cognitive effects of early treatment with phenobarbital. Clin Pediatr 1999; 38:387–394.

Uvebrandt P. Hemiplegic CP. Aetiology and outcome. Acta Paediatr Scand (Suppl.) 1988; 345:5–100.

Vargha-Khadem F, Isaacs E, Van der Werf S et al. Development of intelligence and memory in children with hemiplegic CP. The deleterious consequences of early seizures. Brain 1992; 1115:315–329.

Vining EP, Freeman JM, Ballaban-Gil K et al. A multicenter study of the efficacy of the ketogenic diet. Arch Neurol 1998; 55:1433–1437.

Wong IC, Lhatoo SD. Adverse reactions to new anticonvulsant drugs. Drug Safety 2000; 23:35–56.

Working Group on Status Epilepticus. Treatment of convulsive status epilepticus. Recommendation of the Epilepsy Foundation of America. JAMA 1993; 270:854–859.

Wyllie E, Lüders H, Morris HH et al. The lateralizing significance of versive head and eye movements during epileptic seizures. Neurology 1986; 36:606–611.

Useful websites

In English

Epilepsy Foundation (USA): www.epilepsyfoundation.org.

Epilepsy Therapy Development Project (USA): www.epilepsy.com.

International Bureau for Epilepsy: www.ibe-epilepsy.org.

National Centre for Young People with Epilepsy (UK): www.ncype.org.uk.

National Society for Epilepsy (UK): www.epilepsynse.org.uk.

In French

Bureau français de l'épilepsie: www.bfe.asso.fr.

In Italian

Associazione italiana contro l'epilessia: www.aice-epilessia.it.

Chapter Six

6

Parents' problems

J Bavin • Eva Bower

CHAPTER CONTENTS

The problem of acceptance

No one wants their child to be disabled. We all want fit, handsome, intelligent children who will do well in the competitive society we live in, and be 'a credit to us'. We even have competitions to find the most beautiful baby. It is unsurprising, therefore, that parents worry during pregnancy about what sort of child they are going to have, and become acutely distressed if they give birth to a damaged or imperfect child.

The parents' distress may be, and often is, severe. At first, the feelings of anger, guilt, shame, despair and self-pity may be overwhelming, and give way to the agony of longing for a way out. In some, these feelings may even be accompanied by a resolve to end the child's and their own life. If the distress of meeting the situation is intolerable, there may be total rejection of the child, or denial that there is anything wrong with the child, or a belief that the child belongs to someone else.

Torturing questions flood the mind: 'What did I do wrong? Why did it happen to me? What is wrong with me?' The answers are no less distressing: 'Perhaps I can't produce ordinary children. I damaged its brain because my pelvis is small – "they" said it is. I wish I had never got married. How I hate the other mothers who have ordinary babies.' And then, maybe, more questions such as: 'Oh, why am I thinking these terrible thoughts – what sort of person am I? My child needs a mother to be loved by and we were considering abandoning this child.'

The initial turmoil may give way to sadness, a feeling of desolation and isolation, and a longing for the 'lost', 'ordinary' child. While this mourning process continues, with its slow adjustment to the loss of the child one wanted, the real child – the disabled one – is lying there in its place, requiring daily care.

The way in which parents adjust to this apparently disastrous situation is crucial for the future welfare not only of the disabled child, but of the whole family. It is not surprising that many parents are ambivalent about the child; that is, they sometimes feel they love the child as if he or she were an ordinary child and at other times feel distressed, anxious and even rejecting. This is because they love and want the child, but do not want, and are distressed by, the disabilities. They may try to solve this problem by 'shopping around' for a doctor or hospital which will offer a miraculous cure. Parents who suffer severe guilt may attempt to relieve their distress, and to right the wrongs done to the innocent child, by one of two ways: they may either punish themselves by dedicating their whole life to unremitting slavery in caring for the child, or they may project the guilt on to their doctors, social workers and teachers, and angrily accuse them of neglect or mistakes. Sometimes they do both.

Satisfactory adjustment must rapidly be achieved because otherwise the disabled child will become more disabled, and a family's happiness and social life partly or totally destroyed.

Without skilled help, most distressed parents will tend to make an adjustment which reduces their distress, but at the cost of distorting their relationships with the disabled child and the rest of the family. Ideally these relationships should remain emotionally and socially normal, but extra skills are needed to help the child overcome the disabilities faced as far as is possible.

This means that the child needs to be loved and accepted as an ordinary child would be – accepted as they are, with all their difficulties and problems, whatever they may be. Acceptance in the normal way, so that mutually enjoyable relationships are established between the child and the family, will allow the child's personality to grow in the most favourable environment. In the long run it is the ability to face the world with self-confidence, to be friendly, helpful and useful, so that one is socially acceptable, that matters, not being physically perfect or very intelligent. Whether a child is disabled or not at birth, happiness and a satisfying adult social role, will most easily be achieved if the child is brought up in a happy, contented, united family. Even learning in the strict educational sense is greatly facilitated if the child is happy and secure in first relationships within the family.

Adjustment

The first shock of being told of the child's disabilities is greatly lessened if the telling is done skilfully and with compassion by a doctor who offers to help the family through the early problem period. Many families do not receive this help even today, but things are slowly improving. If parents find they need more help than they are receiving they should contact SCOPE, MENCAP (in England) or a similar voluntary organization, whose local branches may be able to arrange contact with the appropriate professional services.

As the initial distress lessens, the family must take stock in relation to the task of doing the best for the new disabled child. Perhaps the most important asset a family can have is a firmly united partnership between the parents. It is of the highest importance that both parents should accept their full share of the responsibility for the care of their child. Any tendency for one to blame the other or to feel less involved, or on the other hand for one to accept the total responsibility, can be disastrous. Mothers are more likely to accept the full responsibility and fathers to allow this to happen. Mothers nurture the child for 9 months within their body, and are told of all the things they must do to keep their unborn child healthy, and of all the things they must not do in order to prevent damage. Not unnaturally, therefore, they easily fall prey to feelings of guilt or inadequacy as a wife and mother, and believe that they have to suffer alone in caring for the child. Unfortunately, doctors sometimes reinforce this tendency by revealing the news to the father alone, and leave him to tell his wife as best he can, giving the impression that the child is really *her* problem, and the wife's distress is *his* problem.

Ideally both parents should draw closer together, and support each other by resolving to share fully the problems and the joys. Fathers should realize what an enormous comfort it is to their partners if they can speak openly about their attitudes to the child and each other, and if their feelings can be shared. Parents should also try to realize from the beginning that *they*, as well as the child, have needs, and they should not stop enjoying themselves as a couple. They still need each other's companionship, leisure time spent together and separately, friends and social activities, sexual enjoyment and a loving relationship with their other children. Nothing less than a normal family life is satisfactory for the disabled parents themselves. The idea of sacrificing everybody in order to care better for the child should be discouraged. The disabled child who has overburdened and overcaring parents suffers unnecessarily, and so does the rest of the family. At worst, the family may eventually disintegrate under the strain. Fathers who lose their place in their family may resent the disabled child who has replaced them, and may even leave the family to find solace elsewhere. Brothers and sisters may take their pleasures outside a home dominated by the imagined needs of a disabled sibling.

Note: The disabled child has the same emotional and social needs as other children. The child needs love but not smothering; care but not overindulgence; and above all, opportunities for achievement, self-control and social growth towards an independent adult place in society.

Shame, embarrassment and social isolation

One problem facing parents, as soon as they have been told about their child's disabilities, is what to tell relatives, friends and neighbours. The answer is undoubtedly: the truth. You expect your doctor to tell you the truth, and you should do the same. Doctors sometimes misguidedly cover up the truth for fear of distressing parents, and parents often cover up in order to save themselves and their friends from embarrassment. Friends and neighbours are bound to enquire when you take the child home from hospital, and failure to tell them at once of the child's disability will only make it more difficult next time. Tell all enquirers, including your other children, as naturally as you can that the doctors think that the child has weak arms and legs, or is very mentally and/or physically disabled, or that the child has fits, and that treatment has begun. You have nothing to be ashamed of, and few people will fail to be helpful and sympathetic. On the other hand, once you have told someone that your child is 'fine', you have begun to lie, and to build a wall between you and your friends. As time goes by, it will be more and more difficult to meet people, who can see for themselves that something is wrong. They will wonder whether you know, and are too embarrassed to tell them, or whether you do not know, in which case they will not want to be the first to suggest it. Gradually you will become socially isolated, your embarrassment causing them and you to avoid each other.

Of course, some people's attempts to help may be a little misguided. Some may try to persuade you that the diagnosis must be wrong: 'How can they tell at such an early age?' or 'He'll grow out of it'. You must let your friends be sympathetic, as they are trying to be, and then help them to see that wishful thinking is not going to mend anything.

If you tell people in this straightforward way, you will quickly have a circle of helpful friends, relatives, neighbours and other members of the community whose interest, enquiries and offers of help will be of the greatest support to you and your family. The alternative course, leading to gradually increasing social embarrassment, distress at having to face the outside world and eventual social isolation and withdrawal of the family into itself, is harmful. If you maintain and even extend or strengthen your social contacts, you will be secure enough to be able to withstand the occasional rebuff or hurtful remark from the few people who lack understanding, knowledge or sympathy. Let *them* be the odd ones out – not *you*. Do not hate them for hurting you: try to help them to understand. The natural and normal behaviour of parents of disabled children in the community is probably the greatest force we have for informing the public of their needs and dispelling the prejudice and ignorance which still exist.

Accepting help

Parents of older children often complain that no one wants to help. Many people will help, however, if given the chance. Right from the start, encourage them. Do not be too proud to ask for help, or to accept it if it is offered. Do not keep putting off the time when you return to going out in the evening as a couple. Ask a friend to child-sit, and then go out and enjoy yourselves. If you believe no one would want to help in this way, that no one but you can manage to look after your child, that no one else could cope with a fit, or that you must always be with the child in case something happens, in most cases you are already making unnecessary excuses.

You are overburdening yourself without benefit to the child, and jeopardizing the future happiness of the whole family. No family can be happy with a worn-out, overburdened, irritable mother (it is usually mothers who martyr themselves). Find some child-sitters. If you do not know of any, your health visitor, general practitioner or social worker may well be able to recommend one. Perhaps the local parents' group organizes arrangements for looking after one another's children. Explain to the child-sitter what the child's needs are, what may happen and how to cope. Even teenagers are capable of taking on this task (and often do so willingly) given the chance. The community will never really understand the problems of disabled people or be sympathetic and helpful if they are not given the chance to help.

Social acceptance: the ultimate objective

When parents have reached the stage when their distress is diminishing and they have resolved to do everything in their power to help the child, it is time to think carefully about what one is trying to do. The disabled child is going to become an adult. As an adult, happiness will depend on social acceptance. If the child has friends, can live and work in the community and can actively participate in leisure and community activities, the child will be happy. If, on the other hand, the child has no friends and is shunned by acquaintances and strangers alike because of odd, infantile, aggressive or unpleasant behaviour, the child will be unhappy. Nothing is more important for the parents than to realize at the beginning, and to remember all along, that the ultimate objective in rearing your child is to produce an adult who behaves like other adults, as far as this is possible with disabilities – and it is certainly far more possible than most people believe. Any form of bizarre behaviour, especially behaviour which is inappropriate to age, will make real social acceptance difficult or impossible.

But, you may ask, what if the child is not intelligent enough to understand how to behave? The answer is: do not believe it, because it is never true. Socially appropriate behaviour requires very little intelligence for its learning. It requires only consistent training which provides the child with clear-cut learning situations in which no doubt is left as to what is expected.

Establishing the first relationships

Social acceptance begins in the family group, where the child will establish the first and most important relationships. These experiences will colour relationships with other people, and personality growth will be facilitated if the early social experiences are satisfactory. The disabled child's needs, from an emotional and social point of view, are exactly the same as those of other children. The child needs love and care, but not *more* love and care. The child certainly does not need pitying, oversentimental, clinging, smothering, tearful, overprotective stroking and cuddling treatment for the rest of his or her life. At first, of course, the child needs lots of physical contact, lots of gentle vocal stimulation and total physical care. But even this is not likely to be satisfactory unless the child is loved in a relaxed, joyful, accepting way, because children are very sensitive to the mood of the mother, transmitted through her voice and physical handling.

Very quickly, however the child begins to establish themselves as a person in their own right. The child is not just helpless and passive, and if disabled it is very important to observe and notice the little signs that listening and looking are beginning, and that the repetition of familiar experiences is expected. The child is already beginning to learn about you and the world.

The changing relationship

It is very fashionable to talk of *child* development, and to emphasize its importance, but few people talk of *parent* development, which is equally important. It should be obvious that the normal parent–child relationship is constantly changing as time passes. What is appropriate parental behaviour towards a 2-week-old child is not appropriate for a child of 6 months, or even more obviously for a child of 5 years. Beware the tendency to say: 'The child is only a baby', or 'It's time enough for that later', or 'The child can't understand'. It may well be that these remarks stem from a wish to deny the disabilities, with a consequent tendency to 'infantilize' the child, so that the child is thought of as a child (and treated as one) in order to explain the helplessness. Unfortunately such treatment promotes helplessness, so that the child's development is retarded, even in areas where progress could be taking place.

The more the child progresses in areas of development where able, the more the remaining disabilities will be obvious by comparison, and it takes courage to be able to face up to the gradual unveiling of the true picture. On the other hand, to keep the child totally and uniformly helpless in order to hide the disabilities for a long time is to deny the child the right to develop maximal independence. For optimal development of the child, you must gradually be changing your relationship with the child, always gently encouraging every effort the child makes to observe, to vocalize and to explore and manipulate the environment. Month by month and year by year the child should therefore be learning to do things that were previously not possible, and learning under your skilled and caring guidance. This, not keeping your child dependent on you, is true parental love.

One day your child is going to have to live without you, and even if grievously disabled, the child will be better prepared for the parting if the stage in social development has been reached whereby the company of others is needed and enjoyed, and the grown-up child is not still emotionally attached to the parents.

The ultimate objective of adult independence is reached, therefore, by starting from a basis of security resulting from your warm, tender, stimulating care, and moving gradually and steadily, with your encouragement of the child's efforts, towards self-confident achievement.

The mother as teacher

All children need frequent, close and intimate contact with the mother in order to form the social bond which enables the mother, and later others, to influence the child's behaviour. The association between the feeding, warming and comforting tasks which the mother frequently and regularly performs in the early months of the child's life with her actual presence results in the infant starting to regard the mother as the primary source of pleasure. The mother's face, voice, smell and skin contact become highly rewarding and pleasurable in their own right, and therefore motivating. The child therefore looks forward to this stimulation, seeks it, desires it and becomes distressed if it is not frequently forthcoming. The fact that the child's waking moments are often filled with the pleasure of contact with the mother makes the child feel secure, so that a little later the child can begin to investigate the rest of the environment for short periods, secure in the knowledge that the mother is close at hand to help, comfort or protect if the child gets into difficulties.

The importance of this process for the child's social development is obvious, but it is equally important for intellectual development. Learning does not start at 5 years of age in school: it starts at birth (some say before birth). The most important teaching is done by the mother, often spontaneously and unknowingly. The frequent and close imposition of the 'talking face' in front of the child teaches the vital skill of concentrating on one set of meaningful and associated stimuli, rather than vaguely scanning the world in general. The child learns to filter out confusing and irrelevant sensations, and to pay attention to one problem at a time. The child also learns to be alert, to think, to anticipate and later to explore, manipulate and experiment. This is done initially by becoming socially responsive, as the child derives much pleasure from paying attention to the mother's face, which in turn responds to the child, thus rewarding the effort.

This process is essential for laying the foundation of all future learning. It is impossible to learn without paying attention to stimuli in a structured way. This means being able to concentrate on the relevant or linked stimuli, in order to discover the connection between them, without being distracted. The mother's face blots out the rest of the environment by its approach to a very close distance; it does this frequently in a way which nothing else does; it repeats the same pattern day after day, and yet it is moving and interesting; it consists of shapes, colour and the fascination of staring eyes; and it is accompanied by familiar sounds, smell and comforting skin contact. Imagine the contrast which exists for an unwanted child, or one which the mother finds distressing or repulsive. Such a child is left to lie alone for most of the time, not handled tenderly, not spoken to lovingly and not frequently comforted. It is not surprising if such an under-stimulated child becomes apathetic, incurious, miserable and socially unresponsive. Little useful learning will then be possible, and eventually no motivation will activate the child to seek stimulation and experience.

Play

The importance of play for any child's development is well known, but even today few parents receive sufficient help in learning how to play with their children. Play can be defined as a pleasurable exploration of the environment. If a task is interesting and enjoyable, it will be actively pursued without apparent effort. If, on the other hand, it becomes boring, repetitive or too difficult, it will soon seem to be hard work, and require self-discipline, external pressure or reward to continue with it.

The essence of play for the child must be pleasure, a mutual pleasure for parent and child. If the child is smiling and excited by the adult, the child is playing and learning. At first the games most likely to give pleasure are simple physical contact games (cuddling, tickling, stroking, rubbing noses, kissing); visual games (approach and retreat of your face, movements of your mouth, tongue and head, hiding and reappearing); and vocal games (singing, gentle talking, lip and tongue noises, blowing and puffing air). These lead on to simple nursery games of a more structured type, such as 'clap hands' and 'round and round the garden'. We must not forget that fathers also need to play with children. They play differently and more roughly from the beginning – they talk in a deeper voice, look slightly different and engage in antigravity play. This provides the child with excitement and variety of play, as well as getting the child used to males and their different behaviour.

Noisy toys are useful – rattles, paper being crumpled, spoons banged on trays or cups – because it is vital that the child becomes interested in sounds. Always talk when you are with your child – never handle the child silently. Do not try to get the child to imitate single words. Let the child hear the sing-song rhythm of normal speech, and the flow of normal language. Later on the child will try to imitate this, and you will be excited when the child 'scribble-talks' in his or her own 'language'. Even if the cerebral palsy (CP) affects the muscles of the child's throat and mouth, the child will understand more by hearing sentences spoken spontaneously than by listening to words repeated artificially.

When your child makes a noise, imitate it, even a burp or a chuckle. Then wait a little while and repeat the noise again. Later on, the child will listen for your response, and smile on hearing it.

The child is now playing with sounds. Still later the child will make his or her own noise in order to get you to copy, and in this way you are both 'throwing' sounds back and forwards like a ball, with enjoyment. You can then vary the sound and the child will try to follow you, and you are teaching the child to enjoy learning to control the speech organs in order to make the sounds wanted. The child is on the way to acquiring speech.

The point about waiting for a response from the child is an important one during any form of play or learning. It is all too easy to be impatient, and to keep showing a child what you want him or her to do, without giving the child a chance to try. By waiting, after you have shown the child what to do, you increase his or her desire to act in an effort to try independently. You make it clear to the child that you want the child to participate. If and when the child tries to imitate your play or voice, repeat the procedure and wait again, so that the child knows that it is his or her turn. The more disabled the child, mentally or physically (or both), the more one needs to wait in order to encourage participation. Too much hurry or repetition too quickly may deter the child from trying to make an effort. The child may then fall into a pattern of being a passive recipient of your efforts, and merely a spectator.

Self-help skills

The same principles apply here as for play. Every effort should be made to encourage the child to attempt tasks independently. This requires not only patience but time. The child must not be left to struggle too long unaided, so that the child is discouraged by failure, nor must everything be done hurriedly for him or her, the child thus becoming a passive doll. The child must be shown the task, and then helped to go through the movements with his or her own hands or body. After a number of trials like this, the child may be moving with you, or at least offering minimal resistance. At this point you should gradually withdraw your effort, particularly at the end of a sequence of movements, so that the child tends to complete the task independently. For example, when

feeding with a spoon, put your hand over the child's hand when holding the spoon. Then take it to the food, fill it, take it to the mouth and after a few trials withdraw your hand at the last point before the spoon goes into the mouth. The task is therefore easily understood, and the tendency to complete the sequence is maximal. In fact, it would almost require a positive desire to resist in order to avoid completion of the task.

This process of active encouragement of self-help and participation must start at birth. Encourage your child to look at the bottle or breast and to open the mouth when it is touched by the teat or nipple. Do not just force it in. It is so easy to believe that your child is helpless and not able to understand, especially if you know the child is disabled. Failure to interest, stimulate and motivate for exploration is in fact discouragement. The child is learning, whether you like it or not. If the child is not being taught to self-help, the child is being taught to lie helplessly. It may give a parent satisfaction to feel that a child is totally dependent, and will always be so, but this is really a poor substitute for the joy of helping one's child to learn, to struggle and to overcome disabilities.

Guiding principles

During any teaching periods, attention to the following principles may be helpful in making your efforts more effective:

1. The infant or child should be keen to cooperate, and therefore be alert, happy, responsive to you and interested in the task. Teach, therefore, when the child is most highly motivated; for example, feeding is best taught at the beginning of a meal when the child is hungry, not at the end when the child is satisfied and likely to play about or resist.

2. The teaching period should be kept short, and ended at once if boredom or protest of any sort begins.

3. No battling should occur; if it does you will always lose. The session must be fun for both of you.

4. Demonstrate, wait, encourage, wait, demonstrate, and so on. Give the child time to

respond, and as soon as any effort is made, encourage further by praise and smiling.

5. Try to be positive: encourage every effort, rather than criticizing for clumsiness, messiness or failure to complete the whole task. Encouragement and praise for every little effort will help the child to enjoy learning.

6. Gradually work backwards from the end of a sequence. That is, get the child to do the last bit, after you have done the rest; then, when this is well learned, get the child to learn the next-to-last step, and so on, so that the child is working into areas which can already be done, so that the child gets the feeling of achievement as if the whole job had been done by the child.

7. If you meet rebellion, or negativism, do not respond with pressure, but instead terminate the session. Remember: the more important a thing is to you, the more likely the child is to resist. Why? Because the child does not like the pressure to conform to your wishes, and because the child enjoys the power of being able to upset you by resisting. Do not let the child enjoy upsetting you. If the child will not eat a meal, calmly take it away and do not relent later. The child should get nothing till the next meal, so that is clear that the child is upset rather than you. Cruel? Not really, in the long run it is kinder to be firm. If the rules are crystal clear, then they will quickly be learned.

8. You must have both patience and time. Unless the slow, disabled child has plenty of your calm, unhurried time, the child may be unable to respond quickly enough, and may therefore look as if nothing is being understood. This is particularly true if the child is physically disabled, because the physical responses may be slow, difficult or even impossible.

9. If the limbs are completely paralysed, try to develop another way of knowing whether the child understands, such as head-nodding for 'yes', and head-shaking for 'no'.

10. Keep on trying if progress is very slow, and look for very small signs of progress. If you give up teaching your child, then the child has no possibility of learning. If you decide that the child cannot do something, then he or she never will. Remember trying to learn to swim? For months one feels it is impossible, and one cannot understand how people do it, then suddenly it comes, and one cannot understand what the problem was.

Helping now

It is natural that parents should worry about the child's future. They often worry constantly about this, and are preoccupied with questions such as: 'Will my child speak? Will my child walk? Will my child ever be able to work? What will happen to our child when we die?' These questions should obviously be answered truthfully by the family's medical adviser, as far as it is possible to do so. But often they can only be answered in a very guarded fashion, as accurate prediction may be difficult, especially when the child is very young.

It is, however, most important that parents should concentrate on helping the child now, rather than worrying about the future. Worry is often destructive; it may prevent you, the parents, from making the best of present opportunities, and it may also be transmitted to the disabled child, who may become unhappy as a result. What is needed is not even a blind acceptance of the somewhat vague prediction you may have been given of final performance, but a realistic look at the child's present state of development and a determination to help the child develop to the best of his or her capabilities. Nothing is so healing of your distress as the certain knowledge that you are working steadily and expertly, day by day, to help your child overcome disabilities. Progress, even very slow progress, keeps hope alive, realistic hope for another small step in the child's achievement. Read, listen and learn from others about ways of helping your child. You are the principal teacher. The professionals help, but they cannot do your job. Learn from them, so that your child gets the best help all the time, not just for a few hours a week. And do not forget that you did the most expert and important job of all at the beginning, when the child was very young – you taught the child to love people, to concentrate, to be curious, to explore the environment and to want to learn.

Concentrate therefore on the present state of development and what needs to be done to try to reach the next stage, not on whether the child will ever be completely ordinary. Regrets, recriminations, worry, sentimental sympathy or painful longing for miracles are not helpful. Effort is needed: informed, skilled, patient, determined, but relaxed effort, and not an excessive preoccupation with the child to the exclusion of your happiness and that of your family.

The task facing parents is like that of a mountaineer determined to scale Everest: the climber wants to reach the summit but knows well that many have failed, and that he or she may fail. But the climber also knows that it is dangerous not to concentrate on the present position, and on how to overcome the immediate obstacles. The climber may not succeed in reaching the top, but only a meticulous and careful step-by-step approach will ensure that the climber gets as far as is humanly possible in the circumstances.

Discipline

This may sound like a severe and inappropriate subject for discussion in relation to disabled children, but it is not. Disabled children must develop socially appropriate behaviour like everybody else, and they must learn that inconsiderate behaviour causes social disapproval. Even people with very severe mental disabilities can learn to behave normally in social situations, because the learning of simple social behaviour requires little intelligence. It does, however, require consistent behaviour by the adults teaching the developing child, so that the child is in no doubt as to what is expected. If disabled older children or adults still behave in an infantile fashion, it is not because they could not learn to behave like an adult, but because they were taught to remain childish. Sitting still rather than running about; being quiet rather than noisy; leaving things alone rather than touching objects, pulling them down or knocking them over; cooperating with others rather than attacking or annoying them; playing with other children rather than stealing their toys: all of these are largely learned, one way or another.

Discipline, or self-control, is learned gradually and begins early. Try not to think, 'The child can't understand', but instead say to yourself, 'My child has got to learn like other children'. Right from the start the child will begin to form that all-important relationship with you which leads to seeking your approval and avoiding your disapproval. This is all that is required for the child to learn which behaviour is acceptable and which is not acceptable. Disapproval shown by a frown or scowl, and a more severe voice, should be enough to produce inhibition of the forbidden behaviour, and a desire to be restored to a position of friendship. Thus distraction into a more desirable activity is readily achieved, with encouragement facilitating the change. Needless to say, consistency is essential.

This process is used by most parents, but it can easily appear to fail, usually because it is not being properly applied. It only works if the proportion of approval to disapproval is high, so that the child can form a satisfying relationship on the basis of many mutually enjoyed activities. The child then knows he or she is loved, and in turn loves you and you both wish to please each other as much as possible. The child will therefore, at least most of the time, try to avoid doing what displeases you. If, however, the child feels that he or she is always, or very frequently, displeasing you, so that every time you see the child move or hear the child call out you disapprove, the relationship will clearly be mutually painful and disturbing. The child will feel unwanted and unloved. Constant criticism and disapproval will cause retaliation, or withdrawal, or both. The child may become increasingly naughty, and enjoy upsetting and annoying you, or may take avoiding action in a fearful, timid way. In either case useful social learning will not be possible, and the situation may eventually deteriorate to the point where the child cannot be tolerated in the family at all.

On the other hand, a child who receives approval for, say, 95% of actions, and disapproval or no response for 5%, has the opportunity to be able to discriminate right from wrong, while still feeling secure. If the disapproval is consistently and firmly given in relation to particular acts or behaviour, these acts will tend to be avoided. Consistency means that both parents must disapprove of the same behaviour, and the disapproval must be firm and unchanging. It is obviously confusing at best, and totally ineffectual or even cruel at worst, if verbal or other mild disapproval is followed by smiling or other encouragement, or if one parent is treating the child's behaviour in a contradictory way.

It is not always easy to realize that one may be encouraging behaviour which is naughty, unrestrained, inconsiderate or socially inappropriate. It is also easy not to realize that behaviour which is appropriate to one developmental stage is being prolonged inappropriately into a later age by continuing encouragement, when the normal process would entail a gradual cessation of encouragement, followed by the slow development of actual disapproval. Children cannot develop typically unless their parents develop, by which I mean that the parents' behaviour must 'grow up' with the child. In fact, the difficulty faced by the parents of a disabled child can be summarized by saying that the child appears not to be developing, and so the parents may not develop, and if the parents do not develop, the disabled child cannot move forward.

It is therefore important indeed not to stand still in your mutual development with your disabled child, so that you both remain locked firmly in the earliest child–parent relationship, with no changes occurring. Behaviour such as the child scratching your face and pulling your hair may possibly be attractive in a young child. Its encouragement at first by parental smiling and gentle vocal response is appropriate for the development of the social bond between parent and child, and essential for the acquisition of movement skills and for the learning of body awareness. At a later stage, however, the child should learn to be gentle while growing in strength, because the child needs to become aware of other people's feelings, and should be moving on to the exploration of toys, objects and the physical environment. This change is achieved by parental encouragement of these object-centred activities, and disapproval of the unwanted behaviour.

However, it must be emphasized that it is not disapproval which is the most effective means of training social behaviour. It is far more effective to continue to encourage, and to 'move on' in a gradually unfolding sequence, so that the child is not allowed to stand still in development. The introduction of a toy to a child who has previously enjoyed only physical contact games

between him- or herself and the adult immediately changes the relationship into a triangular one, in which part of the attention switches to the toy. Encouragement of interest in the toy, and manipulation of it, causes the child to move on in development, so that the child does not get stuck at the person-to-person relationship stage. Although adult encouragement is still needed, the child does not now demand one's full-time undivided attention, because the child now finds the manipulation of the toy rewarding in itself. The parent is rewarded by observing a gradually developing independence, and an unfolding personality which can adapt to other people and other social situations.

Obstinacy and tantrums

The tendency to carry on letting the child have his or her own way is likely to result in an excessively self-willed child. Eventually the parent may come to feel that the child should behave better, and then suddenly decide to change demands. This abrupt, as opposed to a very gradual change, presents the child with an unpleasant and frustrating situation. The child is suddenly expected to give up some behaviour which has been performed for a long time without correction. It is hardly surprising if the child now objects and gives a show of infantile anger, such as screaming or thrashing the legs about on the floor. If this tantrum meets with success, that is, if the mother changes her mind and gives in for fear of upsetting the child, then tantrums may be used by the child to get his or her own way in continuing the form of behaviour. Prevention requires a gradual expectation of changing behaviour as the child develops, and a calm firmness on insisting that the child conforms to reasonable requests.

If tantrums are already established, they may be difficult to control. It is best to ignore the tantrum and to withdraw from the child to another room or, if a group of people is present, to remove the child to another room for a few minutes until the child has settled. On return to the group the child should not be comforted because of tears of anger, but diverted to a constructive activity the child enjoys, and then immediately encouraged by smiling and talking when cooperating. If the child is relatively helpless physically, it is often enough to withdraw attention while the child is screaming by looking away, and then to restore your interest as soon as there is quietness.

It must be pointed out, however, that if tantrums are well established, the child will go through a period at first of seeming to get worse if a programme of control is started. This is because tantrums have worked previously in getting the child's way, and it is natural for the child to increase efforts using the hitherto successful method. The child may therefore scream louder, and thrash about more fiercely and for longer, at the beginning of your efforts to control. It is essential, therefore, to resolve that one is going through this period in order to achieve improvement later. If you give in again after a prolonged struggle, the situation will be worse, because the child now knows that even in the difficult circumstances when the parents are trying to hold out, the child can win if continuing long enough.

It is also important that one carefully chooses the time and place to start such a programme. Do not start it while out shopping: it is very embarrassing to try ignoring a tantrum in a crowded shop or public place. Begin at home and avoid public situations until some improvement has occurred.

It must be emphasized that this rather fierce method, in which one seems to be exerting a harsh external control over a more helpless person, can be avoided by the gradual teaching of self-control from early childhood in the expectation that the child should behave ordinarily from the beginning. Ignoring tantrums, if they have become a regular feature of behaviour, coupled with placing the child away from social contact if the tantrums become fierce or prolonged, is still far preferable to smacking or physical punishment. The latter is not only more likely to destroy a satisfactory relationship with the child, it also teaches the child to be aggressive, as the child will model him- or herself on you. This may well lead to later fighting and spitefulness towards siblings or other children. Nothing is more irrational that a parent threatening a child with: 'If you hit that child, I shall hit you!' This teaches the child

that aggression is acceptable, and the bigger and stronger person wins.

Obstinacy of the kind where passive resistance is used should be dealt with differently. This is often due to the child having been under pressure to achieve, accompanied by much criticism. In other words, if the child is often criticized for being too stupid or too slow, or for not trying, and the adult is impatient, irritable and frustrated by the fumbling efforts, the relationship will be unpleasant for both, and learning situations particularly painful. Refusal to try is a natural avoidance response, and at its worst is shown by muteness, a bowed head, averted or closed eyes and clenched hands. Only by avoiding impatient, demanding pressure to achieve, and replacing it with gentle, patient encouragement of constructive effort, can this situation be remedied. It often requires the intervention of a teacher, or some other less emotionally involved person, so that the child can more easily start a new teaching relationship free from past painful experiences.

Food fads, toilet training, negativism

The more fiercely a parent holds to the belief that meat, fish, protein or whatever must be eaten each day to ensure health, brain growth or intelligence, the more likely it is that the child will refuse to eat it. The pressure to which the child is subjected makes the child rebel. The rebellion upsets the parent and battle commences – a battle which the parent cannot win. You cannot force a child to eat and retain food; if you try, the child may well vomit it all up immediately afterwards. If the pressure is dropped the battle ceases, and in time the child may well feel that he or she wants what everyone else is having. The child has lost the motivation for refusal, namely to upset you, which is obviously very easy if you are overconcerned with the need to give certain foods.

A similar situation arises when there is pressure to eat more. The child who has had enough will start to play with food, and make a mess. If pressure is exerted to make the child eat more or quicker, the child may rebel in order to upset the parent. If, on the other hand, the child is treated as an individual who knows what is needed, playing can be taken as a signal that the child has had enough. The uneaten food should then be calmly removed, with no retreat from this position, even if the child protests, so that the child goes without until the next usual mealtime. If the child does not protest, then the child did not need any more; if the child does protest, then the child will quickly learn to eat what is wanted without playing about.

For similar reasons toilet training is another common battleground. It may seem so important to a parent that pressure is exerted on the child to oblige, and the child soon realizes that he or she is in control, and can therefore easily upset the parent. A child who refuses to use the pot, or who sits on it for 10 minutes and then soils the nappy just after it has been put on, may well have achieved full bowel control, but is using it for his or her own purpose.

Both the above behavioural problems are forms of negativism, or refusal to cooperate with a too-demanding parent. If you are easily upset by your child's disobedience, your child will enjoy disobeying. If you keep pressing the child to do something, such as eating protein, using the pot or tidying toys away, the child may refuse to cooperate and prefer to be negative. Children have wills of their own which they wish to assert, and if you try to dominate, the child will try to dominate you, and may well succeed. In certain circumstances children have a right to say 'no' (many children acquire this word before any other), and will if you keep pushing them to conform to an unreasonable demand.

Other behavioural problems

In a clinic, children are occasionally seen who exhibit more severe behavioural problems such as screaming at night, head-banging, hand-biting, rocking or overactivity. Such problems need medical investigation as they may indicate an underlying medical condition, but often nothing is found which can be remedied. In that case we must attempt to help the child using educational methods.

Children who receive little attention, stimulation or social contact will tend to occupy themselves with body manipulation, especially if that child has partial or complete loss of vision or hearing, or is more severely mentally disabled. Many stereotyped, repetitive behaviours such as body-rocking, head-rolling, tongue-stroking and complicated movements of the fingers sometimes appear to be substitutes for external stimulation and manipulation. They also seem to comfort the child, who may therefore use such behaviour for this purpose, particularly if distressed. These mannerisms are certainly difficult to eliminate once they are firmly established, because the child becomes absorbed in self-stimulation, and is at the same time relatively unresponsive to social contact.

Trying to stop the mannerisms by a direct disapproving approach alone is bound to fail, so it is necessary to substitute something more interesting and pleasurable. Once these mannerisms are established, only a long, patient, gentle approach to the child by one or two people, who try to join in the child's world rather than forcing other activities on to the child, is likely to succeed in establishing more social responsiveness and interest in the environment. From simple physical person-to-person contact games, progress can be made to physical games using apparatus such as swings and roundabouts, and from there to simple object-centred play such as catching balls or rolling toy cars.

Physically disabled children seem less liable to develop these manneristic behaviours or to become withdrawn, but if they do appear, or you feel your child is unresponsive to you, it is wise to seek expert help early, so that vision and hearing can be checked or rechecked, and advice given regarding play and stimulation.

Other disturbing types of behaviour, such as disruptive rushing about and touching forbidden household objects, are often a means of attracting attention. Mute children, in particular, are likely to develop some disturbing types of behaviour in order to attract the attention of adults, and if the child is physically helpless the child may be forced to use screaming. It is common to believe that talking to, picking up, caressing or taking the child into one's own bed are comforting to the child who is distressed. This is certainly true in infancy, but the child may quickly learn to use screaming as a signal that social contact is wanted. As time goes by, parents may get worn out with the noise, and having to respond to the child's demands, which may even become incessant. They may try to break the pattern by ignoring the screams, but the child often then responds by redoubling efforts. The child therefore screams louder and longer, and the parents may then give in, or smack the child in irritable bad temper. In the latter case they will then probably feel guilty at having caused more distress, and will then comfort the child again.

An ordinary young child obviously needs frequent social contact with an adult, and even casual observation reveals that the child signals to the adult every few minutes by vocalization, eye contact (looking at the adult's face) and physical contact (touching the adult's arm or climbing on to knee), and that a response is obtained from the adult. Unfortunately, the physically disabled child, who has the same social needs, is often less able to signal effectively by these typical methods. If the child cannot move, cannot vocalize, cannot turn the head, and sometimes cannot even turn the eyes, what is the child to do? The child does the only thing possible – cries. If this works, the child goes on using crying as a signal for attention. If the child gets little response, the child may eventually become withdrawn and apathetic.

The remedy may be obvious to some, but is certainly not easy. The parent needs to make a very special effort to keep the infant nearby at first, and in a position where he or she can establish frequent vocal contact, eye-to-eye contact and physical contact. It sounds easy, but it is not. You have to make all the effort because the child is not able to signal needs in the ordinary way. You also have to keep this up for many more months, and in some cases, years, than you would with an ordinary child. This will need great persistence and patience, because there is less reward for your effort.

Another very important point is that you need to be very observant in order to detect the tiny signals which your child, unless very grievously disabled, will soon start to make. If the child does look at you, you must at once look back. Of course, you cannot sit watching all the time, so listen carefully for little vocal sounds, and respond with your voice and interest to these, so that the child quickly learns to 'call' you. If you do not respond to these quieter sounds, the child will be forced to use louder and less desirable ones. Try to remember how frequently an ordinary child keeps on contacting its parent, and that the disabled child has the same needs. It is tiring, yes; mothers frequently and justifiably complain of the strain of responding to the demands of ordinary children, but nevertheless we have to recognize the importance of this social contact for the development of children.

The adult's response will therefore determine which signals the child comes to use by habit, to obtain the attention needed for social development. If the child is using screaming, this indicates that the need for social stimulation is probably being insufficiently recognized when quiet, or when making the early signals of eye contact and gentle vocalization. The child may not need more stimulation than you are giving already in response to the screaming, but may be having to 'shout' loudly before being heard. In other words, it is possible that the child is being ignored unless screaming is used, and then the child gets what is wanted. What is needed is the social stimulation or your response to be given before the child screams. Ideally this is achieved by your heightened sensitivity to the gentle signals which the child is giving. It may also be true that the quality of the social stimulation is inadequate. The response to screaming is often just a comforting, kissing, cuddling, caressing or rocking. What is really needed, certainly after the first few weeks, is the introduction of play activities, and therefore 'peek-a-boo'-type games should be introduced as soon as possible, followed by the use of rattles, paper and other toys and materials, in order to encourage interest in the environment.

The child who is less physically disabled may, because of the same causes, develop head-banging, hand-biting or disruptive overactivity and other disturbing types of behaviour. The more severe and disturbing the behaviour, the more certain it is that it will effectively 'switch on' the adults in the environment to pay attention to the child. The adult therefore tries to stop the child carrying out the disturbing activity, and in doing so provides the child with the rewarding social contact needed, and which is almost certainly not being given at other times. Again one must ignore the disturbing behaviour as much as possible and, most importantly, provide the child with more satisfying and interesting stimulation at other times. It is surprisingly difficult for some adults to be interested in children when they are quiet and constructively occupied, rather than when they are noisy or disruptive. You must be positive in your relationship, like a teacher. You must go to the child to interest the child, encouraging and playing with the child, because you want the child to learn, not chase the child to stop the child doing things you do not like, nor go to the child only when it seems that comforting is needed. Ask yourself: 'When do I talk to my child? When do I touch my child? When do we play together?' If the answer is, usually after screaming or throwing ornaments on the floor, or banging the head, then you are teaching the child to do these very things in order to obtain your interest.

Overattachment

The child who is dependent for a longer than normal time is in danger of overattachment, especially if only one person cares for the child for most of the time. Not only may this make it difficult for the child to adjust later to playgroup, nursery or school, but it may leave the child/person very vulnerable if you become ill and have to go into hospital, or if you die, or if the child has to go into hospital for a period. It is important that both parents, and brothers and sisters, should play a full part in the first year of life, and that other people should be in some contact with the child from time to time.

Being handled by other people should be as routine a part of life as for any typical child of the same age, so that social contact is pleasurable and not frightening. After 2 years of age these contacts will become more important, and

should result in a gradual widening of the child's acquaintances, so that nursery activities are enjoyed at age 3–4 years without any trouble or separation anxiety. If the child has been overprotected, and has therefore become overattached to the mother or to both parents, the introduction to a nursery group will be painful and distressing to both, and this will further convince the parents that the child is too young to leave them, even for a few hours. The child may therefore still stay at home, and the longer this occurs, the more overattached the child and the parents will become. Again, these processes of social development must be gradual, so that the child feels secure within the family at first, and then slowly generalizes this feeling to more and more people and relationships. An overprotective parent does not produce a happy, secure child, but one who is anxious, dependent and frightened of the rest of the world. Remember that your child, like your other children, cannot belong totally to you: your child has a right to grow away from you and towards others, who must be allowed, and encouraged, to share in care and happiness.

Brothers and sisters

It is easy to forget the brothers and sisters (siblings) of a disabled child, but they need special attention in their own right. The birth of a new child can easily cause jealousy in a toddler, especially if all attention suddenly switches to the newcomer. This is even more likely to happen if the new child has medical problems which worry the parents and are time-consuming to deal with. A special effort therefore needs to be made to continue to give time and attention to older siblings, in order to satisfy their needs for play, attention and affection. They must not be allowed to feel forgotten, or even resentful.

It is possible, and helpful, to involve older siblings in the care of a disabled child, thus giving your attention to the needs of both. If you praise the helping children, they will enjoy being useful and develop a caring and loving relationship with the disabled one. Later, questions will be asked about the disabled child's slowness to progress, or inability to sit, talk or walk. These should always be answered truthfully, at a level that the child can understand.

Siblings in their teens may feel embarrassed by a disabled brother or sister, especially when opposite-sex friends are brought home. However, if the parents have always answered questions truthfully and without embarrassment, and generally involved their friends and neighbours in an open and cheerful fashion, it is likely that siblings will also be able to act naturally and with minimal embarrassment.

An important lifelong parental anxiety concerns the care of the disabled child when the parents are themselves old or dead. In the past, siblings were often pressurized by parents to take over the care, sometimes even being forced to promise this at the parent's deathbed. This action often stemmed from a fear of old-fashioned institutional care, but with the development of modern, higher-quality residential care such parental anxieties should be rarer. Disabled children, as they grow into their teens, should be able to experience periods of short-term residential care in modern small homes close to their family home, and the parents' observation of the child's enjoyment of such stays should do much to reassure them, and help them to foster eventual independence.

Many disabled young adults (in England) are familiar with short-term care, and increasingly they should have the opportunity to move out of the parental home when the family feels this is right. As young adults they should have their own home if they wish, with whatever degree of care and supervision is necessary, and their parents should have the normal right to expect a relatively care-free middle age and retirement. Similarly their siblings should expect to form their own new families without having to care full-time for a brother or sister unless they wish to.

Social behaviour

Parents naturally want their physically and possibly mentally disabled child to be able to read, write, count and to make further progress in formal education. But social behaviour is much more important than intellectual achievement, whether for typical or disabled people. For the mentally disabled in particular, with limited abstract learning ability, it is essential to concentrate on the fundamentals for social adaptation, the acquisition of basic self-help skills: feeding, communication, continence, mobility, and the development of a likeable personality, so that behaviour immediately evokes from others a friendly and helpful response. One of the most valuable, and relatively sophisticated, social skills is the ability to put others at ease and to get them to help us or cooperate with us. To be able to approach people in a friendly, outgoing and charming way in order to ask for help, or to offer it, is a great asset. Timidity, awkwardness or fumbling, incoherent approaches on the other hand may be met by rejection, rebuff or humiliating amusement. This in turn is hurtful, and increases the disabled person's social anxiety, clumsiness and misery.

This brings us to the importance of allowing, and encouraging, the disabled person to help others. Full community recognition as valuable members is accorded to those who are seen to be making a valuable contribution to society. The active helpers and doers, 'the pillars of society', have the highest status, whereas those who are dependent and helpless, 'a burden on society', have the lowest. It may seem strange to try to encourage disabled people to help others, but it can often be done. There are many mildly disabled adults who enjoy looking after more severely disabled children, and who give them devoted care. In turn, the severely disabled child may give the adults a loving relationship which they might otherwise never have. Both parties in such a relationship are able to help each other in a way which others may be unable to do for either.

Generally, disabled individuals who might spend most of their life being helped by caring people at home, at school or in sheltered employment or a residential home should be encouraged to give direct personal services to others. The person should be involved in small responsibilities as soon as possible, for you at home, for brothers and sisters, for neighbours and friends. There is no reason why the mildly disabled person should not enjoy helping old people, for example either at the neighbourhood level or by taking part in organized community projects. We must not only aim at encouraging disabled persons to make their own decisions, to exercise choices, to feel the satisfaction of recognized achievement and to enjoy the same variety of opportunity as the rest of us: we must allow them to step into the helping, caring role that we have in the past carefully reserved for ourselves. Only in this way will they really feel part of the adult community.

Conclusion

It is a difficult task to write a helpful chapter for the many different parents of children of different ages with different disabilities. Some problems have been left out, while on the other hand some parents may well feel daunted by the many difficulties which have been presented. It is better, however, to have a quick look at the country ahead, with all its hazards, before setting off on a journey, provided that one is then determined to plan well in order to avoid the worst pitfalls. Being a parent is never an easy job, and none of us is perfect. Luckily children are very resilient, and most parents make a good job of their children's upbringing without instruction or much help. I hope, therefore, that after having skimmed through this chapter, parents will turn back to those parts most applicable to their situation, and then read them more carefully and frequently. If you still have difficulties which do not seem to be easily resolved, and particularly if you remain distressed, anxious or depressed, you should seek additional help. It may be that other parents will be able to help you, either directly from their own experience, or because they know better than anybody the best source of professional help in your locality. Whatever you do, do not try to press on in misery and hopelessness by yourself.

Chapter Seven

7

Learning and behaviour – the psychologist's role

Mary Gardner

If a young child is disabled it is natural that parents and professionals should want to find out exactly what is holding up the child's development so that they can make plans for helping, and seeing how far and in what ways they can reduce the difficulties. In the case of children with more severe cerebral palsy (CP), this process of finding out what is wrong can be quite complicated. This is because CP is due to impairment in parts of the brain. Since the brain is very complex and controls much of behaviour and learning, speech and motor movements and thinking and feeling, it is no simple matter to sort this out and to find out what is causing the difficulties and then to find the most helpful solutions. The joint effort of professionals working in close partnership with parents is very important for this process.

Sometimes such an array of professionals – medical, psychological, therapeutic, educational and social work – seems formidable to parents, but it is helpful to realize that these people exist and have come together for the single purpose of helping the family and their child. The younger the child, the more important it is that help should be channelled through the parents; they are the child's first diagnosticians, therapists and teachers. Their influence is paramount and remains so throughout the early years of the child's life. No matter how much professional help the family is getting, it is the parents who have to cope with the day-to-day problems that arise.

Parents can get most benefit from professionals if they know more about their work and the methods they use. The parents are then in a better position to ask the right questions. Parents should not hesitate to ask questions, and should not worry that their queries may be viewed as criticism. Many professional people like answering questions. It reassures them of the usefulness of their work and helps to reduce the tendency to look at problems only from their professional point of view.

In this chapter the work of one of these professionals, the child psychologist, and their part in supporting the parents and the child with a disability will be discussed. Psychologists are chiefly interested in the processes by which children learn and in their emotional response to the world around them. The more we know about how children learn, the better chance we have of helping a child who has difficulties in learning.

How typical children learn

Children start learning right from birth. For example, a baby or any young creature makes a variety of uncoordinated movements. By chance, some of these movements result in a sensation that may be found enjoyable. The child's waving arms while lying in the cot may for instance encounter a dangling ring which may be held on to with a primitive hand grasp. The child's reactions are too disorganized to grip the ring intentionally but gradually over days and weeks of repeating the same movement the developing brain discerns a pattern which finally results, by the age of around 6 months, in the child being instantly able to grasp the ring whenever it is in view. From this example we can see that, as the nervous system matures, the child learns, by means of repetition, to coordinate hand and eye movements.

In more complex situations repetition and practice may also be important. For example, we have all observed and wondered at the apparently purposeless dropping of toys over the side of a highchair or cot. When the child repeatedly cries for the toy to be picked up, we might be justified in thinking that it is being done merely to annoy. This may be so in an older child, but in younger children who have recently learnt to sit up, the action shows that they are beginning to have the first glimmerings of an idea that objects continue

to exist even though they have disappeared from sight. This is such a novel and fascinating insight that they feel the need to drop the toy over and over again to see if the same thing happens each time. By means of these simple actions children are beginning to appreciate quite complicated ideas of cause and effect and the influence of gravity, of which they need to be aware before tackling more advanced activities such as building with bricks or climbing.

A child also learns about the world by experimenting and trying things out. Telling children constantly 'not to touch' is depriving them of a necessary sensory experience in much the same way as shutting them up in a darkened room. Children learn about the characteristics of things around them by comparing what the eyes and ears tell them with what can be felt with the hands and mouth.

Another way that a child learns is by imitation. One of the earliest imitative behaviours is connected with making sounds. A child babbles spontaneously during the earliest months, but by about 12 months many children will attempt to make the same sounds as the adult who is playing with them. When children are alone these sounds are practised, they listen to themselves doing so and gradually widen their repertoire. A cross-cultural study has shown that, by the age of 18 months, children are beginning to 'specialize' when they babble, in those sounds which are most common in their native language. We can see from this that imitation starts early in a child's life.

These simple examples show the way in which children begin to make sense out of the mass of impressions that bombard them from all sides. They are starting to make sense out of the sounds and sights and the feel of objects around them, moving and manipulating things, vocalizing and talking, gradually increasing their understanding and control of their surroundings.

How does a child with more severe CP learn?

The fundamentals for effective learning are the same for disabled children as for all children with, of course, some important differences of emphasis and timing, depending on the severity of the problems.

In considering the learning process we note that learning involves eagerness and striving to achieve, the drive to explore and seek new experiences, plus the confidence to do so. Confidence is vitally important for learning. Although the drive and eagerness to learn may not be so clearly evident in some children with more severe CP, for the vast majority the urge to learn is there, but may be reduced by frustration and failure. This is likely to occur when the stimulation given to children and the activities expected of them are either too difficult and upsetting or, at the other extreme, too simple and boring, both of which provide them with little sense of achievement. Children may therefore fail to develop a view of themselves as competent persons.

Confidence is increased by parents' encouragement of and praise for their child's efforts, rather than by constantly drawing attention to their inadequacies.

Parents' expectations

Sometimes a child's failures are not really failures but simply a matter of adults setting standards that are too high. Parents' expectations of their child's rate of learning are important. These expectations must be realistic and the goals they expect their child to reach in mobility, handling objects, using communication and reasoning things out must be related to the severity of the child's disabilities physically, intellectually and emotionally.

It is here that the help of the professional team may be useful in setting reasonable expectations and reasonable targets. Otherwise parents may be expecting either too much or too little of their child, who may then become discouraged and show less eagerness when tackling new tasks.

How can we assess learning ability?

Parents, when looking at signs of their child's progress, compare the child with brothers and sisters, or with friends' children. Making allowances for differences in age, they notice how 'quick on the uptake' certain children are compared with others in their daily life and in their play with bricks, toys and books.

The psychologist makes the same sort of comparison, only in a more systematic way and with the help of intelligence tests that have been worked out over many years. These tests give us a fairly accurate idea of what abilities are to be expected of the average 2- or 3-year-old child, and so on. For example, if a child aged 2 years completes the set of simple tasks which are appropriate for this age group, such as building with bricks, naming a certain number of toys and pictures or picking out a particular toy on request, it suggests that the child has a mental age in the region of 2 years. Since this mental age corresponds exactly with the actual age of 2 years, we can say that the child is of average intelligence. Another way of expressing this is to say that the child has an intelligence quotient or IQ of 100.

There is nothing magical about the IQ figure. It is simply a convenient way of expressing the degree to which the intellectual or cognitive age corresponds to the chronological age of the child. The IQ figure is calculated by dividing the intellectual or cognitive age by the actual age and multiplying by 100. In the case of a 4-year-old child who succeeds in the test at a level appropriate to a child of around 3 years, we can say that the child has an intellectual age of 3 years, and therefore an IQ of about 75, which is at the lower end of the normal range of intelligence.

Parents may consider that this kind of measurement might be all right for the average youngster but those with a child with CP may well ask: 'How can you expect my child to show intelligence when he or she cannot use their hands or speak clearly, and has had very little experience with these kinds of activities?' This is where the skill of the child psychologist comes in. It is the child psychologist's job to get through to the child's intellectual abilities, although these may be hidden by the presence of physical and speech disabilities.

The psychologist makes careful observations of the child playing spontaneously, noting what catches the child's interest and how he or she interacts with the family. The degrees of interest and concentration shown when presented with specific tasks are important indicators of the level of development.

Psychologists are also interested in assessing a child's intentions, rather than actual performance in the tests. The child's attempts, however clumsy, to build a tower of graduated bricks, for example, are carefully observed and can provide quite convincing evidence that the child has grasped ideas of size and sequence; the fact that the tower of bricks may keep falling down is not important for this purpose. Many children with CP have sufficient motor control to give a reliable indication of their intentions and of their understanding.

For those children with only a little hand control or speech, however, some specialized tests are available that require practically no motor control or speech. The child merely has to point in the right direction with eyes or hands in response to a series of questions or simply to give some sign which indicates 'yes' or 'no'. For example, in multiple choice tests, given a series of pictures, the psychologist will point to each one in turn, asking the child to give some sort of indication when the picture is reached which represents, say, 'the bed' or 'the thing we sleep in' or 'the one with four legs'.

On the whole, intelligence tests are not as reliable for children with disabilities as they are for typical children, but in the hands of a psychologist who is experienced with disabilities and aware of the strengths and limitations of the tests, useful guidelines can be obtained.

The need for guidelines

The chief purpose of these formal assessments of learning abilities is to provide guidelines. They tell us approximately how far a child has reached in learning, and how much progress may reasonably be expected over the next few years.

We mentioned earlier the importance of adult expectations about what a child may or may not achieve at certain stages in life. If we expect a 5-year-old whose present reasoning level is around

2 years to begin reading and number work, then disappointment is bound to ensue. Both the child and the parents are likely to become extremely frustrated. Alternatively, if we expect too little we may miss the chance of encouraging children's efforts at a stage when they are receptive and ready to learn.

Some studies have indicated that approximately half of the children with CP function within the average or above-average range of intelligence, about a quarter function within the moderately slow learning range, while the remaining quarter are very slow-learning, which means that their intellectual level is rather below that of an average child of half their age. It is these very slow-learning children, who often have more severe physical and speech impairments, who need a great deal of professional educational and therapeutic help.

Encouraging your child's interest in learning

Some people might question the point of trying to improve the performance of a severely disabled child. They might argue that their skills are so limited that the time and effort are scarcely worthwhile. Any parent after a tiring day may well feel the same!

However, anyone who has watched a child struggling with determination and persistence to master some task that he or she has observed others doing and has seen the delight which accompanies success, will realize that achievement is as important to the disabled child as it is to any child. Indeed, one might argue that the smallest steps towards self-help in dressing, feeding and moving around take on a greater significance in the life of a child with CP, whose horizons are necessarily limited. The parents' aim should be to encourage the child's efforts in self-help skills, ensuring that any task is almost within the child's reach so that continued disappointment does not dampen their eagerness. Teaching a new skill is a subtle compromise between you doing too much of what the child could manage, and setting so hard a task that failure is bound to ensue.

We can summarize the most effective ways of encouraging learning as follows:

1. *Interesting tasks*. Some more disabled children do not, in the early years, seem to show much curiosity or eagerness to learn. The parent must therefore work towards stimulating their interest by using large bright toys and materials, including something different each week that has not been seen before or has not been seen for some time, so that an element of curiosity is maintained.

2. *Short sessions*. Set aside one or two periods of say 10–15 minutes each day for carrying out some fairly concentrated learning. This is better than trying to carry on for hours at a time. Children may concentrate and achieve quite a lot in fairly short spurts with rest and relaxation in between.

3. *Set a target*. It helps both parents and child to aim at a goal. It enables us to be aware of progress and to get satisfaction from knowing when we reach a certain goal, or nearly do so. These goals can range from very simple activities such as building with bricks, or putting objects in and taking objects out of containers, to more complicated activities such as matching shapes or coloured cards, completing form boards, and so on.

4. *Small steps*. Choose simple activities and break them down into manageable steps. For example, with a game like Picture Lotto, the matching of pictures can start with a few obviously different pictures, moving gradually to matching those in which differences between them are more subtle. Give plenty of opportunities for practice.

5. *Encouragement*. Give plenty of praise for success, praising for effort as well as for actual accomplishment. Play down failure as much as possible without showing surprise or irritation.

If these general principles are kept in mind, mastering the simplest skill will bring with it much satisfaction to the child. Learning can be enjoyable.

Learning in the child with additional impairments

Visual problems

There are some children with CP who have visual as well as movement problems. Children with poor vision, because they can not see their parents' faces so clearly, will need more in the way of touching and cuddling and singing than the typical child. Children will become aware of affection by the way they are handled and by the tone of the adult's voice, and will gradually be able to recognize familiar people by these means, as well as by the texture and smell of their clothes. They will begin to learn about the world by touching and exploring with their fingers and with the mouth, and will gradually come to appreciate feelings through the sound of laughter or the tone of disapproval in the parent's voice.

But most of all, children with a visual problem will learn by listening to all the wide variety of sounds around them as well as to people talking. Being talked to is of vital importance to the visually impaired child. For instance, it is especially helpful if the parent provides a running commentary while preparing a meal, so that the child may begin to associate the sounds and smell of meal preparation with the feel and taste of the different foods. Similarly with the preparations for a bath or an outing.

Children with limited vision enjoy musical toys and those that make a noise, such as saucepans with lids, trays to bang with a spoon, or friction-drive cars. They may need more than usual encouragement to explore their surroundings, since they may be understandably timid until accustomed to a familiar room and to avoiding obstacles in it. Toys that make a noise such as a ball with a bell inside it may tempt a child to go after it, whether by rolling or crawling.

For the child with milder visual problems it is even more difficult to imagine what it must be like to have only a vague impression of people's faces; to be not quite sure whether one is seeing a frown or a grin. As with more severely impaired children it is the adult's tone of voice that becomes important, and the child needs to be given clear verbal messages, for instance about future activities and what is about to happen.

Even with quite minor visual problems children may not be able to distinguish distant objects: to know, for instance, which is their coat until getting near enough to feel the texture. Tidiness and routine play a major part in the lives of these children and it helps if the household is well organized, otherwise the child will trip over things left lying about or get very frustrated at not finding things in expected places.

When we are outside the house, knowing where we are depends on recognizing a series of familiar landmarks which we 'tick off' in our minds, so to speak, as we go along. For children with poor vision who are being taken out in a buggy or wheelchair, it is especially helpful if they are allowed to touch the hedge or fence as you pass, so that they can recognize where you have got to along a familiar route. It is also helpful if the adult can talk about the interesting buildings or vehicles they are passing, and the reasons for stopping at a particular crossing point. By doing this the visually disabled child will quickly build up a series of clues into an auditory and tactile map of the local neighbourhood. You will thus be able to supplement whatever visual impressions children are able to receive and enhance their understanding of the world around.

Hearing problems

Nearly everybody has occasional hearing problems due to ear blockages and infections, especially after a common cold. These can cause a mild temporary hearing loss known as a conductive loss which usually responds well to medical treatments. A small percentage of children with CP have hearing losses which are not due to blockages but to a defect in the nerve fibres, either within the inner section of the ear or in the nerve pathways to the brain. This is known as a nerve or sensorineural hearing loss which can range from mild to severe, sometimes affecting the hearing of higher rather than lower tones.

The parents are often the first to notice a hearing difficulty, comparing their child's responses to their own responses, and to those of other children, to everyday sounds such as the doorbell, radio or telephone, in situations where their child's attention is not fully engaged in some other activity that completely absorbs the child.

If a hearing loss is suspected, then prompt professional testing is important, so that if a loss is confirmed, its causes and extent can be determined and remedial action planned.

The main effect of a significant and permanent hearing loss is to delay a child's language, communication and social skills, so early advice on training and equipment is important. In England, such advice is obtainable from local audiology units, working in conjunction with medical and educational services.

Hearing aids can help if they can amplify sounds without distorting them too much. Radio aids, through which the speaker uses a microphone and a transmitter, are often considered better.

Lip reading, gestures and sign language such as Makaton should also be encouraged in children with severe hearing losses, using visual cues to compensate for their impaired hearing.

It is particularly important for children with physical disabilities to be properly positioned for good communication: that is, head and trunk well supported, facing the speaker in good light, earpieces for the hearing aid fitting properly and not too much disturbance from movements which can cause unwanted noises through the hearing aid. It is difficult to maintain these proper conditions for good communication all day, but they should be maintained for some periods during each day. This is important to ensure that simple language is absorbed, vocabulary is built up and sentence formation grows. From this input, communication by the child may follow through speech and signing, or by using electronic equipment, including word processors.

Help from a teacher of the hearing-impaired will be important in furthering your child's language and communication skills, on which a great deal of the social skills depend. It is difficult to relate to people if you cannot fully understand what they are saying. This help, during the formative years, will ensure that a child is well prepared for nursery and primary schooling. In England, many schools have the services of a visiting teacher of the hearing-impaired, and some have special units for children with severe hearing losses who require more concentrated help within small groups.

Subtle learning difficulties

Some children with CP who possess adequate intelligence and vision and relatively minor physical problems may nevertheless have unevenly developed learning abilities. For example, they may be good with words, conversing readily, using sentences well at an early age, but may be poor at practical things, such as handling constructional toys or dressing. These children have quite subtle difficulties in their perception of the world around them.

Visual perception is the ability to recognize and distinguish between shapes, such as a circle and a square, to distinguish between the outline of a drawing and its surrounding background and to recognize different directions in space (left and right, up and down), especially in relation to one's own body. Some children are easily confused about which direction to take and how to get their body past obstacles, their arms into sleeves, and so on. They may also have difficulty in relating what they see to what they hear and to what they touch. In other words, their different senses do not hang together well. For example, by 6 months of age most children not only hear a sound but will usually turn their head and look inquiringly, attempting to identify what might be making the noise. Over the months hearing, vision, motor control and intelligence have worked together to accomplish this, whereas a child with perceptual disabilities cannot link these up or rather may be slow in learning to do so.

This linking-up of visual and motor performance is important since we use our visual perception a great deal in everyday life. Indeed, much of the information we receive from our surroundings comes through the eyes and is then interpreted by the brain. We may act on the information we have gained and make some sort of motor or vocal response. In short, we integrate vision with movement. Children start to do this during the first months of life, for example in watching their own hand movements or reaching for a toy.

How to help the child with poor visual perception

In helping children with perceptual problems we need to encourage and teach things that come more or less automatically to the typical child. Otherwise they may tend to shy away from what they find difficult – visual judgement in this case – and 'overdevelop' what might come more easily, such as speech and appreciation of language. In short they may become great talkers and poor doers.

Lots of encouragement and opportunities are needed to help develop a child's appreciation of shape and pattern, and to link these perceptions with the use of the hands. There is plenty of material available for this, such as simple form boards, posting boxes, graduated beakers and boxes of bricks. As emphasized earlier, try to begin with some measure of success by using the simplest posting box or form board with just a few shapes. At first, encourage the child to place just one or two shapes, a circle or square for instance, while you help with the rest. If you start in this gradual way children will be pleased with their success and will want to tackle the whole task as soon as they are confident of a chance of succeeding.

Modern form boards are often in bright colours thought to be attractive to younger children and certainly are helpful to those with a visual problem. Whether plain or highly coloured is not of particular significance but it is the act of selecting the shape, looking at it carefully and comparing it with the hole that is the important thing. Children are discovering that, by scanning the alternatives before making a choice, they will gain more success than by trying the first piece that comes to hand. An important lesson is being learnt here, especially for children who tend to be impulsive and have difficulty in controlling hand and arm movements. Look first, think second and act third.

If children are good with words, use this to help their visual judgement, for example by naming a circle and pointing out its similarity to a football, thus helping the child distinguish between a round and an oval shape. One form board insert could be described as 'like a roof', another 'like a tunnel'. These early experiences with shapes form the basis for later attempts at reading, which is basically a process of distinguishing one slightly different shape from another.

How to help the child with attention problems

Some children show a short attention span and are easily distracted from the task in hand by any extraneous sound, such as a lorry passing, or the sight of a curtain swaying in the wind. With children who are easily diverted a helpful move is to cut down the amount of distraction around.

For teaching and training periods a quiet corner of the room should be used and kept fairly plain and bare, tidying other toys out of sight and presenting children with only a few pieces of equipment at a time. This helps to focus their attention and eventually to get more satisfaction from what is being done, so that eventually, when older, they are more able to cope with ordinary surroundings and distractions.

Many psychologists regard these perceptual and attention disabilities as a kind of time-lag in a child's development, rather than a more permanent impairment; that is, the attention and perception of the disabled child are often at a level appropriate to a younger child. The techniques described above may help to focus and extend concentration.

Alternative forms of communication

We have been considering various factors to do with the way a child learns; the input of impression through the various senses, and the intelligence, perception and attention that enable the child to organize and make sense of these impressions. We will now mention the 'output' from children: their means of expression through speech, hand control and gesture.

Careful consideration needs to be given to those children whose communication difficulties are such that they cannot properly express their thoughts and ideas, either through speech or hand movement, if constant frustration is to be reduced. We have already mentioned some of the ways in which the psychologist communicates with more severely disabled children, such as by providing toys and test situations in which the adult can do the talking and movements, and the child merely has to signal 'yes' or 'no' at the right time.

Parents can practise this sort of communication with their child. For example, a 3- or 4-year-old child without speech or very much hand control can gain stimulation and enjoyment from a simple picture such as a street scene. The parent can talk about it and then ask questions. 'Is this the policeman? Is this the ice cream van?', pointing to various parts of the picture in turn, and waiting for the child to give some sign for 'yes' when the correct illustration is shown. These signs for 'yes' and 'no' are important; any sign will do, such as nodding the head, looking at the speaker to indicate 'yes', looking to one side or grimacing to indicate 'no'. When reliable signs of this kind are established children can begin to express their ideas and preferences, in spite of speech and hand control difficulties.

Some equipment can be provided to extend this expression; a head pointer can be used if hand control is inadequate, or better still, an electronically operated indicator, with the child using a simple switch, that allows the child to control a moving light to express a choice.

Signing is a wider-ranging alternative to speech through hand movements and gestures, as often used by people who are deaf to indicate words. Examples are the Paget–Gorman system and its simplified form, known as Makaton. Makaton signs are also available in the form of symbol boards, which can be operated electronically for children with limited hand control.

For children with a cognitive age of 5 years plus, who are beginning to learn simple reading and spelling, some form of electronic typing is a more advanced form of expression for those with limited speech and hand control; a wide range of computer-based communication aids is available in many places. Keyboards can be in expanded forms or activated by foot controls, vocalizations or even eye movements. Output can be on a video screen, on paper or through a voice synthesizer. Professional advice and proper training in the use of such equipment are important; given this, such communication aids can be of great value. In our experience, they do not interfere with children's efforts to develop their own more natural ways of communicating.

Educational groups

Education, in the broadest sense, begins at home with the family. The family can benefit from professional expertise, but nothing can substitute for their unconditional love and care during the early impressionable years.

Playgroups and schools provide the child with wider horizons, new challenges and stimulation, learning to become accustomed to other adults and children outside the family nest, and to cope with new demands.

The majority of children with CP can benefit by early admission, a few hours each week initially, to an ordinary neighbourhood playgroup or nursery, provided that the staff are alerted well in advance, through the parents and their professional advisers, of the child's special needs, such as in feeding, toileting, seating, communication and mobility arrangements.

Some parents will find that these arrangements are not as complete as they would wish. This is partly because the playgroup staff's time and energy has to be shared among several children. This sharing and turn-taking is an important part of the group's purpose in helping the child to mature socially. Regular contact between staff and parents helps to resolve these issues.

Much depends on the degree of disability. Children with more severe physical communication and learning difficulties may need 'special' rather than ordinary nursery groups; these have the advantage of providing a wider range of teaching, therapy and care facilities 'under one roof'.

More formal education at school from around age 5 years is the rule in England, for which assessment teams of psychologists, doctors, therapists and educationalists provide professional advice on educational facilities, ranging from mainstream schooling with various degrees of extra help, special units attached to ordinary schools, to specialized schools for children with multiple disabilities.

Since parents' commitment to their child's education from birth onwards is usually very strong, their part in the assessment team's deliberations is crucial.

Playgroups and schooling

Once children are 2–3 years old they may need wider opportunities to learn and to engage in exploratory play than can be provided at home. Provision varies: in some areas, a child with visual and motor problems may attend a local nursery group where visiting specialists can advise staff and parents. The ordinary bustling nursery environment may need some adaptation, with attention being given to lighting levels, and the various hazards around. A very gradual introduction with a parent present is usually needed so that the child can get used to the noise and excitement of group activity – something which they often learn to love and look forward to as a highlight.

Although in some communities separate units have been set up for the sensory-disabled, the more recent emphasis is for pupils to be integrated into schools most appropriate to their intellectual or cognitive level. When children attend neighbourhood schools, supportive services of visiting teachers are helpful to give advice about teaching methods and any auxiliary aids to learning. Special aids can range from simple whole-page magnifying lenses to special slow-speed audio recorders and closed-circuit TV magnifiers. Audio recordings and radio programmes can also play an important part.

Formal educational provision

When considering schooling for pupils with any type of disability, the emphasis has changed in England since the Education Acts of the 1980s came into force. Before the Warnock Committee's report, children were categorized according to their disability and then allocated to schools accordingly. The emphasis is now on the assessment of the educational needs of each child who may have a disability; the local education authority along with the parents may make a formal

Statement of Special Educational Need. The aim is to provide an appropriate teaching environment that will cater for each child's particular brand of abilities and difficulties. This may be in a specialized school or unit or in the ordinary classroom, with extra support if necessary.

When planning the style of education best suited for a child in England, those professionals already involved will discuss the various alternatives with the parents and together they will work out what seems most appropriate at each stage in the child's school life. The type of schooling decided upon will, of course, depend on local circumstances, with practical matters such as distance, transport facilities and amount of awkward stairs within the school being taken into account.

Another factor that needs to be considered is the unique qualities of each child: temperament and intellectual capabilities, as well as physical difficulties. For instance, two children with more moderate CP who need to make use of a wheelchair for part of the school day might have quite different requirements. One may be an outgoing child, easily bored with his or her own company and inspired to succeed by the competition of other children; this child may thrive in an ordinary classroom with some additional support. By contrast, a child with similar physical difficulties who is hypersensitive to noise and agitated by stimulation and bustle may respond best in a small unit with a protective and encouraging atmosphere. Small specialized classes within the ordinary neighbourhood school are ideal for these sensitive and sometimes timid children; they gradually become accustomed to larger groups, joining the mainstream class on occasion for story or music sessions.

Many countries are at the planning stage of setting up special facilities for pupils with varying disabilities. It is this variety of provision that is important since it gives families a range of options. An option which is currently favoured in England is the setting-up of small units staffed by specially trained teachers, attached to mainstream schools, so that those with a disability can integrate as appropriate, making use of equipment such as computers, typewriters or science apparatus which is available for the whole school.

In this way pupils can feel part of the larger school community and not isolated in a protective environment, which perhaps does not have much contact with the wider life beyond school.

Emotional factors

I have concentrated in the first part of this chapter on considering how children learn, including learning in children with sensory and perceptual problems. I have stressed how much children's development involves their curiosity about the world and their eagerness to master new tasks; this means that children should have learned a great deal before reaching school age. When their striving to explore and gain some mastery of the environment is held up by physical incapacity, then it is understandable that the child should seek other means of exercising some control and the child may focus instead on controlling the parents and carers!

Being denied the opportunity to satisfy the wish to investigate the surroundings by opening every cupboard, as a toddler loves to do, the young child with CP is particularly prone to boredom.

Relative immobility may mean that the child comes to rely on the parents and brothers and sisters being close at hand to provide entertainment, to make up for the limited range of things that the child can do independently. In the early months, especially if premature and delicate, the mother may carry the child around in a sling most of the time. It does sometimes happen that the child wants this to continue for 24 hours a day, so that the mother's own needs to have a bath, to wash her hair or to get dressed are resented by the child, and a screaming bout may ensue. This is clearly upsetting for all the family, often leading to a build-up of irritation as well as exhaustion.

Even the most patient parents experience resentment mixed in with love at the seemingly overwhelming demands of a young child. These feelings are often exaggerated when a child is slow to develop, partly because such children cannot easily occupy themselves, and partly because of the family's understandable mixture of emotions of sadness, protectiveness and uncertainty as to how to act for the best.

Sharing the care

The situation of the child becoming very dependent on the mother's presence is even more likely to occur in a single-parent family or where the mother is on her own for much of the day. In this case it may be helpful to seek suggestions and support about sharing the child's care from professional people such as a social worker, health visitor or physiotherapist. Friends or members of neighbourhood groups often want to be helpful, but may be hesitant if they doubt their capacity to cope with a child who seems vulnerable.

You may need to pluck up courage and ask for support. When you do, you will find that people are eager to help once you explain the situation.

You will also need to build up their confidence by demonstrating the best ways of undertaking care routines. Begin with brief periods away from your child – otherwise you may become anxious – at first, perhaps, only for as long as it takes to write an important letter, or to make a phone call. Once you and your helper are confident that your child is in good hands, then longer outings can be attempted.

These brief respites give you a chance to consider your own needs and recharge your emotional batteries. Sharing the caring with relatives, friends and voluntary as well as professional helpers very often brings great benefit to the child as well as to the parents. Children need some changes of routine too!

Chapter **Eight**

8

Emotional health

Cathy Laver-Bradbury

From the moment of conception a mother and child are forming a relationship. Living together for 9 months gives the child a chance to experience the emotions of the mother first-hand, albeit with little understanding. It is the start of the relationship. Pregnancies vary depending on many factors. These can include whether the timing of the birth is right and whether the father is supportive and available. Financial pressures affect couples just starting up with a new home. How will they manage with a child? Does the mother go back to work? Who will look after the child? Who do they trust to do so? Are both parents in agreement about these questions?

As the mother feels the child move and kick or sees it on the ultrasound, so the child becomes more of a person, someone to worry about. Routine antenatal care tests influence the parents as they make choices about where and sometimes when the child will be born, who will be present at the birth, who will they call on to help and who they will not. From the very beginning, the influences of friends, family and professionals affect the parental relationship with the child.

The relationship that forms between the father and the child is different from that of the mother. It may be no less strong but it is different. Many men find it hard to express emotions during their partner's pregnancy and find the hormonal roller-coaster hard to understand. Being present at the ultrasound and the birth helps some fathers, but for others it increases their anxieties, as the responsibility of caring for a child can feel daunting. The relationship between partners during a pregnancy can be difficult at times as partners may have different views about how the child should be raised and who should help. Good communication is essential to ensure that both parents' needs are met.

If the parents have experienced a difficult childhood themselves, they may have increased fears and worries during and after the child's birth.

It is a time when many parents say they reflect on their own experiences of childhood and their relationship with their own parents. Some such reflections can have an emotional effect on their new role as parents.

Often children born with cerebral palsy (CP) are not identified as having difficulties until they are a few months old, sometimes later. Parents have often suspected that some part of their child's development is not quite as they think it should be. Many have asked close friends and relatives if they have noticed anything or if the same things happened with their child. Often people have tried to reassure them that things will be all right. The process of accepting that you have a child requiring extra support takes time and varies between parents and relatives. Having a child with CP requires special consideration. All parenting is challenging, and all parents should challenge themselves about their parenting role. It is a crucial role in a person's life and requires much thought. Having a child with CP requires even more consideration, especially when, as a parent, you are being influenced by others and relying on professionals for guidance concerning your child's condition.

The relationship that forms with a child after it is born can take time to develop. If the birth has been difficult or the mother is experiencing physical or emotional difficulties, these may affect how 'available' she is to build a relationship with the child. Having a supportive partner or grandparent around at this time can be helpful. This ensures that the mother and the child are cared for, or at least that the housework is done, whilst the parents spend some time recovering together. If others are caring for the child, it is important that this is carried out near the parents. I add this, as sometimes when parents are under extreme distress they form a protective barrier around their emotional selves, sometimes to such an extent that the child is given to someone else to be cared for, the parents believing that the other carer can make a better job of it. This is rarely the case in reality. Having someone who is gentle but persistent, rather than actually taking over the child's care, helps parents to get back on track in caring for their own child.

All children are born with different temperaments. Some have an easier temperament; others may be more fractious and sensitive. Children with CP are no different in this respect. Children who have a sensitive temperament often find it harder to adapt to the outside world and it may take them longer to find their own body rhythms and understanding of their parents. Children who are sensitive often cry easily and get more upset than other children. They may appear more emotionally sensitive.

The development of a relationship is a two-way process between child and parent. It relies on both being receptive to each other and 'available' to learn each others' needs. This often takes time and patience. It is important to recognize if either the parent's or the child's needs are not being met at as early a stage as possible. A few small steps, such as those described below, may help form the relationship between a parent and child.

If either parent has postnatal depression it can affect the response time of the parent to the child. This is often something that parents are not aware of. Children respond to this in different ways, depending on the temperament of the child. The quiet child may be content to sit and almost to mirror the parent's response, becoming quieter and less responsive. The child with a more active temperament may try to evoke a quicker response by continually crying to force a quicker response from the parent. It is important to seek help for postnatal depression. A variety of treatments, from support groups to medication, are available.

The early days

Practical tips on forming a relationship with your child

1. Spend time together just watching each other. Choose a time when your child is relaxed. Get to know your child's movements and what they may mean.

2. Look at your child in the eyes. Some children avoid eye contact but it is important to keep trying gently. If your child avoids eye contact, follow his or her eyes with yours and try to get

your child to follow yours back. Remember to smile when doing this. This helps to encourage your child more. Do not force eye contact by holding your child's face, as this can cause distress in children with a sensitive temperament. Just gently encourage your child to look at you.

3. Recognize your child's temperament. Children's temperaments may be easy or difficult. If your child has a difficult temperament then he or she may find life a bit harder to adapt to. This means that your child may need to be introduced to new situations gently to help him or her to learn to relax and trust you.

4. Stroke your child. Choose a time when you are both relaxed. In a warm room wrap your child in a towel, unwrap one arm at a time and stroke it gently in light downward strokes. Move to the other arm and then the tummy and legs. If your child does not like being unwrapped it may be due to a sensitive temperament. So start with a foot and gently build up to exposing the whole leg or arm. Some children prefer to be swaddled. It seems to make them feel more secure. In many areas baby massage classes are offered. If there is one near you, try to attend. It is a great way of meeting other mothers and helping your child to learn to relax. Children need to find ways of relaxing, when stressed, early on. This is a good method for them to learn.

5. Recognize your own temperament. Are you shy or extroverted? What is the child's other parent like? Does this child seem to resemble you or the other parent? Children are not copies of their parents but they sometimes do display similarities. Notice these similarities and help your child to learn from you how to manage situations which they may find difficult. If you know that you are a person with an active temperament remember it may be upsetting to your child if they have a quiet temperament.

6. Talk to your child. It does not matter what you say. You can talk about washing or cleaning. Children often like hearing your voice and knowing you are nearby. Give them a chance to respond to you. Communication is a skill that is learned from earliest childhood. Parents and children can hold conversations lasting a few minutes from a very early age. Encourage this. It helps the child's development.

7. Smile at your child. Children mimic adults so if you want them to smile, try to teach them by example.

8. Play with your child; even very young children will respond to baby books and stories, rattles, cuddly toys and brightly coloured objects.

9. Try not to be too rushed. Life is often busy. If possible, slow your pace to that of your child's as often as possible.

10. Try to get into a routine. Even very young children can feel more relaxed and secure when they are in a routine which they can recognize. This does not have to be stuck to rigidly.

11. Do not be afraid to ask for help. Often friends and relatives are more than happy to lend a hand with the ironing or just watching the child while you have some time to yourself.

12. Identify other supportive parents nearby. There will be many people who say they will try to help, but most parents usually only have two or three close friends who really do help. Try to go to postnatal groups and later to toddlers' groups. Take someone with you if it helps you to form contacts.

13. Do not worry if you make a mistake. No one is perfect and no one is a perfect parent. Small children can make parents feel quite inadequate at times.

14. Notice the small changes that happen to your child as he or she develops. If you are able, keep notes of them in a diary. This does not have to be every day but at each milestone, for example when the child first smiles or reaches out to you. You may enjoy sharing these notes with your child in later years.

Crying

For some parents, hearing their child cry is very distressing. Here are some tips to help.

Crying is always difficult for parents to listen to. It can evoke reminders of distress. When young children cry it can be for a number of reasons: hunger, cold, heat, frustration, boredom or as a way of attracting your attention. Most parents find it hard to leave a child to cry. We are correctly designed to respond to our child's needs. Over time most parents learn which type of cry indicates when their child is in distress or when they are just moaning. Being responsive to your young child will provide him or her with comfort and relief. As children grow, parents learn to comfort their children in other ways.

Parents should value each other's skills with the child. This is usually a difficult time when parents may lack confidence. Make sure you build each other's confidence, especially if one parent is with the child more and appears to understand the child's needs more quickly. Each of you will have different skills to help the child. Support each other in these skills.

Take it in turns to respond to distress. Handling a child who cries is very draining. Recognize your limitations and when to ask for help. Children can often sense when an adult is stressed and they can then react by becoming even more distressed. If you recognize that you are stressed, find someone to take over for a while. If no one is available, put the child in a safe place in a cot or a pram. It is better to leave the child to cry for a little while whilst you calm down than to risk hurting him or her.

Some children with special needs cry more, especially if the muscles of their body are affected. For example, some children may present with colic which may be linked to the intestinal muscles being affected. When the child eats it seems to elicit particularly bad colic. If you are worried that this may be the case, seek medical advice. This can happen whether your child is breast- or bottle-fed.

Hold your child close to you. Sensitive children often respond to being held close or carried around when in distress.

Sing or listen to music together with your child. Children respond to many types of music but beware of upbeat music which can act as a stimulant, so it is best not used if trying to get the child to sleep.

The toddler years

These years can be both a magical and a demanding time for parents, watching as their child's personality develops. Toddlers can be both engaging and naughty, often at the same time.

Toddlers with CP can face additional problems, depending on the degree of their physical difficulties and the way in which their understanding is developing.

Being aware of your child's developmental age as opposed to their chronological age is important in helping to structure tasks to help them in their early experience of playing. Some children may need extra help with playing, which is a crucial skill in development. Those children with developmental delay may need more time learning the skills involved in dexterity (using their hands), in coordination (using their movements efficiently), in communication (verbal or non-verbal) and in social skills. These skills are all learned and practised throughout childhood but the toddler years are important for their progression. Toddlers are learning at a very fast rate. They want to be independent without having the skills to ensure they are acting safely. Hence it can be a very tiring time for parents.

Most parents find the challenge of temper tantrums the most difficult in the toddler years. Here are some tips to help:

1. Understand that tantrums are very common in this age group. It is not just your child. Most temper tantrums are normal.

2. Keep calm. It is better if just one of you is having a tantrum.

3. Ensure that the child is safe if throwing him- or herself on the floor, screaming or hitting out. Tantrums can be amazing to watch (though mostly when it's not your child having one).

4. Distract where possible. In the early stages of a tantrum children will often respond to a calm spontaneous distraction, for example, 'Look over there, I can see a duck'. It is better for the distraction not to involve the child. For example, it is probably best not to say 'Everyone is watching you', as this can make the tantrum worse.

5. If the tantrum is happening in a safe place then ignoring it can work well. Toddlers often like to have an audience that reacts to the tantrum. If you ignore it and say little, the tantrum often lasts for a shorter length of time.

6. If your child is very sensitive, try holding him or her (if not kicking out too much). This can calm a sensitive child and help to make him or her feel more secure.

7. If you feel that things are worsening, then 'time out' can help. The purpose of 'time out' is to provide you and your child with a breathing space to calm down. It is not a punishment but a space to think and be calm. 'Time out' involves removing the child to a safe place such as the bottom of the stairs or bedroom. Most 'time out' is short. One minute for each year of the child's age is a good guide. The difficulty can be that the child calms down quite quickly but it can take an adult up to half an hour to feel calm again. This means that things can quickly escalate a second time if you are not careful and do not appreciate how long it takes you to calm down. It is important that once the tantrum is over both you and your child start afresh.

8. 'Time out' for some children is very difficult. They may react intensely to being separated from you by destroying toys or ripping wallpaper off walls. If your child reacts in this way it is better to have a 'calm down' time. This can be achieved by having a small carpet square or mat on which the child has to sit quietly when needing to calm down. Parents can sit with the child during this time reading a book or telling a story but the child has to sit quietly. The useful thing about this 'special mat' is that it can be transported to granny's or elsewhere if necessary.

9. Don't try to reason with your child once he or she is in a temper. Children are the same as adults in this way. Remember when you last lost your temper. Were you able to reason with anyone? It is unlikely.

10. Discussions involving what happened are best done after everyone is calm.

11. Try to pre-empt situations that are likely to be difficult by breaking down the tasks. For example, if you know your child is likely to have to wait, break the waiting time down into tasks. Simple games of matching colours, 'I spy', colouring and silly stories can help.

12. Anxious children will often go into a tantrum as a way of expressing their anxiety. If your child is naturally anxious, look out for this. The child needs to learn other ways of expressing anxiety.

13. If you have said 'no' to something and your child says he or she hates you, do not worry. Just reply: 'I think you are angry with me for saying no but you cannot have this today'. Children will often say they hate you when they cannot have their own way. It is important not to react intensely to this. They are learning to express their feelings. They just need to learn the right feeling to describe. Name the feeling to your child if you can. Most children will learn happy and sad quite quickly. Anger, jealousy, boredom, anxiety and frustration take longer to understand and express.

14. It is important to stick to something that you have decided and not to be persuaded to change your mind if your child goes into a tantrum. However you can change your mind if you think you are being unreasonable. This must be done showing that you are in control by saying something such as 'As you have been such a help to me by picking up your toys [providing the child has] I have decided you can have…'. This way your child knows that you are in charge and for what the reward is being given.

Preparing for playschool and school

Attending playschool and, later, main school are big changes for any child. Stepping out from the security of their own home can be frightening, even with supportive parents present who know them well, and therefore this is a very important stage for a child.

In England children who have special needs are likely to be offered places at nursery schools at a fairly early age. Often areas have home workers who visit to offer their support to parents from the time when their children are very young up until school age. This support often focuses on physical development and communication and can help the parent and child, especially if the child is a first child and the parents have little experience of rearing children, and thus do not know the ages at which children usually reach developmental milestones. Home workers are also a good resource for gaining information that will help to support your child throughout the school years. Often organized by Educational Services, they recognize that children with special needs may require extra support when starting school and identify the ways it may be provided.

Preparation and communication are the keys to successful transition into school. Different children require different approaches. This is again when the parents' knowledge of their child's temperament should guide them in knowing how much and how often they should be away from their child when the child starts nursery or school, or whether it is better for them to stay with their child at first until the child is settled before leaving at all.

Here are some hints or tips about preparing your child for playschool or starting school.

1. Make several trips to the location before the actual starting date so the child knows where he or she will be. If possible, stay for increasing amounts of time to familiarize you and your child with the activities that he or she is likely to do.

2. Identify a worker whom you like, and whom you think your child may like and encourage a relationship between them. Most helpers like to work with parents in helping the child. If your child has difficulty in communicating, let the helpers know how you manage. If language is a difficulty, picture charts often help as children can point to the things they want. The adults involved in their care can also do this and this helps them both understand what happens and when.

3. Establish a routine. Sometimes pictures help. Make a chart that has a picture of the playschool, a snack, a lunch bag and the uniform, if one is used. This may help to familiarize your child with a routine of going to playschool. Weekly charts sometimes help, listing the days of the week and the activities that occur on particular days.

4. If your child appears distressed when you leave, try not to get upset yourself. This is a difficult time. The child is making the first steps towards being independent of you. However if this distress does not settle, be prepared to spend longer preparing the child for leaving you. If your child spends the whole session distressed, he or she is probably not emotionally ready to leave you yet. Think about whether to delay starting nursery, or to spend more time with your child, gradually leaving him or her for increasing amounts of time.

5. Tell your child if you are leaving. Many parents think it is better to sneak off without telling the

child so as not to distress him or her, but often this leads to the child becoming anxious as he or she never knows when mum or dad is likely to disappear and so the child often becomes more clingy. It is better to say: 'Mummy is going to go shopping now and I will be back at … Have fun', and leave quickly. You can always peep in after 10 minutes to check your child has calmed down and is joining in.

Encouraging independence and helping your child to learn

Sometimes when caring for a child with CP, parents feel they are not able to let go of the child just in case someone does not understand what their child needs. It is always hard letting go of your child, but as parents, our role is to prepare children to be independent of us. We have their whole childhood to help them prepare for this, but it takes time – years. Children with special needs are no exception to this. Even if the likelihood is that they will always need help, it may be that this will be in a residential setting, or in assisted-living accommodation. Alternatively they may remain in your care at home. However, the most important thing is for them and for you to have a choice if possible. By preparing them as best you can and allowing them to try certain situations you are helping them with this. So these early situations help in preparation for this later choice.

Do not stop trying new things even if your child does not manage a new task or situation well. Try to find ways of breaking the task down into smaller stages and bit by bit gain the skills to manage the whole task.

Acknowledge your child's strengths and limitations; encouragement helps with both. Strengths help to build self-esteem and confidence; if you are faced with a limitation, try to understand it realistically and find ways around it, if possible. Sometimes supporting the child emotionally whilst he or she comes to understand the disability is crucial.

Seek support for yourselves as parents. If possible, help out on the parent–teachers association or become a governor involved with the school.

All this can help you continue to support your child and others.

Remember to smile when you pick your child up from school. Look forward to seeing your child and hearing about his or her day. Not all children will tell you about their day as soon as they come out from school, but may do so later in the evening. If you ask what pictures they drew or look at what they have brought home you may learn more. Keeping in touch with what they are doing allows you to ask if they have learned (such and such) yet. Remember to praise your child, however small the achievement. This really builds self-esteem. Even if you think something should be better, children try harder with praise than criticism.

Praise, praise and more praise. Children thrive on praise and encouragement. Let your child over-hear you tell somebody else how good he or she has been and what he or she has achieved; it is an excellent way to boost confidence.

Help your child to learn by including him or her in everyday tasks. It is important that your child learns from you. Take into account his or her development and give tasks your child can achieve easily at first to build up confidence. Then grad-ually introduce more difficult tasks. Do not step in too early to help. Let your child try different things independently and if you do have to help, keep it to a minimum. There is nothing more rewarding than achieving things yourself.

Supporting children emotionally through diffi-cult times can be hard to do. Children with CP can be subjected to bullying and teasing, which upsets them. Helping your child to develop a 'protective emotional overcoat' can help. Doing this often requires listening to your child's distress and then helping to find ways of dealing with it. It is tempting to fight your child's battles and some-times it is necessary. Knowing when to step in is always difficult. If physical abuse is taking place than parental intervention is necessary. If it is occasional teasing or name-calling it may be that your child will learn to ignore it or laugh it off. This does not make light of it and your child will need parents to offload to. But it may also give your child a sense of achievement when his or her own actions cause it to stop. All this can be very upsetting for parents. Listening and seeing your child upset is emotionally painful. It is also often difficult to put on a brave face while listening but it is helpful for the child if the parents are helping to solve problems rather than resorting to anger or crying. However parents can say how they feel. This is helpful for their children in acknowledging their own distress.

Children fall in and out of friendships regu-larly. They can hate someone one week and be best friends the next. Help them to see that friendships can be like this and, if they have a falling out, try not to let it involve other friends within the friendship group. This helps to stop children being isolated when they have upsets as other group members learn to help them make up rather than take sides in an argument.

Play

Play is crucial to all children It may seem all too simple but play is a really good way of helping your child. Children often rush through play and as a result do not learn how to play well. Play is very important to children as it helps them learn about many aspects of life – how to interact with other people and so to improve their social skills. Play can take many forms, from imaginative play to educational play. It is important that children have the opportunity to benefit from as many types of play as possible. Listed below are some hints and tips on how to encourage your child's play and in turn to improve their concentration.

1. Helping your child learn to play may really help your child. He or she may learn how to get on with friends. Try to help your child learn to play for longer periods by using language to expand your child's ideas. Describing what your child is doing often helps prolong play and adds to enjoyment.

2. Pace the play to your child's developmental level. Children develop at different rates. Find a toy that your child can play with easily and then build on to this by adding things that gently challenge the child.

3. Follow your child's lead. Let your child choose what he or she wants to play.

4. Do not compete (you are an adult who has learned the skill: your child is not).

5. Engage in role play and make believe with your child.

6. Laugh and have fun.

7. Reward quiet play with your attention.

8. Praise and encourage your child's ideas and creativity. Do not criticize.

9. Do not give too much help. Encourage your child's problem solving.

10. Tell your child when you have enjoyed time with him or her.

Remember: 10 minutes a day will help your child learn through play!

Behavioural problems

If your child is displaying behavioural problems it may seem strange to concentrate on play. However we have learned from research and from other parents that children with behavioural difficulties often miss out on learning how to play and therefore how to communicate their emotional needs. Children learn to communicate through play. It is a way that they can learn to express their difficulties or act them out in play rather than in the supermarket. When playing with your child it is very important that your child controls the play and not you. Many parents get carried away with 'playing properly'. When playing, the idea is that your child controls what you do, so it does not matter if the drawing is not perfect or the furniture in the doll's house is upside down. This is your child learning. By shifting the balance of control from you as a parent to the child, the child gets to know that their ideas are good and worthwhile. Playing is a situation where it is safe for the child to control the parent. If children lead in play they do not need to try to lead or control in other situations.

If you have tried most of the above and things still remain difficult, it may be helpful to seek advice. It is not always easy to know when is the right time to involve someone else. Below are some pointers.

When to seek help

It is always difficult to know when to seek help. The following is a guide, but the most important consideration is whether you feel either you or your child need help.

1. If a behaviour is impairing either your or your child's quality of life.

2. If you consider your child is likely to self-harm or harm others, for example, if your child is sad or expressing thoughts of self-harm or suicide. Often young children say they want to die. If this is a reaction to being told off, check it out with them 'Is it because you have been told off?' If they say 'yes' it is probably an anger reaction. If, however, your child is sad and says, 'I wish I was dead and I am going to jump off the wall and kill myself', you need to explore this further and to seek help.

3. If your child is upset and cries more than usual and for longer than usual.

4. If your child appears not to be making progress at school.

5. When you are worried about your child's behaviour.

6. When others are expressing concern regarding your child's behaviour.

7. When you know that life events are having a detrimental effect on your relationship with your child.

8. When you know that your own mental health is having a detrimental effect on your child.

9. If the behaviour problem is persisting despite having tried different things to help.

Asking for help can be difficult for many parents. We are often told by parents they feel they have failed by having to ask for help. Remember that it could be argued that the opposite is true, and that by asking for help parents recognize when things are not progressing as they should be.

It can be difficult finding out what kind of help you feel would be a benefit to you and your child. When seeking help it is worth clarifying with the person you see what ranges of treatment options are available within that professional's service. The person you first see may not be the person who will be the most helpful, but he or she could act as a signpost to help you access the help you or your child need.

Be honest with the person you work with. If you disagree with something the professional says, tell him or her and say why you feel you will not be able to use this advice. In practice professionals often have a range of strategies they can discuss and only by being told can they work out with you those which might help.

If you do not feel you can relate to the person you are seeing, ask to see someone else. We cannot all get along with everyone. It is better to ask to see someone else than to stop going because you do not relate to the person you are seeing. If you feel that you cannot ask, then see if someone else will do this for you. Relatives and friends are often happy to do this and on occasion general practitioners will write to support a change.

If you really do not feel you are making progress, ask for a second opinion. Some services will offer this if they feel things are not improving as they should be. Sometimes the professionals themselves ask to bring in other professionals to review the situation. Two heads can often be better than one and a fresh look at a difficulty can bring in new ideas.

Be prepared for some hard work. Changing a difficult behaviour is hard for the parent and the child. Changes rarely happen overnight. Stick with strategies even if they do not appear to be working at first. Sometimes it is 'hanging in there' that eventually works.

There is nothing more frustrating for parents than being offered advice when you just want someone to listen. If you want to get something off your chest or talk about your worries, tell the person you are seeing that you need him or her to listen today and not offer any advice. Then the professional knows what you need from the session. This can save a lot of frustration on both sides.

Preschool attention deficit hyperactivity disorder (PS-ADHD)

This can be called hyperactivity, attention deficit hyperactivity disorder (ADHD) or overactivity.

Many children will have symptoms of ADHD in the preschool years and a number of children with PS-ADHD will require help with the disorder.

PS-ADHD emerges early in children, often from birth, runs in families and children have a variety of symptoms. These include having lots of energy and constantly being on the go. They may have a poor sleeping and/or eating pattern. They are easily distracted, hate waiting, get bored easily, have difficulty taking turns and have short-term memory problems.

Children with CP are not excluded from PS-ADHD. In fact, a number of the disorders of childhood have the symptoms of this disorder. As a parent, it is important to recognize the symptoms and seek help. Particular behavioural strategies are very effective in the preschool years in helping children with PS-ADHD and the earlier the parents and children are helped, the better. However, parents need to understand the underlying effects of the disorder to be able to target the behaviours needing intervention in their child.

Here are some of the strategies to help the child with PS-ADHD:

1. Remember it is not your fault or your child's fault that he or she has PS-ADHD.

2. Active children receive approximately nine times more criticism than children who are not active. Try to reverse this. Praise little and often for all small tasks achieved, for example pulling on shoes or socks. These children respond well to praise.

3. Only give short messages, not more than a sentence. The child will not remember any more.

4. Get eye contact by gently holding the child's face. Do this initially when praising the child. When your child is used to looking at you, start to give instructions this way.

5. Break any waiting time down into manageable chunks and reward each waiting time.

6. Distract temper outbursts. Do not make threats you cannot keep and keep any punishments short, repeatable and realistic.

7. Help your child to problem-solve. If you have told your child off, it is important that he or she learns what to do to stop being in trouble.

8. Try to help your child learn to relax. Massage and quiet times are good ways of learning this.

9. Practise difficult situations in small stages, for example if the weekly shop with the child is a nightmare, try not to take your child. Make time to go shopping together for a short time using a list of items that the child can collect independently, even if in a wheelchair – preferably tins or something unbreakable.

The aim of this chapter is to provide an insight into children's and their parents' emotional health, detailing how they are interlinked during the child's development, acknowledging some of the factors that affect this and suggesting when to seek help if needed.

This is an introduction. There are many articles and websites dedicated to helping children and parents. I have listed a few below.

Further reading

Barnes J, Freude-Lagevardi A. From pregnancy to early childhood: early interventions to enhance the mental health of children and families. Mental Health Foundation, UCL, London, 2002.

Cooper H, Thompson M. Parenting packages: child and adolescent mental health: theory and practice. Hodder Arnold, London, 2005.

Polke L, Thompson M. The crying child. Southampton University Hospitals Community Unit, Southampton, 1994.

Polke L, Thompson M. Temper tantrums. Southampton University Hospitals Community Unit, Southampton, 1994.

Polke L, Thompson M. Overactive children. Southampton University Hospitals Community Unit, Southampton, 1994.

Sonuga-Barke EJS, Daley D, Thompson M et al. Parent based therapies for pre-school attention-deficit hyperactivity disorder: a randomised controlled trial with a community sample. Am Acad Child Adolesc Psychiatry 2001; 40:402–408.

Thompson M, Laver-Bradbury C, Weeks A. The new forest parenting package for preschool ADHD children (updated version). Southampton City Primary Care Trust, 2007.

Thompson M, Laver-Bradbury C, Weeks C. On the go: the hyperactive child – a DVD for parents and professionals. University of Southampton Media Services, Southampton, 2008.

Useful websites

Mental Health Foundation: http://www.mentalhealth.org.uk.

Royal College of Psychiatrists: http://www.rcpsych.ac.uk.

Young Minds: http://www.youngminds.org.uk.

Chapter Nine

Parents' contribution to early learning – developing a dialogue using touch, sight, hearing and communication

9

Revised by Eva Bower

It is universally recognized that parents have an important role as educators of their child, especially during the early formative years. In this chapter we will look at the ways in which a child learns during the early months, with particular reference to the part that the mother plays in this early learning process while she tends to the child's needs throughout the day. This is a time in which a partnership grows between mother and child, providing both with an opportunity to share and learn together, each guiding and modifying the development of the other.

A dialogue develops very early on between a mother and her child while she feeds, baths, changes nappies, dresses, undresses and carries her child. As she holds and moves her child she automatically gives visual, tactile and auditory clues. Later, in everyday routine situations, she will encourage her child to develop functional and communication skills, all of which will be based on this fabric of early learning, with part of one

skill being integrated with another until a more complex task is achieved.

Naturally she is not alone in this task for, although a father's interaction is different from a mother's, and that of siblings and other family members, each in his or her own way provides opportunities and encouragement for learning. It is through continuous and progressive interaction with parents and various other members of the family, in secure and familiar surroundings, that a child learns and grows, experimenting and practising new abilities and skills while at the same time maturing both emotionally and socially.

Clearly the child with cerebral palsy (CP) is just as dependent on this early learning/inter-action, but the movement disorder and abnormal responses may interfere with the natural process, creating barriers to learning basic skills. It is also possible that sometimes the apparent emphasis on the movement aspects of development may mask or detract from the importance of other aspects of early learning.

In the following paragraphs I have outlined how a mother typically interacts with her child and in later chapters how this may be integrated with techniques in the total management of the child with CP.

It is generally accepted that all children at birth share common characteristics on which future personality and attainment will be based. That is, while every child is born with the capacity to learn, the rate of development is influenced to a certain extent by personality. Some children are vigorous and active, others placid and slow, all progressing at their own pace, with considerable variation in motivation and drive.

The child with CP, although sharing these same common characteristics, will possibly lack the spontaneous behaviour and ability necessary to interact as positively with the mother and the environment. The mother therefore will need to be aware of how much holding and moving her child can tolerate, and, guided by visual signals, facial expression and body movements, balance more carefully the intensity of her input. In this way she, too, will be able to build up a social ritual with her child.

The child with CP is also born with the same ability to learn and interact with his or her mother during routine situations as any other child, but the pace of progress and the future potential will depend upon the severity of the disability, including any associated problems that may be present. The child will need help for a longer period of time in organizing movements, and any sensory input will have to be timed and graded more carefully, while reactions are carefully monitored.

After a few weeks of repeating the same procedures day after day, every mother develops a routine and methods of holding and moving her child. These will be those that she feels most comfortable with and which meet the needs of her child.

As so much of a child's learning is dependent upon the early interaction and dialogue that exist between the child and the mother as she sees to daily needs, it follows logically that any treatment/management programme for the child with CP should be incorporated into this daily routine. Working in this way has advantages for both mother and child, giving the mother the opportunity to combine specific techniques of holding and moving her child with her own mothering skills. The child, when held and moved, becomes aware of the body parts when feeling pressure through the skin, muscles and joints in different positions, later learning to self-orient in space. As this sensory input is vital if the child is to progress smoothly from gross activities to fine motor skills, it may be helpful to look briefly at a mother's

role in providing sensory input during the early months. For the sake of clarity I have separated discussion of the different sensory inputs from the development of the motor system. It should be emphasized, however, that in function the sensory motor systems are inseparably linked. That is, interacting one with the other, they enable the child, if able, to become mobile against gravity and finally to attain an upright position and use the hands for functional activities.

How does a child learn?

A child learns by: (1) touching; (2) looking; and (3) listening and communicating.

Touching

The tactile system is one of the most mature systems the child has at birth, providing the child with a means of early communication with the mother, when experiencing the feeling of body weight against the mother during her support. To begin with, most of a child's reactions to sensory stimulation will be reflex in nature, some elicited automatically by the mother as she holds and moves the child. If, for example, she touches the side or middle of the lips, the child moves towards the part that is stimulated; in this way the child roots to find the nipple (rooting reflex). If a finger is placed in the mouth the child sucks automatically (sucking reflex). If one strokes, or puts a finger in the palm of the child's hand, the feeling of touch and pressure will cause the child immediately to close the fingers around it (hand grasp).

All children vary in the type of tactile stimulation they enjoy. For example, some like the pressures and warmth of being cuddled and rocked, whereas others prefer the sensation of being gently stroked, a preference a mother recognizes early on, and so we see the beginnings of early social interaction emerging. When a child has sufficient voluntary control actively to put the thumb or fingers into the mouth, for the first time the child has a means of self-comfort as and when the child pleases. The child can suck the thumb or fingers to self-console when tired, unhappy or bored or, when happy and contented, to enjoy the sensory experience it gives.

If the child is able to maintain the head in alignment with the body and has developed sufficient trunk and shoulder girdle stability, the child is able to bring the arms forward off the support, and through tactile stimulation explore and become familiar with various parts of the body.

At first, the child enjoys the tactile experience of clasping and unclasping the hands, pressing the palms together, moving the fingers and wrists, then putting the fingers back into the mouth to suck, although at this stage with hardly any visual attention. Gradually, as the child becomes more competent visually, the child will start to look at the hands while moving them, initially holding them immediately in front of the face, then moving them away and watching the movement of the fingers before sucking them once again. Although unable to reach and grasp a rattle, if one is put into the hand the child is able to hold it, taking it immediately to the mouth to explore with the lips and tongue. The tactile stimulation of mouthing the rattle provides the child with information regarding its texture and taste and at the same time gives the child an opportunity to exercise the musculature of the oral area, developing patterns of movement that may be used later for eating and speech.

A child also enjoys the sensation of rubbing one foot against the other and against various surfaces, and crossing and uncrossing the ankles, often rubbing one foot against the shin of the other leg, which serves a useful purpose, that of desensitizing the soles of the feet.

So we can see that, although a child's control over voluntary movements is at this stage minimal, the child is still able to build up an awareness of the body parts through the sensory experiences of touch and visual clues. As the child gains more voluntary control and becomes more proficient at using the hands, further exploration will be possible. The child becomes aware of how parts of the body relate to one another, and the relationship of self in space and to surrounding objects. This eventually helps the child to understand 'what is me' and 'what is not me'.

Looking

From the child's birth a mother gradually enters her child's visual world, providing them both with an ideal opportunity to interact one with the other. Visual contact occurs at a distance of around 18–21 cm (7–8 inches) during these early weeks. The child's most frequent visual contact with the mother at this time takes place during feeds, when from time to time the child will pause between bursts of sucking and gaze at her intently, attracted by the variations of light and shade, her hair and facial outline, and in time being able to focus on other distinguishing features.

It takes time for a child's eyes to develop physically; the first eye movements occur in response to changes in the position, as the mother sees to daily needs. At first the eye movements lag behind those of the head, but in quite a short time they will adjust to both head and body movements, following the direction of the movement. The combination of touch, change in position and the visual cues the child receives provide sensory information about any changes in position that takes place.

During the early weeks, when placed on the back a child often lies with the head turned to the side, the arms in a 'fencing' position, which is a position imposed by one of the primitive reactions, a posture that from time to time brings the child's hand into the field of vision.

As the head becomes steadier, the child begins to fixate on a stationary object and it has been shown that at this time the child responds more readily to black and white, and shades of dark and light, rather than colour, and to simple designs rather than complex ones. When the child first starts to scan this is done by moving the head and the eyes together, the eyes moving in rather a jerky manner, at first horizontally then vertically, as the child selects what holds the attention. Finally the visual organization is such that the child is able to track a moving object. As the eye sensitivity increases and the child starts to accommodate to distance, the child becomes competent at picking out details of people and objects at a distance. It is known that children reach out with their eyes long before they have the ability to reach out with their hands to grasp, so the choice of cot toys is important.

When a child first starts to smile, a new and exciting dialogue develops between mother and child, through turn-taking. Fascinated by the mother's face, the child at this stage, rather than looking at one feature as done previously, will look up and down repeatedly from her hairline to her smiling mouth, her eyes and chin.

As the mother speaks to her child, the child responds by smiling, cooing, shouting and wriggling, at first moving the hands and fingers, later with 'signalling' movements of the arms which take on a repetitive pattern in a rhythm of bursts and pauses. It has been shown that during this time of prespeech and vocalization, not only are there movements of the head and whole body but there are also more complex movements of the fingers, which include pointing of the index finger. This type of behaviour is in contrast to the stillness of the posture and the seriousness of the expression when looking at a stationary object. With the development of head control the child now has the ability to avert the gaze at will, and so becomes an active partner in this social play. This non-verbal communication forms the basis of an important two-way relationship between mother and child.

As the link between auditory and visual stimuli develops the child will begin to recognize that voices and faces go together, that father and mother look and sound different and that both differ from strangers. The dialogue with adults will rapidly grow and change in character, as we will see when discussing the beginnings of communication, below.

Listening and communicating

Following studies of the various ways in which a child reacts to sound from an early age, it has been established that the child is able to distinguish between the sounds heard. While the child will remain calm and still when spoken to softly in short repetitive sentences, changes in levels of sound and very high or low sounds will startle and may make the child cry. Continuous gentle sounds or singing, on the other hand, may be found comforting.

At first, the child enjoys repeating the sounds made and begins to imitate the sounds of the mother and other adults. The child then learns how both to start and end a 'conversation' at will, by remaining still and silent or by just looking away, perhaps reminding us that the art of communication is also to be a good listener. These early 'conversations' normally start as a result of the child's spontaneous behaviour, with the mother's coming in to support and elaborate the responses and then waiting for the child to resume. In this way a rhythm of turn-taking takes place, the child now having a means of being an active participant in the dialogue, and by the response it is clear that at this stage the child's preference is for the mother to imitate the sounds the child makes. A favourite pastime now is copying and 'blowing raspberries', at which the child soon becomes adept, using it as a ploy to attract attention.

Although joining in and interacting well with the mother at this time, the child will not necessarily be looking at her while she is speaking. It will be at around 2 years of age when visual and vocal activities become well coordinated.

As the child develops sufficient inhibition to remain still and pay attention, and has an understanding of what comes next, anticipatory games such as 'round and round the garden', 'this little piggy goes to market' and 'pop goes the weasel' become favourites. The child enjoys the sound and rhythm of these songs, responding by smiling, gurgling and shouting, and later clapping the hands, encouraging us to repeat the game.

In the beginning the dialogue between a mother and her child will obviously be one-sided, her conversation directed at the child, often interpreting how the child may feel in different situations. For example, expecting the child to anticipate what is going to happen as she prepares the bottle: 'You know what is going to happen next?' Wanting bath time to be a happy experience, she will say, 'This is fun, now is the time to kick and splash'. Well aware that the child is going to scream when she cleans the ears, she says, 'You don't like this bit'. A few months later her response to the same situation has changed to: 'It wasn't so awful, was it?' As soon as she is free of the responsibility of moving her child from one position to another and no longer has to give support when the child sits, she directs the child's behaviour using verbal control, urging cooperation, at first by gesture and speech and later by speech alone. For example, 'Lift up your arms so I can take your sweater off', 'Push your foot into your shoe', 'Hold on tight and you won't fall', 'Let go of the flannel so I can wash your face', 'Sit still while I zip up your jacket'.

I have emphasized the importance of early communication, as not only does it play an important role in the child's social development, but speech is also an important tool for organizing and reinforcing movement, often used by a child later when learning new skills. When a child has CP, this is an area that can so easily be ignored during the early years, either because we feel that the child does not understand and we become frustrated because progress is so slow, or we feel that we must concentrate all our efforts on helping the child to move. However, as stated above, speech is a very useful tool in learning motor tasks.

If a child with CP does not have the opportunity to listen to speech and be spoken to throughout the day, how is the child ever going to learn to imitate speech and expand the language experiences? Different facets of language and communications skills should not be in addition to, but part of any child's treatment/management programme introduced throughout the day and in various situations. Your speech and language therapist will of course advise you on the basic skills necessary at the different stages in your child's development, and in the event that your child has a particular problem with speech, feeding or language development, will provide specific advice and treatment.

In this chapter I have tried to illustrate how the naturally occurring sensory inputs of touching, looking and listening are used by the child as building blocks in the development of gross and fine motor skills, each of these interlocking with the other and with the development of the motor system so that the child continually expands the sphere of competence as able. I have also tried to help parents to make the most of each opportunity as it is presented throughout each and every day.

In other chapters on dressing, bathing and all the other routine repetitive activities of daily life, this theme is repeated and specific ways of modifying holding and moving to help the child with CP make the most of this learning experience are described.

Chapter Ten

Understanding movement, both typical and in the child with cerebral palsy

Revised by Eva Bower

This chapter is intended to help the reader understand how we move and the difficulties experienced by a child with cerebral palsy (CP). In order to reach this understanding it is helpful to know how we develop from being relatively defenceless creatures at birth with movements characterized as spontaneous and random, sometimes interfered with by involuntary reflex activity, to adults capable of performing complex, voluntary and purposeful tasks.

In order to help the child with CP to reach a more useful level in functional activities, we may try to modify and modulate the child's abnormalities by holding and moving the child in ways that may make it easier for both the child and the carer to undertake routine functional activities. These ways are described in Chapter 11. The information provided in this chapter is intended as a background to understanding the difficulties children with CP experience in maintaining postural control against gravity in different positions and how this varies according to the distribution and type of abnormal postural tone present and the position the child is in, all of which may interfere with the child's ability to move into and out of different positions.

Movement

If we are to understand changing problems in the physical development of the child with CP it is helpful if we first know something of the physical development of the typical child. If we observe and understand how we move it may make it easier to assess why the child with CP moves in a particular way and what is interfering with the child's movements.

Our muscles work in groups and the brain responds to our intention by making groups of muscles work to achieve a required posture or movement. As adults we never consciously think which component of a movement is going to occur first or which muscles do the work. The highly complex centres in our brain are constantly working to coordinate the vast amount of information arriving by sensory pathways that provide information on, amongst other things, where we are in space, the position of our limbs and trunk and the state of readiness of our muscles. Our eyes and ears provide additional sensory information.

The centres in our brain filter the information and constantly update the control centre which in turn sends out messages (neural signals) along motor pathways to the muscles of our body to make the fine adjustments necessary to maintain a position. When we signal to our brain an intention to perform a particular activity the control centres instantaneously compute which joints need to move, in which order and sequence, and by how much, at the same time making all the other adjustments necessary to maintain our body in balance.

If you consider an activity such as drinking a cup of tea, you realize that not only are you able to pick up the cup and take it to your mouth without spilling the contents, but also as you drink and reduce the weight of the cup you are still able to move the cup in a smooth coordinated way. This achievement is in part due to the mechanisms already described, but in addition there is the muscle or force factor. The main purpose of muscles is to generate force. The extent to which the force is generated and released is again controlled by the centres in the brain.

Types of muscle activity

To complete this simple introduction to movement it is necessary to explain briefly about the different types of muscle work. Consider the everyday task of writing. Once the pen is held between your fingers and thumb, small bending (flexion) and stretching (extending) movements of your fingers enable you to form letters. These controlled but fluid movements are only possible because your wrist is extended and firm and your elbow and shoulder stable. It becomes obvious that in order for your fingers to bend, the muscles on the palm side must contract, becoming shorter than those over the back of your fingers, the extensors, which become longer. The balance is perfect and we refer to the active, shortening muscles as the agonists and those muscles that oppose a movement, in this case the extensors, as the antagonists. The muscles of the wrist, however, are working in synergy to provide stability; the flexors and extensors are co-contracting at different lengths but with equal force.

Muscles are composed of bundles of fibres with cells. During muscle activity these fibres or at least the structures within them slide on each other to effect the shortening or lengthening. The bundles of fibres are bound together and finally a sheath surrounds the whole muscle and this sheath extends to become the muscle tendon which is specialized fibrous tissue that connects muscle to skeletal bone. An example of this is the large tendon at the heel, the tendo-Achilles, which connects the big, powerful muscle of the calf (gastrocnemius) to the foot.

The underlying systems which allow us voluntarily to conceive and execute highly complex movements in a smooth, coordinated manner, all without conscious thought, are complex and precise.

The child with cerebral palsy

In the child with CP the early insult to the developing nervous system has damaged different parts of the centres and pathways described above. The exact manifestation of the lesion will depend on many factors, some of which are:

1. When the insult occurred – before, during or after birth, or the timing of the damage.

2. The size of the lesion: how big it was.

3. What type of lesion it was, for example, haemorrhagic (bleeding) or anoxic (lack of oxygen).

4. The location in the brain of the lesion or which structures were damaged.

These factors are likely to determine whether the child is described as having hemiplegia (one-sided involvement), diplegia (legs more affected than arms) or total body involvement (quadriplegia, in which the legs, arms and trunk are all involved). These factors may further determine whether the child has increased postural tone (hypertonia or spasticity), decreased postural tone (hypotonia), fluctuating tone (athetosis), a mixture of these (dystonia) or tremor (ataxia). The expression of these lesions will mean that the child with CP will display atypical postures and movements. The exact presentation will also be influenced by the extent to which more general maturation and development have been delayed or arrested.

The child with CP, in common with other children, acquires a movement by 'feeling' it and trying it out. Whereas typical children have a natural or built-in ability for adapting movements to their own satisfaction, children with CP are limited, to a varying extent, to fewer and more inadequate postures and movements which become stereotyped, and on which the child will place whatever functional or motor skills may be acquired later on. If a child is unable to initiate movements by first changing posture and is limited in the variety of postures and normal movements, there is a probability that deformities may develop. That is why the objective of early holding and moving (handling) is often to moderate abnormal posture and movement and try to establish greater postural control. Eventually in this way it is hoped to encourage the child towards a wider choice of postures and movements. Figure 10.1 illustrates normally developing movement and Figure 10.2 shows an example of stereotyped developing movement in a child with CP. The background or

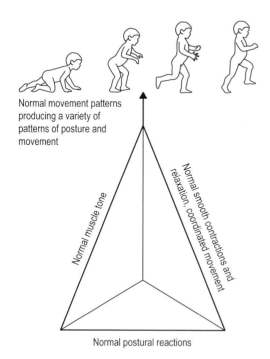

Normal movement patterns producing a variety of patterns of posture and movement

Normal muscle tone

Normal smooth contractions and relaxation, coordinated movement

Normal postural reactions

Figure 10.1 • The background of *normal* muscle tone and postural reactions necessary for normal movement, producing a variety of postures and movements.

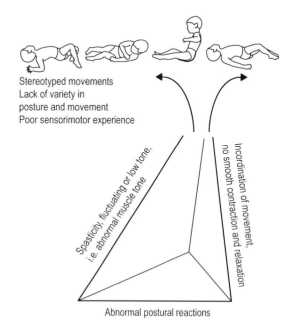

Stereotyped movements
Lack of variety in posture and movement
Poor sensorimotor experience

Spasticity, fluctuating or low tone, i.e. abnormal muscle tone

Incoordination of movement, no smooth contraction and relaxation

Abnormal postural reactions

Figure 10.2 • With an *abnormal* background of muscle tone, postural reactions and movement will be stereotyped and lack variety.

matrix of early infantile reactions (primitive reactions) which serve as a platform for the development of movement are described next.

Primitive reactions, early infantile reactions

In this section I shall describe a few of the early primitive reactions, also known as infantile reactions, present at birth, and the typical automatic postural reactions which are essential for the development of coordinated movements and underlie all our voluntary motor activities.

Children are born with a number of immature responses which take place against a background of normal postural tone. These responses are evoked automatically following a specific stimulus or experience and are called primitive reactions. Some of these primitive reactions, such as rooting, hand grasp and Moro reflex, disappear completely during maturation, whereas others are modified, and a few remain for life.

It is important that one is aware of the difference between the immature primitive reactions of the typical child and the persistent pathological primitive reactions of children with CP.

When these primitive reactions are elicited in the young child they are spontaneous and variable but when present in the child with CP, although the response seems similar, it is often a pathological and obligatory response against a background of abnormal postural tone, a pathological response that continues to be repeated in the same way each time (stereotyped).

A number of these primitive reactions, together with the stimulus that cause them to happen and the child's response, are shown in Table 10.1.

Normal postural tone

Normal postural tone provides the background on which movement is based: high enough to withstand gravity, low enough for easy movement.

Both posture and movement are dynamic and interact to such an extent that they cannot be separated. Postural changes are part of every movement and movements themselves are in effect changes in posture.

During the first year of life on a background of normal postural tone, the primitive reactions become gradually moderated and integrated into the child's voluntary coordinated movements, enabling a group of mature reactions to develop. These are called postural reactions and remain with us throughout life. Gravity affects all our movements from birth onwards but these reactions help the child to master gravity in conjunction with increasingly organized, coordinated and purposeful movements developed during the child's early years. These reactions help the child to master gravity, in time enabling the child to stand and walk.

Postural reactions or automatic reactions

Postural reactions provide the child with a stable postural base so that the child can maintain and adapt the body's position against gravity, keep the body in alignment and, with the weight evenly distributed and sufficient stability at the shoulder and pelvic girdles, move the limbs independently. This truncal stability also enables the child to shift the body weight against gravity.

Righting reactions

These reactions form the basis of future coordinated movements. When a child is moved or moves independently the child maintains the typical position of the head in space and the typical position of the head in relation to the body trunk and limbs. Righting reactions underlie many of a child's movement activities such as rolling over, sitting up, getting on to the hands and knees and kneeling up – all sequences of movements which will enable the child to stand in time.

These reactions become integrated with the balance or equilibrium reactions.

Equilibrium reactions (balance)

The function of the equilibrium reactions is as an automatic rapid response to a loss of balance.

Table 10.1 Primitive reactions, their stimuli and the child's responses

Name of reaction	Stimulus	Response
Rooting	The side of the mouth or cheek is lightly brushed with a finger	The bottom lip goes forward to that side; the tongue moves towards the stimulus
Moro	Held at an angle of 45° from the support, the head is allowed to fall back suddenly a short way	The arms are extended away from the body with open hands followed by the arms coming in towards the body in an 'embrace'
Asymmetrical tonic neck	The head is passively turned to one side	Extension of arm and leg on face side with flexion of arm and leg on skull side
Hand grasp	An object or finger is introduced into the palm of the hand from the ulnar (little-finger) side	The fingers flex and grasp (release is not possible)
Foot grasp	A finger is pressed against the ball of the foot, behind the toes	The toes grasp (curl) around the finger
Placing the lower limbs	The front of the shin and foot is brought up against the edge of the table	The leg bends and the child takes a step; the foot is placed flat on the table
Placing the upper limbs	The front of the forearm and back of the hand are brought up against the edge of the table	The arm is raised and the hand is placed on the table
Automatic walking	Supported under the arms, hands coming round the chest, the child is tilted forwards	Automatic stepping follows, with the feet coming down flat on the support
Neck righting	Lying in the supine position (on the back), the head is turned passively or may be turned actively by the child	The body turns as a whole in the same direction as the head

Equilibrium reactions help the child to maintain and to regain balance, thus making free and independent movements of the head, body and limbs possible in all positions.

Saving reactions

Very sudden or unexpected loss of balance elicits saving reactions. Their purpose is primarily to protect the face and head. If the child should lose balance and fall, the arms are thrust out, usually with straight elbows and open hands, which are placed on the nearest supporting surface to protect the head and face from injury.

In the child with CP these mature automatic postural reactions will often be absent, incomplete or exaggerated.

Differences between typical sequences of movement and sequences of movement in a child with CP

In this section I shall discuss the sequences of movement that enable a child when lying (1) in the supine position (on the back) and (2) in the prone position (on the front) to move away from these positions in a smooth coordinated manner plus make brief references to rolling, standing and walking and the reasons why the child with CP either cannot or may have difficulties in both initiating and carrying out these sequences of movements.

Sitting up from the supine position

The child with typical movements

Before children sit up the first thing that they will probably do is to automatically adjust their position so that they are lying symmetrically with the head, trunk and pelvis in alignment and the limbs lying in a symmetrical, relaxed position.

The body weight will be evenly distributed so that if, for example, someone tried to put their hands under the child's shoulders or pelvis, they would not be able to do so as both would be in contact with the supporting surface.

The way in which children come up to sitting from lying supine will depend on how fit they are and the strength of their abdominal muscles. Assuming that children have good abdominal muscles, they would sit up by lifting and bending their head forwards, chin tucked in and at the same time rounding their spine, bringing their shoulders and arms forwards, hips flexing as the body moves over the legs. Depending upon the strength of the abdominal muscles the legs would either remain on the supporting surface throughout the movement or be slightly bent, straightening just before the child attains the sitting position. Figures 10.3 and 10.4 illustrate the typical child sitting up from the supine position.

If you think this is not what you do when you sit up, I suggest you try the following: lie on your

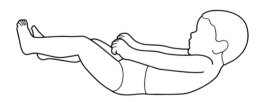

Figure 10.3 • First stage of sitting up from the supine position.

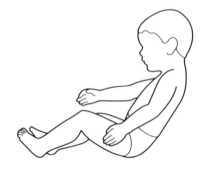

Figure 10.4 • Second stage of sitting up from the supine position. Raising the head forwards and at the same time bringing the arms and shoulders forwards, hips and knees bent.

back and lift your head, wait a second and then lift your arms. Now try and sit up. It is difficult.

The child with cerebral palsy

Let us now consider the difficulties that confront the child with CP: firstly the child with more severe involvement and secondly the child with more moderate involvement.

The child with more severe CP is vulnerable when lying on the back as the pathological reflex activity and abnormal motor postures present are strong in this position. Lacking antigravity flexor tone and unable to make the necessary postural adjustments to get the body into alignment, the child is either unable or limited in the ability to sit up, that is to lift the head and trunk against gravity and at the same time flex the hips. Figures 10.5–10.7 illustrate the problems faced by such a child when attempting to sit up from the supine lying position.

Although the child with moderate CP is able to sit up, the way in which this is achieved may vary from the norm. These variations may be due to the developmental level the child has reached, the distribution of abnormal postural tone and the absence of postural reactions. In addition, whether the arms are more involved than the legs or vice versa or, in some children, whether the muscle tone increases on effort may also influence the ability to sit up from lying on the back.

An example is a child with hemiplegia (one-sided involvement). The child's posture is asymmetrical

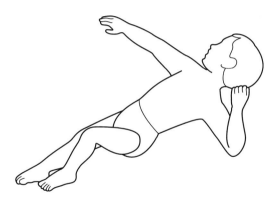

Figure 10.5 • The head, shoulders and arms pushing back make it difficult or nearly impossible to move in or away from these positions. The position of the arms often increases the extension of the hips and legs.

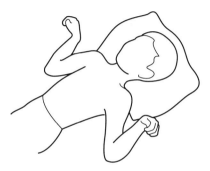

Figure 10.6 • The head, shoulders and arms pushing back make it difficult or nearly impossible to move in or away from these positions. The position of the arms often increases the extension of the hips and legs.

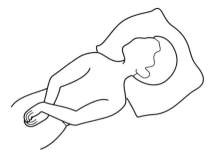

Figure 10.7 • The head pushes back, the shoulders forwards (protracted), internally rotated and extended. The adduction and inward rotation of the arms often increase adduction and inward rotation of the legs.

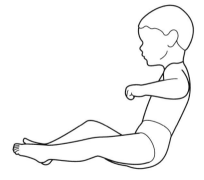

Figure 10.8 • Weight taken on unaffected side but effort involved may increase muscle tone on that side.

and unstable when lying on the back, with the greatest amount of weight taken on the unaffected side so that the only way the child can sit up is by pushing on the hand on the unaffected side. The effort involved in doing so usually increases the tone in both the arm and leg on the unaffected side. Figure 10.8 illustrates the problems faced by a child with one-sided (hemiplegia) involvement when sitting up from the lying position.

Getting into sitting from the prone position

The child with typical movements

Starting from a symmetrical, stable position the child will lift the head, extending the spine and hips. Then bringing the arms towards the body the child will push on the hands at the same time as turning the body to move into a sitting position, that is movement taking place between the pelvis and shoulder girdles. Figures 10.9 and 10.10

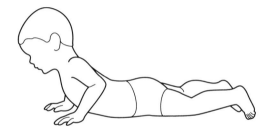

Figure 10.9 • First stage of sitting up from the prone position.

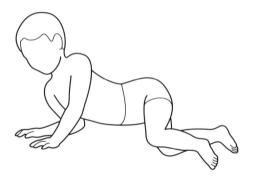

Figure 10.10 • Second stage of sitting up from the prone position.

illustrate the typical child sitting up from the prone position.

The child with cerebral palsy

Figures 10.11 and 10.12 illustrate a typical posture adopted by a child with more severe CP in the prone position. As a result of the child's abnormal postural tone, asymmetrical unstable posture and lack of antigravity extensor ability, the child is unable to move in or away from the prone position.

The majority of children with more moderate involvement are able to get from prone to sitting. An example is a child with good head control, whose legs are more affected than the arms, with limbs on one side more affected than the other;

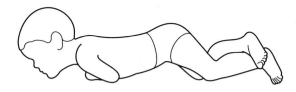

Figure 10.11 • Posture which may be adopted by a child with cerebral palsy in prone position.

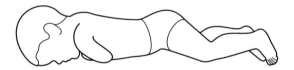

Figure 10.12 • Attempts at extension may result in hips flexing, weight going forwards and arms retracting.

that is, a child with asymmetric diplegia. These children often present with asymmetry of flexion when lying in the prone position. One leg is more flexed than the other and the pelvis is raised on the side of the flexed leg, so that not only does the child lack stability or mobility at the pelvis, but the body weight is shifted to one side. This will inevitably mean that any movement away from this position will be asymmetrical and trunk rotation will be either not possible or limited. To overcome this problem children often resort to pushing themselves back on to their knees, usually ending up in a 'W' asymmetrical sitting posture with their bottom between their legs. Although often discouraged by therapists, this position can be a very stable sitting position in which children are able to use their hands freely.

Any child with CP who cannot sit independently and use their hands for functional activities and play needs to be given an appropriate supportive chair with a tray at the same age as a child without disability is able to sit and use the hands, which is usually at about 6–8 months. If not given this opportunity to sit and use the hands, the child with CP may lose out both socially and in terms of manual abilities.

Rolling from supine to prone

The child with typical movements

The way in which children roll over can be influenced by their muscle power and habit. Rolling is a movement in which there seems to be endless variations. Children start from a symmetrical, stable position and initiate the movement by lifting the head and shoulders off the support with varying degrees of trunk rotation. Some children lead from the head and shoulders, others from the pelvis and legs; some keep their top leg bent and their under-leg straight, others keep both legs straight. The position of the arms as children roll over will also vary. Figure 10.13 illustrates one of the ways many children roll over.

The child with cerebral palsy

The child with more moderate involvement also rolls over in a number of different ways. The

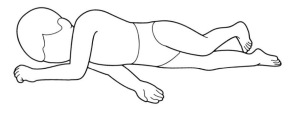

Figure 10.13 • Rolling from supine to prone: movement takes place between pelvic and shoulder girdles using rotation.

manner in which the child rolls over will be dictated by how severely the child is affected, the abnormal postural tone and the absence of postural reactions; later it may also be modified as a result of the presence of deformity. Most children with a certain amount of asymmetry will roll to a preferred side and rotation will be absent.

The child with more moderate involvement, that is, the child with diplegia, often initiates rolling by using flexion from the head, upper trunk and arms. This use of flexion of the upper trunk often results in the under-arm becoming trapped beneath the body, as illustrated in Figure 10.14.

The child with fluctuating tone and involuntary movements initiates rolling from the hips

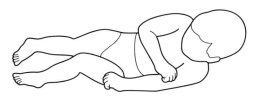

Figure 10.14 • Possible effect on the pelvis and lower limbs when rolling is initiated with excessive flexion of the head, upper limbs and trunk.

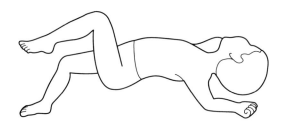

Figure 10.15 • Possible increased extension of the head, upper limbs and trunk when rolling is initiated by movement from the pelvis and lower limbs.

and legs, which tends to increase the extension of the head and trunk, retraction of the shoulders and outward rotation of the arms, as illustrated in Figure 10.15.

The child with low truncal tone will roll in a primitive manner by using total extension. A minimal amount of movement takes place between the shoulders and pelvis.

Movements which may be possible for the child with cerebral palsy, but are abnormally performed

These are the movements which, if continually repeated, may affect a child's ability to develop smooth, well-coordinated movements and fine motor skills at a later stage. Although we need to do all we can to encourage a child with CP to move independently, and the fact that the child does so is a great achievement, nevertheless some therapists suggest trying to avoid encouraging the child to move in a way that may lead to deformity and pain in later life.

Bridging and pushing along backwards on the floor

The child with typical movements

At around 5 months a child will often be seen practising a movement called 'bridging'. Keeping the head on the support, with the chin tucked in, the child shifts the weight back on to the shoulders, bends the knees and, by pushing the feet against the floor, lifts and holds the bottom in the air. At times the child shifts the weight from one foot to the other. Later, using the same sequence of movements, the child is able to push backwards along the floor, as illustrated in Figure 10.16.

The child with cerebral palsy

A child with severe involvement as a result of abnormally extended and adducted legs, lack of pelvic stability or mobility and the inability to isolate movements at the knees and feet is usually

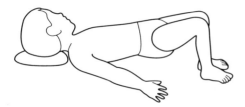

Figure 10.16 • Bridging and pushing backwards along the floor.

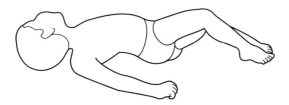

Figure 10.17 • In a child with spasticity excessive extension may be increased as the child pushes backwards with the toes.

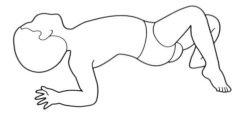

Figure 10.18 • In a child with fluctuating tone and involuntary movements, the head may extend with the chin up, shoulders retracted and with little pelvic stability, so that the child may push along asymmetrically.

unable either to bridge or push backwards. The child will however sometimes try to, and does so by pushing against a wall or the end of the bath, as shown in Figure 10.17. Many therapists discourage such movement as it tends to increase abnormal extensor tone. Children with mild or moderate involvement associated with hemiplegic or diplegic CP usually have sufficient abdominal, trunk or pelvic control to manage a semi-bridge. This means that, as they push themselves backwards, they do so asymmetrically. Many therapists will try to introduce an alternative method of mobility to these children, possibly including a mobility device.

The child with fluctuating tone and involuntary movements usually lies on the back with the head extended, chin up and shoulders retracted. The hips and legs are flexed, abducted and outwardly rotated, as illustrated in Figure 10.18. As it is difficult for such a child to take weight on the arms and creep, pushing backwards is a form of locomotion often favoured. Lacking extension and stability at the hips, the child pushes the feet against the floor, reinforcing the extension of the head and trunk plus the retraction of the arms. It may therefore be

helpful to encourage other means of locomotion in such a child in the form of a mobility device.

Creeping or commando crawling

The child with typical movements

Once a child has sufficient head control, trunk extension and stability at the shoulder and pelvic girdles to shift the weight from side to side in the prone position, the child will often propel forwards, by creeping on the tummy. The child does this by shifting the weight on to the chest and forearm while reaching forward with the other hand to pull forwards. At the same time the child shifts the weight in the lower part of the body, the pelvis rotating on the opposite side, so that the child can flex the leg and push forward. In this way a diagonal movement takes place between the shoulder and pelvic girdles with trunk rotation, as shown in Figure 10.19.

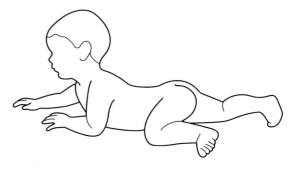

Figure 10.19 • Creeping on the tummy forwards along the floor using trunk rotation between the shoulder and pelvic girdles.

The child with cerebral palsy

The group of children with more moderate involvement, although able to propel forwards, cannot do so by creeping as described above. To understand the reasons for this, let us first look at the method of moving used by the child whose arms are less affected than the legs, i.e. spastic diplegia, and then at a child whose arms and legs are involved on one side only, i.e. spastic hemiplegia.

If you look at Figure 10.20 you will see that, although the child with spastic diplegia can lift the head up, the neck is hyperextended and the chin is in the air, jaw pushed forward. The child props on the arms, but they are close to the child's sides with the shoulders raised to help to stabilize the head. This is a position which makes it impossible for the child to transfer the weight on to one arm, freeing the other to reach and pull forwards. If you look at the child's back and hips you will see that they are overextended and adducted, the pelvis tilted posteriorly and the feet plantarflexed. Lacking mobility at the hips, trunk and pelvis, disassociated movements at the hips cannot take place. Therefore the only way in which the child can move forward is by lifting and pulling both arms towards the body, the legs remaining straight. The effort of using the arms in this way increases the extension of the hips and legs.

The child with spastic hemiplegia, although able to propel forwards, will do so with an asymmetrical or lopsided movement as the child lacks the ability to stabilize and shift the weight on to the affected side. The child moves forwards by turning towards the unaffected side, the affected arm remaining bent and the legs straight.

Children with fluctuating tone and involuntary movements, although able to extend against gravity but resulting from inadequate head and trunk control plus inadequate pelvic stability, dislike lying in the prone position. Unable to propel themselves forwards, they resort to rolling or pushing themselves along on their backs, as described above and shown in Figure 10.18.

Moving backwards and forwards in a sitting position may be an effective means of locomotion for some of these children if they are able to sit on the floor with their hips flexed, back straight supporting themselves on extended arms.

To move backwards the child sits taking the weight on extended arms, with the legs flexed. Keeping the body forwards, the child pushes on the heels, the bottom passing back between the arms as the child straightens, and then bends the legs, as shown in Figure 10.21.

To move forwards, the child sits taking weight on extended arms while keeping the trunk forwards. As the bottom passes between the arms, the child bends and then straightens the legs, as shown in Figure 10.22.

Bunny hopping

The child with typical movements

When playing on the floor many children like to 'bunny hop', but unlike the child with CP, it will be one of many strategies used to move around. Children do so by tucking both legs under their bottom and often play sitting in this position.

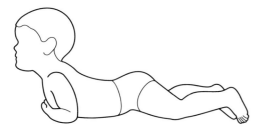

Figure 10.20 • The abnormal posture may prevent the child taking weight on the forearms and shifting the weight to enable forward propulsion.

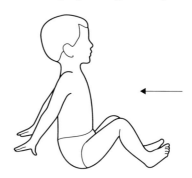

Figure 10.21 • Pushing backwards with weight taken on extended arms and pushing with the heels, then pushing the bottom back and straightening the legs to move backwards.

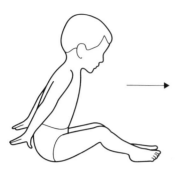

Figure 10.22 • Pushing forwards with weight taken on extended arms and moving the trunk forwards with bent legs, then pushing bottom forwards, straightening legs to move forwards.

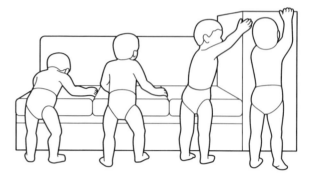

Figure 10.23 • Trunk, arm and hand support used in standing at various stages of motor development before achieving standing balance.

The child with cerebral palsy

The child with spasticity, on the other hand, sits and moves forwards with the bottom between the legs, which are flexed and turned in at the hips (internally rotated), usually taking weight more on one leg than the other. This can be an efficient means of mobility for the child with CP and is a very stable sitting position in which the child may be able to use the hands freely. It is difficult to discourage, except perhaps by providing an alternative aid for mobility and supported sitting. These children do require monitoring for the development of deformity, especially at the hips.

The child with fluctuating tone and involuntary movements also sits with the bottom between the legs when bunny hopping. Lacking trunk and hip stability, the child bunny hops by taking weight forwards on the arms and extending the head, then drawing both legs together towards the arms.

Standing

The child with typical movement

There is considerable variation regarding the age at which a child first pulls up to stand, later usually cruising and then walking. A number of children prefer to 'bottom shuffle' or crawl and then one day just get up on to their feet and walk.

It is usual that a child pulls to stand before having perfected balance in sitting, cruises before having perfected balance in standing and walks before having perfected balance in standing.

When the child first pulls up to stand the child relies on the hands to stabilize and to compensate for lack of stability and control in the trunk and pelvis. Activity in the lower limbs at this time is confined to bending and straightening the legs. Gradually as the child gains more control the child experiments with different methods of getting to standing, eventually managing to do so through kneeling and later half-kneeling.

The methods of supporting oneself in standing also develop in stages. To begin with the child takes weight on the forearms, then on extended arms and finally on one arm only, as shown in Figure 10.23.

Figure 10.24 illustrates the posture that the child adopts when first starting to stand independently. To overcome a lack of trunk and pelvic stability and immature balance reactions in the upright position, the child stands with:

1. Legs apart, hips and knees bent.
2. Pelvis tilted forwards (anteriorly) with a marked lordosis (hollow back).
3. Feet apt to splay outwards with weight taken on the inner borders of the feet.
4. Arms flexed and abducted.

Cruising

The child with typical movement

A child first moves in the upright position by cruising, usually facing in the direction in which

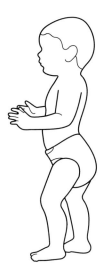

Figure 10.24 • Early standing position of a typical child.

the child wants to go, only moving sideways when becoming more adept at transferring the weight sideways from one leg to the other. As the child becomes more adventurous the child will cruise from one area to another, at times letting go, and at first just flopping down on to the bottom, then gradually learning to lower gently into a squatting position. At this stage the child is able to move at speed while cruising but loses this ability when starting to walk forwards.

Walking

The child with typical movement

When a child takes the first walking steps the child holds the arms abducted and flexed in a position described as 'high guard'. Holding the arms in this position helps the child to stabilize the trunk and enables the child to have more mobility at the hips. The child walks using excessive movements of the trunk with a waddling gait which might remind one of the way a sailor walks when first coming ashore after a long time away at sea.

The child with cerebral palsy

Regardless of the severity of a child's disability, early weight-bearing should be encouraged at the same age as the child without CP would be

expected to stand, that is, at about 9–12 months, even if the child has to be placed in a standing position. Some form of standing system may be needed, varying according to the severity, height and weight of the child.

The postural abnormalities seen in both standing and walking of children with moderate spasticity are due to the adjustment that they have to make in their trunk and limbs to enable them to maintain their centre of gravity or, to put it another way, to compensate for their lack of balance in the upright position.

Figure 10.25 illustrates one of the standing postures of a child whose legs are more involved than the arms (spastic diplegia). The posture is one of flexion, the child having to extend the neck, chin poked forward and up in an attempt to compensate for the lack of extension in the trunk, hips and knees. This is a posture that the child adopts to stop falling forwards. The pelvis is tilted backwards (posteriorly), legs turned in at the hips (internally rotated) and drawn together (adducted) and the weight taken on the inner borders of the feet (valgus position).

When such a child is walked held under the armpits or by the hands with arms flexed, lacking balance and sufficient extensor tone against gravity, the child tends to fall forwards from one leg to the other, the weight falling more and more on

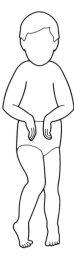

Figure 10.25 • One possible standing position of a child with spastic diplegia.

to the toes. This may result in the legs becoming increasingly stiff and often crossing.

Figure 10.26 illustrates a standing posture often adopted by children whose arms show little involvement but who flex at their hips with hyperextended knees and the pelvis tilted anteriorly. To overcome the flexion at the hips they extend the lower spine (lumbar lordosis).

Figure 10.27 illustrates the standing posture of a child with one side of the body involved (spastic hemiplegia). The child's posture is asymmetrical with all the weight being taken on the unaffected leg, which the child places in front. The pelvis on the affected side is pulled up and back, the leg turned in at the hip and extended with the foot in an equinus and turned-in position. The shoulder is pulled back, the arm flexed and forearm pronated wrist flexed. The position of the arm often becomes more pronounced when the child walks quickly or runs.

Depending upon the severity of the spasticity present, the child will take a step either by flexing the hip and hyperextending the knee to get the foot on to the ground or to take the leg out to the side (abduct) and swing the leg forward, often with the toes contacting the ground first with the foot turned in.

A child with fluctuating tone and involuntary movements lacks postural control and stability and therefore has difficulty in maintaining an upright position. As the balance reactions are often exaggerated, the child may be unable to shift the body weight from side to side or forwards.

When placed on the feet the child has a tendency either to go into total extension and fall backwards, or total flexion and collapse. If one leg is lifted, the weight-bearing leg often flexes involuntarily and the child falls. However if the child learns to extend both arms forwards and to maintain a sustained grasp, the child is often able to gain sufficient postural control to stabilize and flex the hips, which enables the child to shift the weight both sideways and forwards. Figure 10.28 illustrates one of the ways that a child may do this by extending both arms forwards and clasping the hands together.

Table 10.1 lists automatic walking as a reaction present at birth. A more descriptive term might be 'high stepping', for when the sole of one foot touches something solid, one leg bends and the other extends, giving the appearance of walking. If you walk a child with fluctuating tone and involuntary movements, the walking posture is often very similar to this high-stepping gait.

The child who has fairly good arms and can maintain a sustained grasp is often able to stand and walk independently if an appropriate walking aid is given. It is useful to appreciate that principally

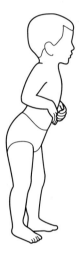

Figure 10.26 • Another possible standing position of a child with diplegia.

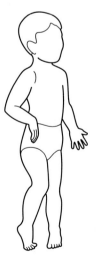

Figure 10.27 • Possible standing position of a child with spastic hemiplegia.

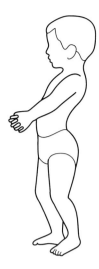

Figure 10.28 • Possible standing position of a child with fluctuating tone and involuntary movements.

a walking aid compensates for a lack of balance and does not usually alter the child's underlying gait problem or enable the child to walk typically. Children with less involvement may of course be able to walk independently.

Understanding early sensorimotor development in the child with typical movement

Throughout this book there is an emphasis on the need for head control, symmetry, stability and sensory input when holding and moving a child with CP. So it might be helpful to describe briefly how sensorimotor development progresses in a child with typical postural tone and reactions.

The stages described below occur at around 4 and 6 months of age in the supine, prone and sitting positions. However within 'normal' or 'typical' there is a naturally occurring wide spectrum of achievement, as no child develops in accordance with a strictly stereotyped course. A wider description of early sensorimotor development can be found in Appendix 1.

Sensorimotor development at around 4 months (head control and midline orientation)

Postural control

1. Symmetry: the child keeps the head, trunk and pelvis in alignment.

2. Postural stability: the child's weight is evenly distributed throughout the body, i.e. head, trunk and pelvis.

3. Weight shift: the child starts to transfer weight to the side (laterally) in the trunk, enabling the limbs to move independently of the trunk. The ability to move the upper limbs in advance of the lower limbs usually occurs.

Muscle control

There is an increased control of the flexor muscles so that they are beginning to balance the strong antigravity extensor muscles. The child also practises extension against gravity in prone.

Sensory input

1. Head in midline, chin tucked in: this encourages the child in visual and auditory communication and social interaction.

2. Hands together in midline: this provides the child with further visual and tactile cues and information regarding the position of the arms and hands in space.

3. Moving the arms independently of the trunk plus the ability to flex and extend the elbows increases the child's body awareness and encourages exploration.

Gross motor movements

These provide additional sensory input through touch and pressure from the skin, joints and muscles.

Figures 10.29 and 10.30 illustrate sensorimotor development in supine at 4 months of age. Figures 10.31 and 10.32 illustrate sensorimotor development in prone at 4 months of age.

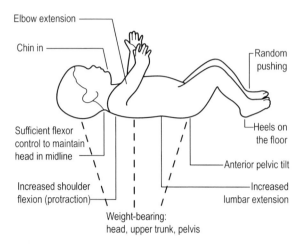

Figure 10.29 • Sensorimotor development in supine at 4 months.

Labels: Elbow extension — Chin in — Random pushing — Sufficient flexor control to maintain head in midline — Heels on the floor — Anterior pelvic tilt — Increased shoulder flexion (protraction) — Increased lumbar extension — Weight-bearing: head, upper trunk, pelvis

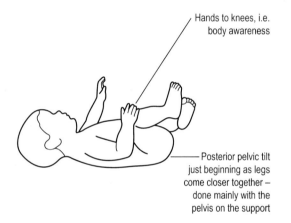

Figure 10.30 • Sensorimotor development in supine at 4 months.

Labels: Hands to knees, i.e. body awareness — Posterior pelvic tilt just beginning as legs come closer together – done mainly with the pelvis on the support

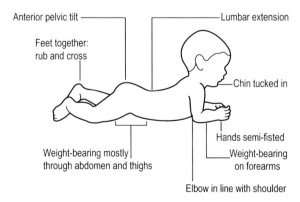

Figure 10.31 • Sensorimotor development in prone at 4 months.

Labels: Anterior pelvic tilt — Lumbar extension — Feet together: rub and cross — Chin tucked in — Hands semi-fisted — Weight-bearing mostly through abdomen and thighs — Weight-bearing on forearms — Elbow in line with shoulder

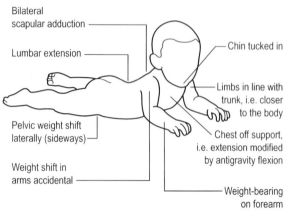

Figures 10.32 • Sensorimotor development in prone at 4 months.

Labels: Bilateral scapular adduction — Chin tucked in — Lumbar extension — Limbs in line with trunk, i.e. closer to the body — Pelvic weight shift laterally (sideways) — Chest off support, i.e. extension modified by antigravity flexion — Weight shift in arms accidental — Weight-bearing on forearm

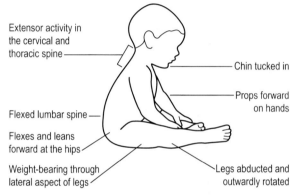

Figure 10.33 • Sensorimotor development in sitting at 4 months.

Labels: Extensor activity in the cervical and thoracic spine — Chin tucked in — Props forward on hands — Flexed lumbar spine — Flexes and leans forward at the hips — Weight-bearing through lateral aspect of legs — Legs abducted and outwardly rotated

In sitting

The only balance between the flexor and extensor muscles in sitting at this age is seen in the head, neck and upper spine of the child. The supporting base is wide, with the child propping on the hands. Figure 10.33 illustrates sensorimotor development in sitting at 4 months of age.

Sensorimotor development at around 6 months (balance between flexor and extensor activity)

Postural control

1. Symmetry: the child is now able to readjust the position if it gets out of alignment. Good

head control against gravity is seen in all positions.

2. Postural stability: in both supine and prone the child takes weight evenly through the head, shoulder and pelvic girdles or through the trunk only.

   There is increased shoulder control so that weight-bearing on the extended arms and protective extension is now possible for the child.

   The child has good stability and mobility in the lumbar pelvic region.

3. Weight shift: the child shifts the weight anteriorly, posteriorly and laterally (sideways) now.

Muscle control

The child now has good balance between flexor and extensor muscles in supine and prone.

Sensory input

In both supine and prone the child starts to integrate the sensory development of the previous months with purposeful movements.

Gross motor movements

In prone extension predominates; the child pushes back on extended arms but when transferring weight on to one arm still weight-bears on a flexed arm for stability.

In supine equilibrium reactions are beginning to appear.

The child rolls from supine to prone and vice versa.

Figures 10.34–10.36 illustrate sensorimotor development in supine and prone at 6 months.

In sitting

The child reaches forward to grasp and manipulate toys, rotates (turns trunk) but falls sideways and backwards if it moves out off the base.

The child still rests with the hands on the knees or supporting forwards if need be, although forward protective extension is usually developed. Figure 10.37 illustrates sensorimotor development in sitting at 6 months.

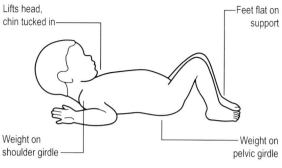

Figure 10.34 • Sensorimotor development in supine at 6 months.

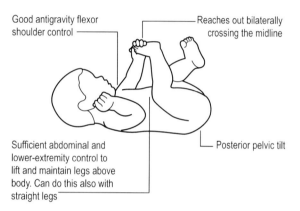

Figure 10.35 • Sensorimotor development in supine at 6 months.

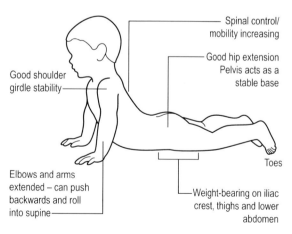

Figure 10.36 • Sensorimotor development in prone at 6 months.

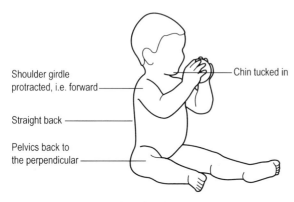

Maintains an upright position, head in alignment with trunk

Chin tucked in

Shoulder girdle protracted, i.e. forward

Straight back

Pelvics back to the perpendicular

Wide base helps maintain balance. One leg flexed, outwardly rotated and abducted, the other extended

Figure 10.37 • Sensorimotor development in sitting at 6 months.

An overview of the first five stages of sensorimotor development in the child with typical movement can be found in Appendix 1.

Chapter Eleven

11

Handling

Revised by Eva Bower

The child with cerebral palsy (CP) often displays atypical postures and movements which may restrict the child's ability to perform purposeful and skilled movement. Appropriate handling may help both the child and the parent. But what do I mean by the word 'handling'? Handling is concerned with the positioning, holding and moving of the child by another person using mainly the hands, although parts of the body may also be used to position and/or support the child. Occasionally equipment may be involved. Good handling should make it physically easier for the parent or 'handler' and child to carry out functional tasks, in contrast to bad handling, which usually makes it physically more difficult for the parent and child to carry out tasks.

In a child with increased tone or stiffness it may be helpful for the parent to position the child as symmetrically and typically aligned as possible.

For example, if the child is habitually in an abnormally straight or extended position in lying it may be helpful to put a child into a more bent or more flexed, symmetrical position. This might help such a child to look at and use two hands for a task at a table placed in front.

If the child is habitually in an abnormally bent or flexed position in sitting it may be helpful to put the child into a straighter or more extended, symmetrical, high-kneeling position. Again this might help such a child to use the eyes and two hands for a task at a table placed in front.

Good handling should help to relax a stiff child.

Handling children is often most effectively achieved by holding the child at, and moving the child from, proximal body points – the head, shoulders, trunk and pelvis.

In a child with decreased tone or floppiness it may be helpful for the parent or handler to apply support at proximal body points similar to those listed above, thus giving the child the needed stability or fixation to undertake functional activities more easily.

Good handling should help to support a floppy child.

An important point to appreciate is that, although the child may look and feel more normal when well handled and be better able to carry out functional activities, when the parents' hands and/or support are taken away the child very often reverts back to the original difficulties. There is no guaranteed carry-over after good handling. Carry-over is most likely to be determined by the severity of the child's problems. Quite often a child may be able to maintain an imposed, improved position but may not be able to move in or out of that position with ease.

Nancie Finnie, when she wrote the first edition of this book, included a number of strategies for the handling of children with CP which, however effective, are no longer socially acceptable. For example, when bathing a child who cannot sit a parent may get in the bath with the child and support the child in sitting by placing the child between the legs. I have endeavoured to take all current (2008) thinking into account in view of the higher profile of the question of physical and sexual abuse of children. Nevertheless, over the years to come some of the strategies I am advocating may suffer a similar fate and this must always be borne in mind.

Using our hands

Two important factors when handling your child with CP, particularly in the early years, are firstly to be sensitive to the varying problems and abnormalities under the hands and secondly to develop the ability to use the hands effectively and economically.

To help appreciate the differences in the *feeling* and *reactions* to handling a limb that offers no resistance and one that does, try the following.

Take an unaffected child's arm and move it in different directions, then let it go. You will find that the arm *feels light* as you move it and offers *no resistance*. When you let it go there is a momentary pause before the arm falls to the child's side. This is because, even though you moved the arm *passively*, the child was able to follow the movement *actively* by controlling and making adjustments to their posture quickly and automatically in response to the movement.

Now move the arm of a child who has increased tone or stiffness in the same way. You will find that the arm *feels heavy* and presses down against your hand and that as you move it there is *resistance*. When you let it go the arm drops immediately to the child's side.

The resistance offered by the child who has intermittent spasms and involuntary movements when an arm is moved will differ in that, although there will be an *initial resistance*, the arm will then *suddenly give*. When you let it go the arm will *fly away* before dropping to the child's side.

A measure of a child's stiffness can be gauged by the amount of resistance to both passive and active movement. For example, when trying to bring the arms forward in an attempt to sit the child up, the degree of resistance that you feel will enable you to judge the difficulties with which the child is faced and whether or not the movement is beyond the capabilities of the child. In other words you should know how much physical cooperation you can really expect and how much of the movement the child should be able to do alone.

When handling your child it is important to take away your support as soon as it is not needed. When *you* are holding and moving your child *you* are doing the movement. The aim is to encourage the child to move actively without help and your child can only do that if you take away your hand or hands at the right moment and encourage your child to move independently. The importance of the speed of handling and the possible gradual taking-over of a movement by your child should be demonstrated to you by your therapist.

Learning to feel confident when using specific techniques of handling takes time. It is *not possible* to learn to use your hands *by just watching*. Ask your therapist to demonstrate and then let *you* do it. There are some children who cooperate better when their parents are not present, but even so, whenever possible do spend at least some of most sessions in the room with your child and your therapist.

Figures 11.1–11.5 illustrate some of the abnormal postures influenced by the position of the head adopted by children with CP. These postures may affect the whole body and the development of righting and balance abilities. The postures are likely to be more permanent in a child with increased tone and stiffness, intermittent in a

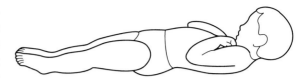

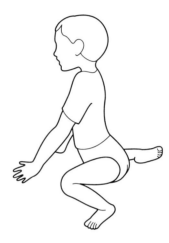

Figure 11.3 • The head is pulled forwards, the arms are bent and pulled over the chest, the hips and legs stiffen. If the child shows this posture lying on the back, the posture will be even more accentuated lying on the tummy.

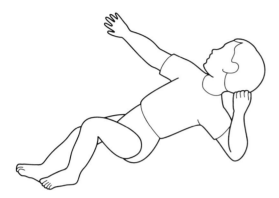

Figure 11.1 • The child turns the head, which may also be bent to the side, and in the more severe child pulled back. The arm and leg towards which the face is turned are straight and the hand open, the other arm and leg are bent and the hand is fisted. This posture is seen most clearly when the child lies on the back or stands but is often present, although modified, when the child is lying on the tummy or in sitting.

Figure 11.4 • Lifting the head up and back results in the arms extending stiffly and the hips, knees and ankles bending. Often the child will sit between the legs. Between-legs sitting, although encouraging an abnormal posture of the hips and legs, is not always a bad position if it enables a child to sit securely and use the upper limbs independently. This is not the case in this illustration.

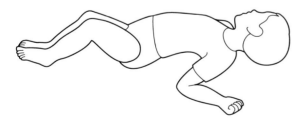

Figure 11.2 • The head and shoulders are pulled back and the back arches. In the child with fluctuating tone and involuntary movements the legs may remain bent but in the child with increased tone and stiffness the legs will be straight and stiff. A more severely affected child may show the same posture when lying on the tummy.

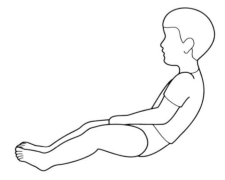

Figure 11.5 • Bending the head has the opposite effect. The arms bend and the hips and knees extend.

child with fluctuating tone and involuntary movement and seen on the affected side in the child with unilateral or hemiplegic involvement.

Figures 11.6–11.11 illustrate some of the difficulties experienced by children with CP with head position and some of the ways in which these may be overcome.

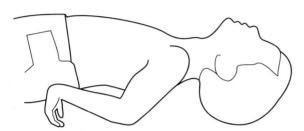

Figure 11.6 • Some children with cerebral palsy push their head back and at the same time bring their shoulders up and forward. It is better not to try to improve the position of the head by putting a hand on the back of the head as this will only cause the child to push back more.

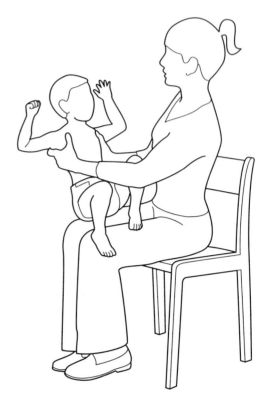

Figure 11.8 • When a young child is held without adequate control, the child often pushes back when sitting, as shown, although at this stage the legs are usually flexed and apart.

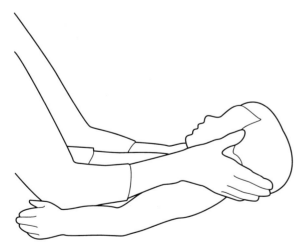

Figure 11.7 • It may be better to place your hands on each side of the head and push upwards, giving the child a long neck. As you do this, push the shoulders down with your forearms.

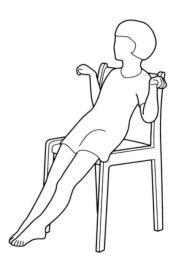

Figure 11.9 • If the young child continues to do this, in time it is likely that the hips and legs will extend and become stiff.

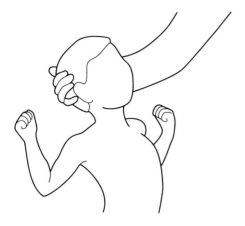

Figure 11.10 • It is better not to try to stop a child pushing the head back by putting your hand on the back of the head as this will only increase the abnormal extensor tone.

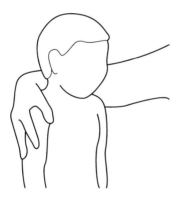

Figure 11.11 • Both the neck and shoulder retraction may be controlled by holding the child as shown, which should encourage head flexion and the bringing-forward of the arms towards the midline.

Figures 11.12–11.14 illustrate some of the difficulties experienced by children with CP with low postural tone and a way of stabilizing the shoulder girdle which may overcome some of the difficulties.

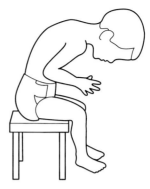

Figure 11.12 • When placed in the sitting position these children tend to flop forwards at the hips.

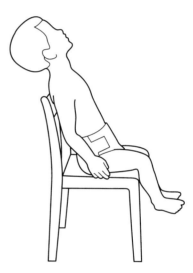

Figure 11.13 • When the trunk is supported, the head falls either back or forwards on to the chest.

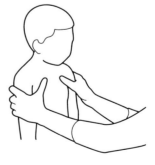

Figure 11.14 • Holding the child firmly around the top of the arms and pulling the shoulders down and forwards should stabilize the shoulder girdle and help the child to keep the head up in midline with the chin tucked in.

Figures 11.15–11.17 illustrate some of the difficulties experienced by children with CP with increased postural tone and a method of encouraging the lifting of the head and straightening of the spine.

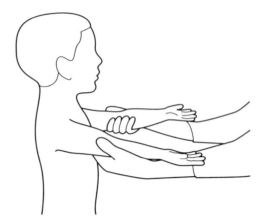

Figure 11.17 • With one movement lift and turn the arms out as you bring the child towards you. By handling the child in this way you may encourage the lifting of the head, straightening of the spine and bending of the hips.

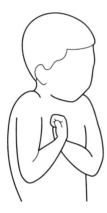

Figure 11.15 • A typical posture of flexion often seen in the child with increased tone and stiffness. The arms are turned in at the shoulders. This is generally accompanied by straight hips.

Figures 11.18 and 11.19 illustrate some of the difficulties experienced by children with CP and low postural tone and a way of encouraging the coming-forwards of the head.

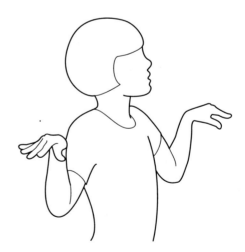

Figure 11.18 • A posture of the head and arms sometimes seen in older children when sitting who have fluctuating tone and intermittent spasms. The arms are flexed and shoulders hunched and turned out. The legs are either flexed and turned out at the hips or extended and turned in at the hips.

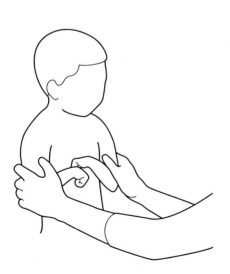

Figure 11.16 • Hold the child over the outsides of the elbows and the tops of the arms.

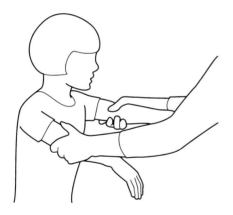

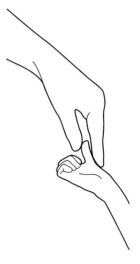

Figure 11.19 • With one movement, turn the shoulders in and down, extending the child's arms as you bring the child forwards towards you. Handling in this way may encourage the head to come forwards with a straight spine and flexed hips.

Figures 11.20–11.24 illustrate some of the difficulties experienced by children with unilateral increased tone in the upper limb and ways which may overcome some of the difficulties.

Figure 11.21 • It is better not to extend the wrist and fingers by pulling on the thumbs, as shown, as this is likely to increase the flexion of the wrist and fingers and there is also a danger that the thumb joints may become damaged.

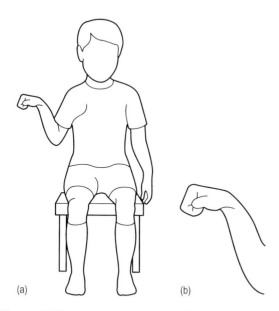

(a)   (b)

Figure 11.20 • An arm posture sometimes seen in children with unilateral, hemiplegic, increased tone and stiffness. The arm is flexed and turned in at the shoulder, which presses down. The forearm is turned in or pronated so that the hand faces down with wrist and fingers flexed and thumb across the palm (see (b)).

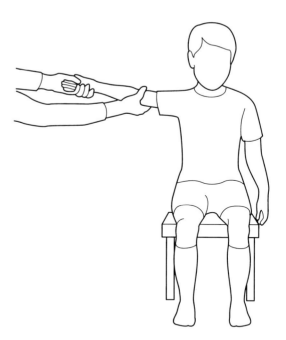

Figure 11.22 • It may be better to extend the arm, wrist and fingers by turning the arm out at the shoulder, with elbow straight and the forearm and palm facing up. This should encourage the extension of the wrist and fingers, making it easier to keep the thumb away from the palm.

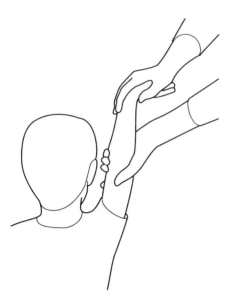

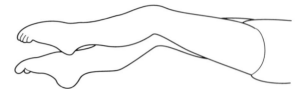

Figure 11.25 • A typically extended posture of hips and legs of a child with increased tone and stiffness when lying on the back.

Figure 11.23 • Raising the arm in outward rotation may discourage the flexor increase in tone and stiffness and the downward pressure of the arm and shoulder girdle. The abduction of the thumb with the arm in supination and outward rotation plus extension of the arm and wrist should encourage opening of all the fingers.

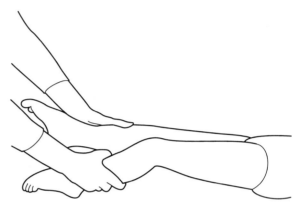

Figure 11.26 • It is better not to try to part the legs by pulling them close together in adduction as this is likely to increase further the turning-in of the legs.

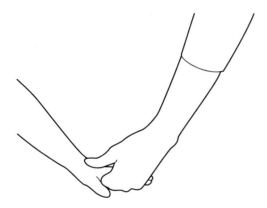

Figure 11.24 • A helpful grasp to use when encouraging a child to self-support is an open hand with an extended arm.

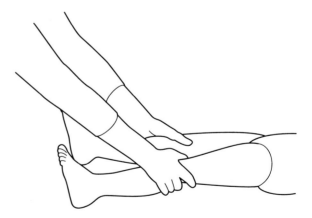

Figure 11.27 • It may be better to part the legs by turning them out at the hips, controlling the legs over or just above the knee joints. The outward rotation of the legs in extension may encourage abduction and dorsiflexion of the ankles.

Figures 11.25–11.30 illustrate some of the difficulties experienced by children with increased tone in the lower limbs and some ways which may overcome the difficulties.

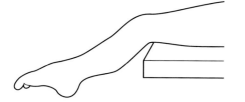

Figure 11.28 • When a child's foot is plantarflexed, as shown (see Figure 11.29).

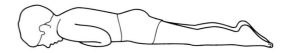

Figure 11.31 • A child with increased tone and stiffness who lies on the tummy, as shown, should find it easier to lift the head and take weight on flexed arms with shoulders protracted if put on a wedge.

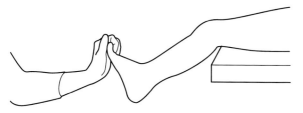

Figure 11.29 • It is better not to try to bend the foot up into dorsiflexion by pushing on the ball of the foot.

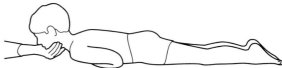

Figure 11.32 • It is better not to put the child on a wedge by lifting the head first and then trying to bring the arms forward as this will probably increase the pulling-down and flexion of the arms and extension of the legs.

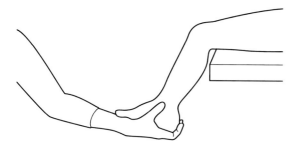

Figure 11.30 • It may be better to hold the knee bent with one hand, grasping the heel and foot with the other hand, keeping the foot in midline and gently bending the foot up as far as is possible.

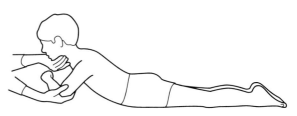

Figure 11.33 • It may be better to lift the head at the same time as you start to bring the arm forward.

Figures 11.31–11.36 illustrate some of the difficulties experienced by a child with increased postural tone when lying on the tummy and some ways which may overcome the difficulties when placing the child on a wedge.

There are other techniques of extending the more severely involved child before putting the child into the prone position which can be demonstrated to you by your therapist.

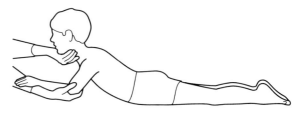

Figure 11.34 • With your hand over the elbow, turn the shoulder out as you lift and straighten the arm.

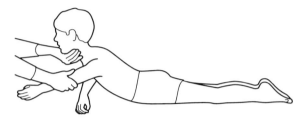

Figure 11.35 • Hold the head, keeping the arm extended and off the support until it feels less heavy and no longer presses down so much at the shoulder. Then place the arm on the support. Follow the same procedure with the other arm, not letting the head flex. Raising the child's head as you extend the arm should encourage the extension of the spine, hips and legs.

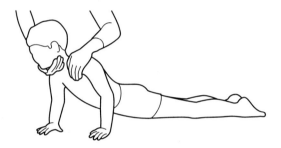

Figure 11.36 • Lifting the shoulder up and over while at the same time rotating the trunk may be sufficient to encourage bringing the arm forward with a child who has less increased tone and stiffness.

Figures 11.37 and 11.38 illustrate a way of putting a child over a roll and encouraging head and trunk extension.

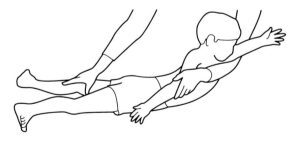

Figure 11.37 • Before putting a child over a roll it may be a good idea to extend the child first. You can help the child to maintain the extension by placing your hands as shown, keeping the legs straight and turned out at the hips.

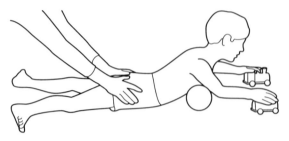

Figure 11.38 • When the child is on the roll and if the child has difficulties controlling the position of the arms, you could encourage trunk and head extension by placing your hands each side of the child's pelvis. With gentle but firm pressure towards yourself, give the child a point of fixation or stability from which to extend.

Figures 11.39–11.41 show various ways of giving a child stability so that the child may be encouraged to keep the head in midline and trunk extended when beginning to take the weight on open hands or using the hands to play. When placing your hands on the child's pelvis, ensure that it is in a neutral but slightly forward position and apply pressure downwards. Do not apply pressure with your thumbs on the lower part of the child's back or lumbar region to tilt the pelvis forwards.

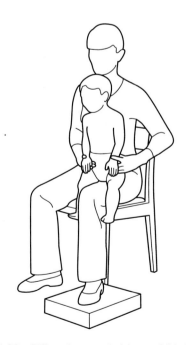

Figure 11.39 • Different ways of giving a child stability.

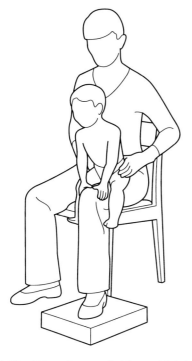

Figure 11.40 • Different ways of giving a child stability.

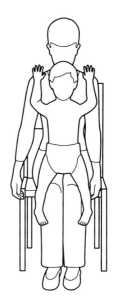

Figure 11.42 • Too wide a sitting base may increase the extension and inward rotation at the hips and legs of a child who pushes back when sitting, affecting the whole posture, but the arms more so than the legs.

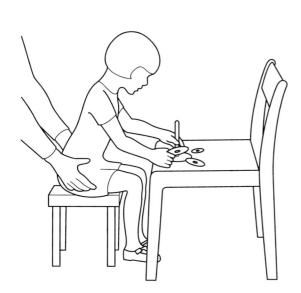

Figure 11.41 • Different ways of giving a child stability.

Figures 11.42–11.45 illustrate some of the difficulties experienced by a child in sitting and a way which may overcome the difficulties.

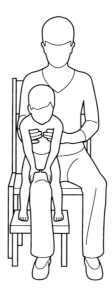

Figure 11.43 • A narrow sitting base may keep the hips outwardly rotated with hips, knees and ankles flexed. The arms and head are controlled by the shoulders, which are lifted and turned in with slight pressure on the chest. The inward rotation at the shoulders with pronation of the elbows may control the retraction and outward rotation of the arms. Weight-bearing with the arms extended on your knee should be encouraged.

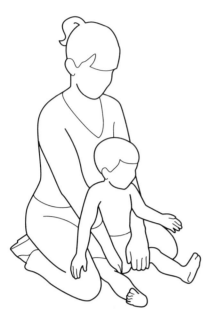

Figures 11.46 and 11.47 illustrate some of the difficulties experienced by a child with fluctuating tone in sitting and a way which may overcome the difficulties.

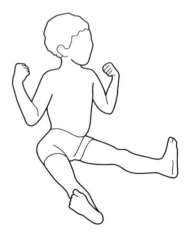

Figure 11.44 • When placing a child with increased tone on the floor in long sitting, it is better not to sit the child on the floor and then try to bend the hips. It may be better to pull the child towards you by the seat of the pants so that the weight of the child's trunk is over the sitting base, and keep the legs turned out and apart.

Figure 11.46 • A child with fluctuating tone is often able to sit in long sitting as a result of a wide sitting base but frequently does so with excessive flexion at the hips, compensating by extending the head and trunk with retraction of the arms. This makes it difficult for the child to move over the sitting base to self-support or to reach forwards to use the hands.

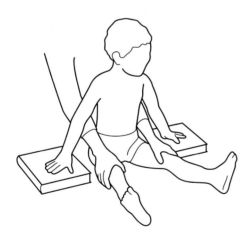

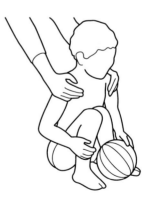

Figure 11.45 • Once a child is able to sit forward independently, keeping the legs straight, encourage the child to self-support, first forwards and then at the sides. It is often felt that long sitting is an inappropriate position for children who can only sit in this position by taking weight on the sacrum, that is, with the pelvis tilted backwards and a rounded back. Such children are usually more secure sitting on a chair with their feet supported.

Figure 11.47 • The child sits with legs flexed and together, arms forward with firm pressure given over shoulders, which are protracted. The child may then be encouraged to maintain a sustained grip on an object. A good way to get a child to hold this position independently is by getting the child to hold the legs together by wrapping the arms round them.

Figures 11.48 and 11.49 illustrate two of the many sitting positions children use when playing on the floor. Note the wide bases and erect spines. Although cross-legged sitting is often recommended for children with CP, it needs to be remembered that it is an asymmetrical position with more weight taken on the under-leg and with weight being taken on the outside of the feet, a position of the feet that some children have a tendency to develop later, causing gait difficulties.

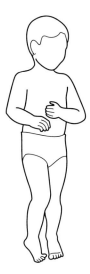

Figure 11.50 • A typical standing posture of a child with increased tone. Hips and knee are flexed with a flat lower back at the lumbar spine and the pelvis tilted back or posteriorly. The standing base is small, with the weight being taken on the inner sides of the feet, making it very difficult to take weight evenly on both feet or to transfer weight sideways on to one foot to take a step.

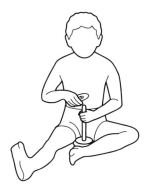

Figure 11.48 • A different sitting position children may use when on the floor.

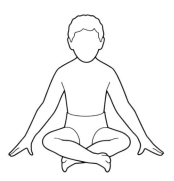

Figure 11.49 • A different sitting position children may use when on the floor.

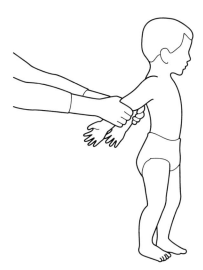

Figure 11.51 • One of the ways of encouraging hip and trunk extension in standing and even weight distribution plus weight shift from one foot to the other. The child's arms are extended diagonally backwards with outward rotation at the shoulders, which are pushed up and forwards. Care must be taken to see that the child's weight is taken forward over the standing base.

Figures 11.50 and 11.51 illustrate some of the difficulties experienced by a child with increased tone in standing and a way in which these difficulties may be overcome.

It may be helpful for a parent or handler to try out many of these positions and manoeuvres on themselves first before trying them out with their child.

Non-recommended handling and the reasons why

It should be recognized that as we handle a child there is as much positive input in the avoidance of certain movements as there is in the performance of others, provided that the reasons for avoiding them are clearly understood.

The following examples illustrate how by our handling of the child we may inadvertently increase tone, intermittent spasms and involuntary movements and the consequential development of postural deformities.

Pulling a young child up to sitting from lying on the back

The typical young child in Figure 11.52 is symmetrical, the head is in alignment with the trunk, the pelvis stable, hips and legs flexed and outwardly rotated. The young child has sufficient control of the flexor muscles to lift the head off the support and with help to assist in pulling up to a sitting position. Slightly later the child should be able to come to sitting, keeping both legs extended on the support.

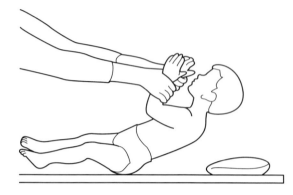

Figure 11.53 • A child with asymmetry and stiffness pulling up to sitting.

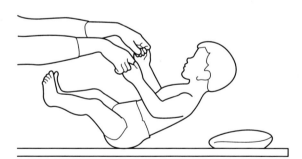

Figure 11.52 • A typical young child pulling up to sitting from lying on the back.

The child with increased tone and stiffness

The child in Figure 11.53, on the other hand, is slightly asymmetrical, the pelvis is unstable and the weight is taken over to one side. Although the child has some head control it is not sufficient to control the flexor muscles and to overcome the pull of gravity and therefore even with help the child is limited in the amount of movement able to be undertaken.

The mother, by encouraging her child to grasp her hands while her arms are flexed, has possibly increased the flexor tone in the arms so that the child has to lift the shoulder to stabilize the head, at the same time rounding the upper part of the spine. By doing this the child has reinforced the hyperextension in the neck, making it difficult for the child to flex the head forward with the chin tucked in.

This posture of flexion in the upper part of the body may reinforce extension, adduction and internal rotation at the hips and legs.

If you have such a child, ask your therapist for a better method of getting your child from lying to sitting.

The child with fluctuating tone and involuntary movements

The child in Figure 11.54 is asymmetrical, the head and trunk control is poor and the child is unable to stabilize the shoulder and pelvic girdles. The child cannot reach forward with extended arms or maintain a sustained grasp.

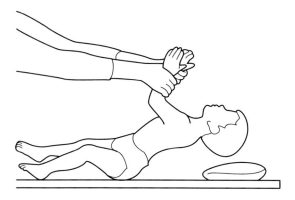

Figure 11.54 • A child with fluctuating tone and involuntary movements pulling up to sitting.

Pulling the child up to sitting by holding the child as shown has increased the extension of the neck and trunk and the retraction of the shoulders. This posture of extension of the upper part of the body may reinforce the hyperextension of the lumbar spine or the bottom of the spine and the posture of flexion, abduction and outward rotation at the hips and legs.

If you have such a child, ask your therapist for a better method of getting your child from lying to sitting.

Bouncing on the floor

Figure 11.55 illustrates how a typical child when bounced on the floor is normally able to keep the head in alignment and the arms forward. As the child is lifted into the air the child bends the legs, straightening them a little just before the feet touch the ground. Eventually as the child grows older the legs will straighten in the air and the feet will be in a position to take weight.

The child with stiffness and low truncal tone

To overcome the lack of extension the child in Figure 11.56 extends the head, chin poked forwards, arms flexed, shoulders protracted or forward and elbows back. The child does this to compensate for the poor truncal tone and lack of shoulder and pelvic stability. In an attempt to

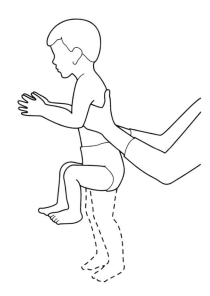

Figure 11.55 • A typical child being bounced on the floor.

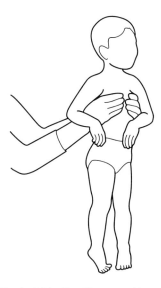

Figure 11.56 • A child with stiffness and low truncal tone being bounced on the floor.

get the feet on the ground, the child has to flex the hips, legs extended and feet plantarflexed. The child is consequently taking the weight on plantarflexed feet, that is, on the toes.

The child with fluctuating tone and involuntary movements

As shown in Figure 11.57, these children when lifted in the air may either draw their legs up into flexion or extend them and then when their feet touch the ground, unable to support their weight, they collapse. If in addition they have strong intermittent spasms, when their feet touch the ground they may extend their head, arms and trunk, standing momentarily on their toes, then collapse or make continuous stepping movements.

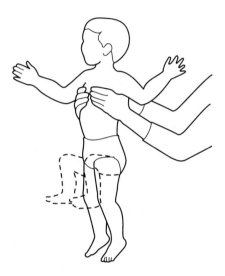

Figure 11.57 • A child with fluctuating tone and involuntary movements being bounced on the floor.

Baby bouncers

At around 7 months of age a typical young child when stood often starts to *bounce* by bending and straightening the legs. The child does so when standing on the parent's lap, in the cot or on the floor, holding on to acquire extra support and stability. If the child is put in a 'baby bouncer', because the child has good head and trunk control plus hip stability, the child is able to keep the head and body in alignment over mobile legs, putting the feet flat on the ground while bouncing. To a certain extent the child is in control of the bouncer and can stop and start bouncing at will.

The child with CP on the other hand has no such control and is therefore controlled by the movement of the bouncer itself, with any asymmetry of posture and movement accentuated.

The child with increased tone when taking weight on the toes will increase the tendency to extend, internally rotate and adduct the legs and the equinus position of the feet will be reinforced both in the air and when they come into contact with the ground.

The child with intermittent spasms and involuntary movements when the feet come into contact with the ground will either draw them both up in a total posture of flexion or draw one leg up in flexion with the other stiffly extending. The child is also likely to push the body back into extension.

I therefore do not recommend the use of baby bouncers for children with CP as the excitement, stimulation and movement may increase any abnormalities in postural tone and movement.

Kicking

When we talk and play with a young child who has CP and the child responds by kicking, we quite naturally want to encourage the child to continue doing so. I would, however, advise you to watch carefully to see the way the child kicks as it is easy without realizing it to reinforce an abnormal kicking posture.

Does the child, for example, kick with only one leg, or pull one leg up into flexion while at the same time pushing the other down into extension? When kicking with both legs, does the child extend them, internally rotating the hips and legs with the feet in plantarflexion or pointing the toes?

Your therapist will be able to show you ways of handling that encourage kicking while taking into account your child's particular problems.

Vigorous play

The majority of children love being thrown in the air and caught again, whirled round and round and joining in rough and tumble. But all parents need to exercise care so that they do not harm their children and are not accused of abuse. Shaking movements in particular are thought to cause harm. In addition the excitement of stimulation and movements in children with CP may cause fear and increase tone or involuntary movements.

Figures 11.58–11.60 illustrate ways of enabling a child with CP to enjoy this important aspect of rough play by controlling the child's postures.

Handling during routine activities

Bathing, dressing and undressing a typical child is normally comparatively easy as the child moves with you rather than against you. If, for example, you lift the child's arm or leg when bathing you will feel no resistance. When you put a tee-shirt on over the child's head the child will automatically

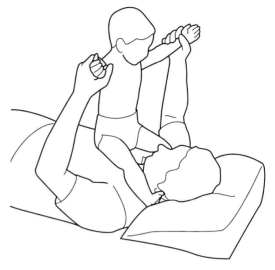

Figure 11.59 • To help the child keep the back straight and bend forward at the hips, as the father moves the child in different directions, he holds the child's hands with wrists extended and arms in extension and outward rotation.

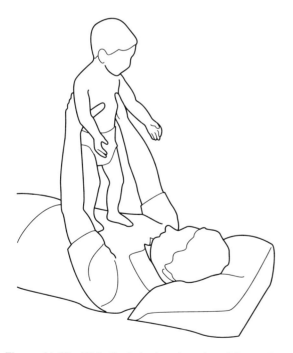

Figure 11.58 • While the baby bends and straightens the legs the father keeps the child's trunk in alignment and weight forward by keeping the child's shoulders up and the arms forward.

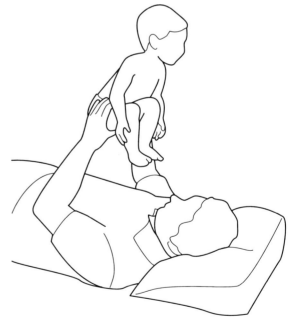

Figure 11.60 • To prevent the child pushing back as the father swings the child in the air, the father stabilizes the pelvis, keeping the hips flexed and weight forward.

push the head up through the opening. The child's natural self-protective reactions and the ability to balance when being handled enable the child to adjust position and, if uncomfortable, to move or alternatively push the mother away.

The child with CP, in contrast, often feels insecure when bathed, dressed and undressed. A child with increased tone and stiffness is limited in movements and is therefore unable to adjust when being moved. A child with intermittent spasms and involuntary movements, although more able to move, lacks stability. It is therefore important before dressing and undressing, for example, to make sure that the child is in a position in which the child feels secure and is symmetrical, that is, the head, trunk and pelvis are in alignment and the weight is evenly distributed. Suggestions of ways of doing this are discussed in the relevant chapters.

Once your child has achieved a new motor skill, make sure that you use every opportunity for the child to practise this skill during handling in everyday situations, during play times and when you are practising self-help tasks together.

Summary

When handling a child with CP one should:

1. Remember that physical, communication and intellectual skills cannot be learned in isolation.

2. Understand the reasons for a child's difficulties in moving and how these may vary.

3. Know how abnormalities of posture and movement may affect the whole body and which techniques of handling may minimize or change these difficulties.

4. Be sensitive to the changes under one's hands, taking away support as soon as it is no longer required.

5. Give a child every opportunity to practise any new skill achieved when handled in everyday situations.

6. Ensure that none of the handling techniques used can be interpreted as dangerous or abuse of the child.

7. Recognize the fact that there may not be any positive carry-over from handling when the hands and support are removed from the child.

Chapter Twelve

12

Sleeping

Jasia Beaumont

CHAPTER CONTENTS

Sleep is necessary for all of us. It refreshes and restores us and we function better, both mentally and physically, if we sleep well. Sleep disturbance in under-5-year-olds is very common and children with cerebral palsy (CP) are no different in this respect.

Their parents, too, have all the usual demands of parenthood plus the additional ones of having a child with CP; consequently the child with CP who does not sleep well presents parents with additional challenges. Having difficult nights is not easy for the child, and a lack of sleep usually means that parents are unable to get their rest and therefore they too may suffer. Exhaustion can worsen adult depression and lead to marital discord which will have adverse effects on the whole family. All in all, the child who does not have good, restorative sleep at night is at a disadvantage and so are the parents.

The child may appear overtired and miserable during the day and become easily upset. Concentration may be affected and behaviour difficult to manage. It is easy to presume that all of these problems are caused by the CP, and certainly to some extent this may be true, but a sleep-deprived child with CP will have even greater struggles with the condition and the ability to function.

Parents of a child with CP want to do all they can to maximize the potential of their child and improve the chances of their child leading a happy, fulfilled life. They are aware that their child's ability to learn, develop physically and function may be affected by the condition. Over time they are likely to realize that the child needs to come to terms with the disability, which may cause distress and even anger to the child. One thing that can have a positive effect on all of these factors is the child's ability to have good, regular sleep at night. It should, in addition, have positive effects on parents' own chances of sleeping well and so improve the quality of life for the whole family. The importance of sleep in a child with CP cannot be overestimated.

In this chapter we shall examine what happens to us when we sleep, considering some of the normal events that can happen during sleep which sometimes worry and concern parents, before moving on to explore ways of improving a child's sleep pattern if night-time difficulties have developed.

The process of sleep

We now know more about sleep and what happens to our bodies during sleep than we did 50 years ago, but there is still much to discover. If your child has difficulties with sleep, whether settling down at bedtime, during the night or early morning, it helps to have some knowledge about sleep.

Sleep is a complex process and not a state of nothingness. During sleep all sorts of events are happening to our bodies. Some of the brain activity can be shown on an electroencephalogram (EEG). The body's muscles may be observed visually, whether tense or relaxed. The regularity of the heart's function can be shown on an electrocardiogram (ECG). Whatever the actual functions of sleep are, we do know that it is vital for life.

Our brains produce a hormone called melatonin which helps us to fall asleep at the start of the night. It does not keep us asleep but helps to begin the sleeping process. We need to experience the daily contrasts of daylight and darkness for optimum melatonin production, so totally blind children may produce very limited amounts or no melatonin. It can be prescribed for short-term use

in conjunction with sensible evening and bedtime routines, but it is not a wonder drug. It does not work for everyone, and there are few reliable scientific studies to enable us to have a clear idea of the effect of its long-term use (Phillips and Appleton 2004). On a short-term basis, it may help to reset the body clock if a child's brain has become accustomed to falling asleep very late at night and then sleeping late into the morning. There are some suggestions that long-term use could possibly have an effect on the reproductive system. More information concerning treatment with melatonin can be found in Jan and Freeman (2004).

Our nightly sleep is divided up into stages and each stage seems to have a different purpose. These stages of sleep are described as rapid eye movement (REM) and non-REM sleep (Table 12.1). Certainly, different events occur according to which stage of sleep we are experiencing. We know that dreams usually happen during REM sleep. This is when the eyes can be seen moving beneath the closed eyelids. This is the stage during which our brain processes information and sorts out what has happened to us during the day. For children with CP this is an extremely important stage, as they may have even more to process and understand than typically functioning children. Our muscles are usually very relaxed during this stage, but with CP the muscles are more likely to be tense or in spasm.

Throughout the night we all pass through light sleep and down into deep sleep and then back

Table 12.1 Typical features of rapid eye movement (REM) and non-REM sleep

Features	REM sleep	Non-REM sleep
Electroencephalogram (EEG)	Low-voltage waves	Big slow waves
Eyes	Rapid eye movements	Quiescent eyes
Throat muscles	Relaxed	Tense
Possible associated behaviours	Nightmares	Sleep-walking

up to light sleep again. The brain regularly moves from one stage to another in well-organized cycles, each lasting between 50 and 90 minutes. One of the interesting things about the cyclical nature of sleep is that, as the brain moves up into light sleep, several times each night, it becomes partially awake. These small arousals are very short and most of us quietly drift back down to a level of deeper sleep. However they may be significant for parents as many worry about what it is that causes their child to come to wakefulness several times each night.

It can be reassuring to realize that it is the very nature of sleep itself that causes the momentary wakefulness and does not always signify that a child who wakes frequently is in pain or suffering some other upset. Of course the possibility of your child being unwell or uncomfortable must always be investigated and, if necessary, dealt with.

This may help parents to realize that children need to fall asleep in the same place where they have these partial wakenings or fully wake up. These arousals cannot be prevented. It can be made easier for your child to drift back down to a deeper level of sleep if your child sees his or her own bed and room in exactly the same state as when the child first settled down to sleep at bedtime. It is not difficult to see a connection between what happens at bedtime and where it happens, and what happens during the night.

Sleep-time events which may occur in any child

There are other events happening during specific stages of sleep over which we have little or no control. They are normal and part of the sleep process. Knowing about them can clarify exactly what is happening to your child at night and often point the way to dealing with them.

Sleep-talking, sleep-walking and tooth-grinding

Such events can occur in any child, usually during the first half of the night, rarely indicating that the child has a psychological problem. These problems often run in families and usually require no intervention from the medical profession. Children have been known to do bizarre things while sleep-walking and hurt themselves. It is therefore important that all measures are taken to ensure your sleep-walking child is safe and that any potentially dangerous objects (kitchen knives, house keys, etc.) are locked away each evening. Your child just needs to be guided calmly back to bed and not woken. There will be no memory of the event next morning, as your child was asleep while it was happening.

Talking in one's sleep and tooth-grinding often pass unnoticed and are of no great significance, rarely requiring intervention. Constant tooth-grinding that persists may indicate dental problems and require a visit to the dentist.

Nightmares

Children may cry out at night and the parent of a child with CP will want to ensure that it is not physical discomfort that is causing distress. Nightmares are unpleasant dreams that we all experience. They usually happen well on into the night or early in the morning. If your child is able to talk, your child will describe them, and be fearful of returning to sleep. Late-evening television may trigger them. Calm reassurance and attempting to reduce any obvious triggers are all that is necessary. Your child should be kept in bed, quietly and briefly reassured, and encouraged to settle back to sleep.

Night/sleep terrors

These are also events which may occur in any child, happening in sleep, and common in children under 7 years old. As the child appears very frightened and is difficult to comfort, night terrors can be very worrying for parents.

Typically, during the first part of the night, the child lets out a piercing scream. The child will be found sitting up in bed, or if unable to sit, lying down with eyes wide open, sweating and apparently frightened. The child will push the parent away and resist cuddling, generally appearing incoherent. A mobile child may try to leave the room. The whole event usually recurs at approximately the same time each night, and can cause distress for a parent, but the child will have no knowledge of it next morning.

There is a theory that night terrors occur as the brain is moving from very deep sleep into a light sleep. Some parts of the brain become almost awake, while others are still in deep sleep. Certainly the child is totally unaware of what is happening. Such terrors seem to be more frequent when the child is overtired.

Management of night/sleep terrors

1. Keep a record of the timing of the event for several weeks and work out the average time at which it happens.

2. Twenty to thirty minutes before the anticipated night terror, go in and gently wake your child. If possible, prepare your child during the day by saying that you are coming in to 'tuck you in'. Once your child acknowledges your presence, quietly and quickly kiss your child and leave so that your child can return to sleep.

3. This management seems to bypass the terror and needs to be repeated every night for at least 1 month.

4. If the terrors recur, a further month of anticipatory wakening may improve things.

5. If night/sleep terrors are infrequent, the only treatment necessary is to stay calmly near to your child without touching, but ensuring that your child does not hurt himself. The terrors rarely last longer than 20 minutes and then your child returns to quiet sleep. Your child is oblivious to the whole event, although the parent may feel quite wretched until the correct diagnosis and explanation are given. Most children outgrow night terrors, but if they persist and resist management, medical help should be sought.

Rolling, rocking and head-banging at sleep onset and during the night

Other sleep phenomena, common in any child under 5 years old, are rhythmic movement disorders. Children with some sort of damage to parts of their brain do seem slightly more susceptible to these rhythmic disorders. The child with CP may have only limited movement, so it may be difficult at first to be sure what is happening. If a child with CP frequently exhibits brief, regular, rhythmic movements prior to sleep, shows no sign of distress and then falls asleep, this phenomenon should be considered.

Side-to-side head movements, head-banging or upper-body rolling can be normal and may begin towards the end of the child's first year. Most movements are outgrown by around 7 years of age and actually seem to help the child relax into sleep. They may also occur during the night after a brief wakening.

Head-banging can be distressing and disturbing for a parent to witness and it is understandable that some parents presume that their child has a headache or is frustrated. Intervening to try to stop this behaviour often makes it worse, so padding the cot or headboard and, if necessary, the wall near the bed helps to prevent bruising. Fire-resistant padding must be used.

Parents may worry that head-banging will induce an epileptic seizure and often feel they must do something. Calm instructions to settle down, although difficult to do, should be all that is necessary. It is rare to see this behaviour in a child with severe CP, but this often normal behaviour is worth ruling out when dealing with a child who is not distressed but apparently restless in a regular fashion prior to sleep.

The behaviour usually ends with the child falling asleep, and often the more a parent gets involved, the longer it lasts. Ensuring that the child is safe and can come to no serious harm is paramount. It may be necessary to accept that short periods of rocking or head-rolling can lead to peaceful sleep. There is no current medical evidence of such behaviour on the part of the child causing serious, long-term injury, but bruising can occasionally occur.

Conditions associated with cerebral palsy which can affect a child's sleep

Children with CP may have a range of associated conditions. These conditions in themselves may not be the cause of poor sleeping but they often do not help. If any of these are present they cannot be ignored and need full investigation, monitoring and, if necessary, treatment. The associated conditions may make it difficult to achieve a good night's sleep, but once the condition is managed at an optimum level, such as through medication for seizure control, then good sleeping habits can begin to be established.

Breathing disturbances

Quiet, regular, relaxed breathing at night supplies the child with oxygen. The child who is a regular, persistent snorer, and who has long pauses in breathing and then gasps to restart breathing, will not be sleeping well. Floppy muscles in the throat may make it more difficult to breathe when asleep and enlarged adenoids can reduce the size of the airway. If loud snoring and gasping are nightly events, then requesting to see an ear, nose and throat surgeon for discussion concerning the possible removal of adenoids may be a first step towards improving the child's breathing at night. Children whose swallow is affected and who aspirate fluid into their lungs may also sleep badly and this situation needs to be addressed.

Seizures

The fear of having a seizure, the seizure itself and even the medication to control it may affect sleep. Epilepsy needs active management and both the child's and parents' fears are real and should not be ignored. Good communication between parents and medical staff, with time to ask questions, may allay parents' anxieties and lead to calmer management of night seizures. Not all night seizures can be prevented, but calm management will help your child return to sleep in his or her own bed after the seizure has passed. After one seizure, fear and anxiety that your child will continue to have repeated night-time seizures occur in many parents. Talking through every possibility with a doctor and/or nurse and planning how to manage the night-time seizures may be of great value. The parent may develop a calmer and more practical approach to night seizures, which may be

comforting for the child and enable the child to relax, sure in the knowledge that the parent will cope, that the child will be all right and that it is safe to try to return to sleep.

Problems connected with the digestive system

Reflux of the stomach contents into the oesophagus (the food pipe) causes pain and discomfort and can be worsened by lying down. Late-evening feeds or milky drinks at bedtime often set the problem off and if possible should be avoided. Medication and occasionally surgery can help and thus make a difference to the child's sleep as the child will no longer wake with pain 2–3 hours after falling asleep.

Difficulties remaining comfortable at night

During the night people move and change position and rearrange their limbs for maximum comfort. In the child with CP this ability may be compromised and cause the child to wake, or to sleep only lightly. Children with breathing difficulties at night also move their head, neck and trunk to enable them to breathe more efficiently. All of these movements can be difficult for the child with CP and affect both quality and quantity of sleep.

Management of sleeping positions

Unless for any special medical reason your child needs to be put down to sleep in a certain way, it is often best to encourage sleeping on the side until the child can roll over independently and choose the most comfortable position. This may, of course, not be possible with a child with CP either because it is too difficult to flex the child sufficiently to place the child on the side and once there the child may immediately extend, pushing on to the back, or because, lacking stability, the child just flops on to the back.

It is not suggested that you put your child to sleep in a position which, although good for the child, is uncomfortable, but, rather, that having observed the preferred sleeping position, you may then use supports or aids in order to reinforce the good aspects of the position and discourage the bad aspects, in this way hoping to minimize future problems. In the meantime it may be helpful to get the child accustomed to lying on the side during daytime activities.

Body position at night

Over the last 20 years much thought and awareness have developed concerning the physical positioning of the child with CP throughout a 24-hour period, particularly throughout the night (Goldsmith 2000). Daytime body positioning using special seating, limb and head supports and standing frames all help to keep the body in good alignment when the child is awake. Holding the body in correct positions and undertaking regular gentle limb exercises may help joints, bones and muscles to develop more correctly and may help to prevent the painful deformities which often occur (Pountney and Mandy 1999).

Current thinking is now focusing increasingly on positioning at night as well as during the day. Children may spend almost half the time lying in bed so good, comfortable positioning and postural support to keep the body properly aligned at night should be considered. A child with CP is likely to have abnormal muscle tone and may tend to lie in unusual positions. Legs may flop outwards or to one side, and the joints, bones and muscles may become fixed in abnormal positions. The vital internal organs may also become adversely affected.

Some of the more common positions that a child with CP can adopt and remain in, while lying in bed, are:

1. Holding the head to one side so that it is at an angle to the trunk.

2. Holding the hips and knees so that they turn inwards (Figure 12.1), outwards (Figure 12.2), or both to one side at an angle to the trunk (Figure 12.3).

3. Holding the whole body in an asymmetrical position or flexed forwards or extended backwards.

The child is not fully able to control the way the body positions itself and the asymmetrical

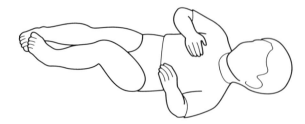

Figure 12.1 • Lying with hips and knees turned inwards.

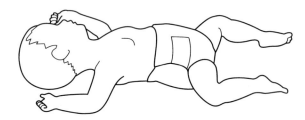

Figure 12.2 • Lying with hips and knees turned outwards.

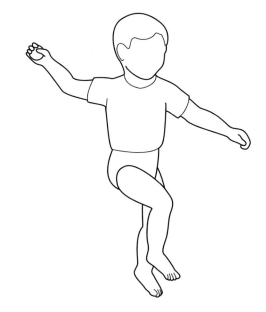

Figure 12.3 • Lying with hips and knees both turned to one side at an angle to the trunk.

postures, if maintained regularly throughout the night, can have long-term consequences for both body development and comfortable sleep. It is therefore helpful if the child is encouraged to lie in as symmetrical a position as is comfortable, with the head and limbs supported and positioned as near to normal as is reasonable for the condition. Figures 12.4 and 12.5 show a child lying in corrected side-lying positions using equipment.

There are systems commercially available to encourage symmetrical positioning which may help towards preventing destructive postures. The help and advice of a physiotherapist may be invaluable when working out what is best for the child, and what the body can safely tolerate and be comfortable with. Whatever position the child sleeps in, the child is likely to remain in it for long periods and may become stiff. A full sleep assessment undertaken by a paediatrician experienced in this field to avoid complications such as hypoxia is recommended before using sleep systems (Gericke 2006). If comfortable, warm and relaxed, the child is less likely to require parental attention during the night.

Severe sight and hearing problems

If a child's sight is so seriously affected that the child cannot distinguish light and dark, then the body clock may be affected. Regular bedtime routines, clear verbal messages and clothes plus soft toys kept just for bed all help your child realize it is sleep time. The body's own production of the night hormone melatonin may be reduced, so getting off to sleep can be a problem. Melatonin may be prescribed for short periods to help reset the child's body clock until the child learns the social cues associated with bedtime.

The severely deaf child who wears hearing aids during the day can feel isolated at night without them. Such a child cannot pick up the normal household sounds and feel reassured that he or she is not alone. Again, regular routines, familiar bedtime environments, a small night light and soft bedtime toys kept only for sleep time use can all help your child to know that it is night.

Daytime naps

The toddler with CP needs short naps to be able to get through the day, like any other toddler. Most children outgrow these naps around 3–4 years. The timing and the length of the nap can influence bedtime settling. Too long or too late a nap may mean that the child is not ready for bed by 7 or 8 p.m., but making the child go without a daytime nap often means that the overtired child is unable to relax and 'let go' at bedtime. Regular naps of

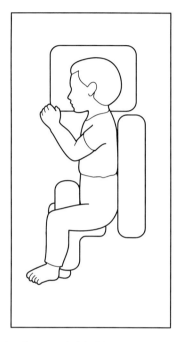

Figure 12.4 • Corrected side-lying position using fireproof foam rolls and pillows.

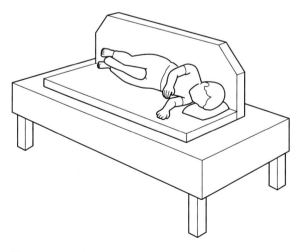

Figure 12.5 • Corrected side-lying position using a side-lying board.

Table 12.2 Average number of hours of sleep required by a typical child per 24 hours

Age in months	Average hours of sleep per night	Average hours of sleep during the day (on one or more occasions depending on age)
1	8.5	7
3	10	5
6	11	3.5
9	11	3
12	11.5	2.75
18	11.5	2.5
24	11.5	1.5
36	11	1
48	11.5	0
60	11	0

turn predominantly one way can be encouraged to look in the opposite direction towards the door or to a favourite toy. Figures 12.6 and 12.7 show bedroom layouts which may help your child to sleep well.

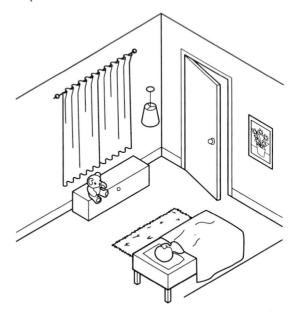

Figure 12.6 • A bedroom layout which may help your child to settle and sleep more easily.

about an hour that finish by early afternoon are beneficial to all toddlers (Table 12.2). Such naps need to be in their bed or cot to encourage even greater association with bed and sleep.

The bedroom

Children relax and sleep better in a bedroom that is warm, comfortable and well ventilated. It is tempting to fill it with bright colours, patterns and pictures of favourite cartoon characters but it is worth remembering that a room that is exciting and stimulating may not be conducive to sleep. If possible keep the decor fairly calm, using only two or three soft colours and try to provide as much storage as possible so that toys can be put away out of sight at bedtime. A well-organized bedroom with most toys put away before bathtime, low lighting and soft colours is a gentle reminder that playtime is over and it is time for sleep.

The bed itself needs careful positioning in the room if size allows. A child whose head tends to

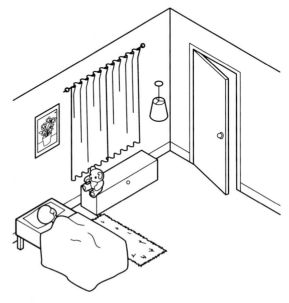

Figure 12.7 • A bedroom layout which may help your child to settle and sleep more easily.

The cot or bed

Cots and beds need to be big enough and have firm, supportive mattresses. Too soft a mattress will make it more difficult for the child to move and may cause discomfort. A full-length board beneath a very soft mattress can provide a cheap, effective solution. Safety is also an issue, particularly if the child makes large involuntary movements. Foam padding can be attached to cot sides but bed guards and padded headboards are preferable. The height of the bed or cot may need to be adjusted to enable carers to lift and manoeuvre the child comfortably and safely without strain to themselves. In the UK, social services and occupational therapists can advise and sometimes provide hoists and rails to facilitate transfer from wheelchair to bed. There are a number of devices available, according to age, weight and degree of disability. Occupational therapists are able to advise where these may be obtained.

Bed clothes

Parents will be aware that their child may be unable to throw off or pull on bed covers and sleep suits may help on cold nights. Light-weight, warm coverings that will not press heavily on limbs or trunk are the best.

Bedroom sharing

Lots of children share a bedroom with one or more siblings. This may help to establish close bonds between them. In addition it may provide an early-morning playmate and a reassuring presence during times of anxiety. Parents often worry about the disruption it may cause to the sleep of the other child if they need to attend to the child with CP. One way of managing possible disturbances is to be frank about the child's condition to the sibling and to discuss the likelihood of night-time intervention. These generalized, low-key conversations are best carried out during the day and the child is then prepared for any night-time event. Even very young children can pick up calm tones and manner when seizures and repositioning

are discussed openly and without anxiety. Every child needs to feel that their parents are in control and can cope. Two-way baby alarms and the now comparatively inexpensive home closed-circuit television (CCTV) systems can help parents monitor the children and provide reassurance to all.

Techniques which may help to prevent later sleep problems in any child

Sleep problems in young children often have their beginnings in what happens to the very young baby. Whether the diagnosis of CP is made early on in infancy or later, there are several useful techniques which may help prevent major sleep problems later. They can be slightly difficult for an inexperienced mother to use but if the reasons are explained and there is a supportive person around for encouragement, then they are certainly worth attempting and may pave the way for the development of good sleep habits:

1. Try to put your young baby down to sleep while still awake, albeit sleepy, at least three times in each 24 hours. It is tempting always to feed and hold your baby until he or she falls asleep in your arms, but this can lead to your baby never learning to go to sleep independently.

2. When your baby stirs in sleep, try to wait a few moments to see if your baby will resettle. Your baby may not always need feeding or nappy changing or comfort. This provides the baby with the chance to come to partial wakefulness then to return to sleep without help from a parent – a good skill to master for later on.

3. Try to settle your baby down in the room where he or she will eventually wake up. This prevents your baby from being startled on waking because surroundings have changed and encourages a sense of security. If your baby is calm, try not always to remain in the room until your baby is deeply asleep, but confidently and calmly leave your baby to settle alone.

4. If possible, try to create a clear difference between night and day. Night feeds can be done

quietly in a dimly lit bedroom and your baby can be calmly returned to the cot. Daytime feeding can be accompanied by light and family hubbub and often followed by a time for play and amusement.

These techniques apply to all babies, not just babies with CP. Over 50% of all children under 5 will experience sleep difficulties at some time, therefore it is worth encouraging good sleep habits from early on.

Optimizing the chance of a good night's sleep for a child with cerebral palsy

Feeling happily tired and sleepy at bedtime is a good way to maximize the chances of everyone having a restful night. To achieve comfortable tiredness the child's daytime activities need to be considered. The child needs to be able to explore, to be stimulated and to interact with loving people. Everything that can be done to enable the child to move, stretch, reach, sit up and play needs to be encouraged. Good postural management may enable the child to play and do more and so use up energy, as well as giving your child a real sense of achievement. Towards the end of the first year, if physically able, your child should have very short periods of playing alone, either in a supportive chair or on the floor, with a parent nearby. Encouraging your child to enjoy his or her own company for brief periods during the day, within the familiar home environment, is a good preparation for being alone at night. Your child should also learn to wait by not having all needs met instantly. Parents can respond verbally but hold back for a few moments before retrieving a lost toy or getting a drink. These are very small tasks, but enable the child to develop a degree of independence and self-reliance which will help the child cope during the night. Later on, attending playgroups where difficulties are accepted and children are encouraged to participate at their own level may improve their feelings of independence and self-worth. It also helps parents to realize that other people can share in the care of their child and that their child

can survive happily for a short time without them. This developing confidence in both the child and parents will help to improve the likelihood of achieving peaceful bedtimes and nights.

Evening routines

Children need to know the order of the day and what is likely to happen next, and children with CP are no exception. A calm, regular evening routine that the child understands and accepts helps to achieve a feeling of security.

Suggested bedtime routine

1. An evening meal followed by playtime, possibly involving both parents and siblings.

2. Busy play can lead on to quiet, calm play, preferably without the family TV being on.

3. Some indicator that playtime is over – perhaps a small drink on dad's lap, or evening medication.

4. Bathtime. This can be a lovely time for your child as the water is relaxing and supportive to disordered limbs. There is a whole range of special supports and seats to enable your child to be well supported and to prevent back strain in parents. Bathtime will then become a particularly special and enjoyable end to the day.

5. Drying and dressing should preferably be done in the child's bedroom. Going back into the living room gives the wrong message to your child, as your child has just been playing there. This time of drying and putting on nightclothes can be very enjoyable for you and your child and can include cuddles and hugs and even a short massage.

6. Position your child comfortably and symmetrically in the bed.

7. Read a short story or spend time with a picture book, with the parent sitting close to, but not on, the bed.

8. All lights need to be very low and the room previously tidied of toys that stimulate. No TV, video or music. This is a room for sleep now, not play and activity.

9. You then leave your child to settle alone or sit in the darkened room and calmly ignore your child. This is not the time for questions, discussions or any conversations, just 'time to sleep'.

If you decide to remain in the child's room until the child is asleep then, over a period of weeks, your chair can be moved gradually nearer and nearer to the bedroom door and eventually out on to the landing. This teaches your child that he or she can go off to sleep with you at a distance and eventually, out of sight. Your child is not abandoned and left to cry but calmly and lovingly ignored and expected to fall asleep.

Night waking

As mentioned earlier, all children wake at night for brief moments. It is easy to presume that for your child with CP it is because the child is uncomfortable or unwell. If this is so, then the cause needs to be established and dealt with. If there is no apparent reason for waking, your child should be gently reminded that it is dark, quiet and still night. Your child can be left to resettle, as at bedtime. If a parent is still remaining in the room at bedtime, this method will need to be repeated. Providing yourself with a comfortable chair and blankets makes this more bearable and the temptation to carry your child into the parental bed can be resisted. Your child should learn that, whatever happens, your child will remain in his or her own room at night.

Even when interaction is necessary, such as during a seizure or painful muscle spasm, your child can be dealt with in his or her own room and encouraged to return to sleep once the event has passed. Any treatment or repositioning can be done with your child remaining in bed and should be regarded as an interruption to the night's sleep, not the end of it. Dealing with night-time interruptions quietly and with a minimum of fuss

teaches the child that there is nothing to be anxious about. Parents will cope and everyone can return to sleep. Room-sharing siblings can learn to sleep through such events. The next morning the event of the previous night can be mentioned, with no overlay of anxiety or emotion and the child and siblings will begin to learn to come to terms with it. Dealing with established sleep problems takes a lot of hard work and demands even greater effort from parents who are already tired. It helps if one can enlist support from a professional who knows you and your child and who has some experience of this sort of night-time management.

Choosing a good time to start making changes is very important. When you and your child are both well and the family is in a relatively stable phase is best. You should then plan how to tackle the problems. Try to enlist some extra daytime support and help for yourself. Begin with establishing the suggested bedtime routine and plan each stage clearly. Write down your plan and how you will cope with unexpected events, such as your child being sick. Involve helpful friends and family to support both you and your child. Try reviewing your progress at weekly intervals as improvements take time and it is easy to become disheartened. Above all, do not give up. The idea that your child has sleep difficulties because of CP and that therefore nothing can be done is unreasonable and you do not have to resign yourself to such a conclusion. There is almost always something that can be changed to improve your child's sleep. You may not achieve perfection, but you can improve on the current situation. Your child will still have CP but by improving the night's sleep you know that you are doing all you can to assist the child's development and your enjoyment as a parent.

References

Gericke T. et al. Postural management for children with cerebral palsy: consensus statement. Dev Med Child Neurol 2006; 48:244.

Goldsmith S. The Mansfield project. Postural care at night within a community setting. Physiotherapy 2000; 86:10.

Jan JE, Freeman RD. Melatonin therapy for circadian rhythm sleep disorders in children with multiple disabilities: what

have we learnt in the last decade? Dev Med Child Neurol 2004; 46:776–782.

Phillips L, Appleton RE. Systematic review of melatonin treatment in children with neurodevelopmental disabilities and sleep impairment. Dev Med Child Neurol 2004; 46:771–775.

Pountney T, Mandy A. Postural management and clinical effectiveness. Association of Paediatric Chartered Physiotherapists, London, 1999.

Further reading

Durand VM. Sleep better, 1998. Paul Brookes, Baltimore, 1998.

Martin P. Counting sheep. Flamingo, London, 2003.

Quine L. Solving children's sleep problems. Beckett and Karlson, Peterborough, 1997.

Stores G, Wiggs L. Sleep disturbance in children and adolescents with disorders of development: its significance and management. Cambridge University Press, Cambridge, 2001.

Chapter Thirteen

Feeding

Helen Cockerill

The complexity of the skills involved in eating and drinking is not immediately obvious because it is such a commonplace activity. It is an activity of daily life we take for granted until its development is disrupted. As a disorder of posture and movement, cerebral palsy (CP) can result in significant feeding difficulties. The management of eating and drinking difficulties may require the involvement of several professionals, including doctors, speech and language therapists, dieticians and physiotherapists. Parents are usually the main care-givers of a young child with CP and are therefore the key players in this area of development.

Feeding is a skill involving several body systems: it depends on intact anatomy; control and coordination of the muscles involved in sucking, biting, chewing and swallowing; sensory perception; gut function; heart and lung support; and neurological integration of all these different aspects.

Food is also central to family and cultural life. Early feeding can be an emotional experience for both parents and children. Although feeding can involve closeness and opportunities for positive communication, it can also be a potential battleground. Up to two-thirds of parents of typically developing toddlers report feeding problems, e.g. eating too little, restricted diets, difficult behaviour at mealtimes. With additional problems due to CP this can make mealtimes unhappy experiences. However, most parents become highly skilled in feeding their child with CP, achieving safe feeding, good nutrition and helping the child develop skills to the best of the child's ability.

Developmental stages: early breast- or bottle-feeding

Feeding in infants is largely driven by the reflexes that are present at birth. Although there is some refinement over the first few weeks of life, most children born at term can feed well enough to gain weight and grow. Some of the reflexes involved include *rooting* (turning towards stimulation around the mouth, which is helpful in finding the nipple or teat), *sucking* (on nipple/teat/finger/dummy placed in the mouth) and *gagging* (if things are placed beyond the front of the mouth, thus preventing foreign bodies entering the airway). The feeding of very small children generally shows strong rhythmic cycles: they usually suck, swallow and then breathe at a rate of around 1 cycle per second. As they mature they may adopt a suck–suck–swallow–breathe rhythm.

Children who are born prematurely may also establish good feeding from 32 weeks' gestation onwards. There is some evidence that children's skills mature significantly between 34 and 40 weeks' gestation, so some premature children need time to develop their skills. Until skills mature they may need tube feeding: usually nasogastric tube feeding, i.e. a tube is passed into the nose, through the throat and gullet, and into the stomach (see Figure 13.9a, page 160).

For many young children with CP early feeding is unproblematic as it depends primarily on infant reflexes. Some young children with neurological problems will show poor coordination of the suck–swallow–breathe cycle, resulting in coughing, tears in the eyes, reddening of the face, irregular breathing patterns, flaring of the nostrils, pulling away from the nipple and dribbling of the feed.

The swallowing mechanism

In order to understand the possible risk involved if a child has swallow coordination difficulties it may be helpful to understand the complexity of the swallowing mechanism. Figure 13.1 includes the main parts of the anatomy involved in swallowing.

When a young child sucks on the breast (or bottle) the child holds the nipple in the mouth, grooving the tongue around it. The child also uses the lips to create a seal against the breast or wider part of the teat. When the child pulls the tongue backwards and upwards within the mouth, this draws milk from the nipple. The milk enters the valleculae and this triggers the swallow. The swallow involves highly coordinated sets of movements, including lifting the larynx (voice box), closing the vocal folds in the larynx, pulling down the epiglottis, lifting the soft palate (to stop milk going up into the nose), opening the sphincter at the top of the oesophagus (gullet) and squeezing

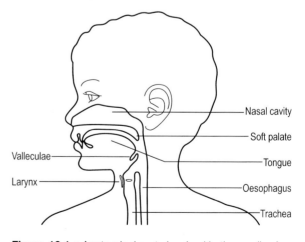

Figure 13.1 • Anatomical parts involved in the swallowing mechanism.

the pharynx (throat) so that the milk enters the oesophagus (gullet) and not the trachea (windpipe). Immediately after the swallow the child breathes out, again protecting the airway. All these movements happen quickly and automatically. Occasionally children with CP have specific problems with swallow coordination, resulting in the risk of aspiration (milk going the wrong way, into the windpipe, and possibly down into the lungs). Excessive coughing during feeding or bubbly-sounding during breathing or after feeds may indicate the need for professional assessment of swallow safety by a speech and language therapist.

Managing early feeding problems

There is a range of simple techniques that can help children with CP who are struggling with one or more aspects of early feeding.

Positioning

Typically developing children are often fed in a semi-reclined position, but become more upright as they develop head control. Children with good suck–swallow–breathe coordination are able to protect their airway in this position. Children with CP who have poor coordination may be helped by more upright but supported positioning. Because children give subtle signals of being uncomfortable or stressed, ideally the feeder should be able to see the child's face. This can be achieved by propping the child on a pillow in a semi-upright position, facing the feeder, or in side-lying (Figure 13.2).

Jaw support

Supporting the child's jaw, by placing a finger under the bony point of the chin, may assist more effective tongue movement and help lip seal on the teat. Additional cheek support may also improve sucking (Figure 13.3).

Pacing

Giving the child a few seconds' break to recover breath every few sucks may help to maintain breath

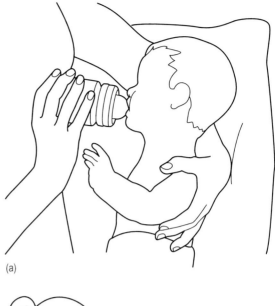
(a)

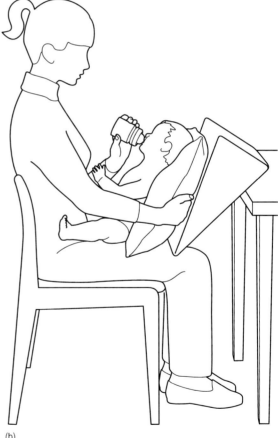
(b)

Figure 13.2 • (a) Side-lying; (b) facing the feeder.

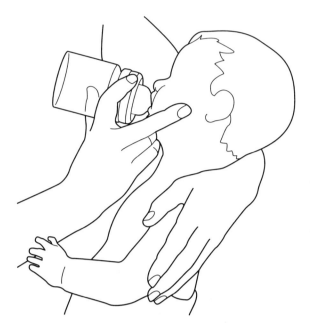

Figure 13.3 • Jaw and cheek support.

support for feeding. It may be necessary to remove the teat or break the seal on the nipple by slightly opening the child's mouth. Many children learn to take a break independently by pulling away.

Thickener

Thickening the feed may help it move more slowly through the child's mouth, giving the child time to organize a safe swallow, and avoid coughing. Advice on this should be sought from a speech and language therapist.

Supplementation

Children who are not achieving their required intake can be supported by concentrating the feeds so they gain maximum energy intake for minimum effort. A dietician will be able to advise on appropriate feeds.

Cup feeding

Some children who have difficulty with sucking may benefit from the introduction of a cup. This is a common technique in some Asian countries for children who are unable to breast-feed, and is increasingly used in special care child units to give children expressed breast milk until breast-feeding is established.

Positive oral experience

If children are tube-fed, have reflux or are experiencing difficulty with oral feeding, it may be necessary to counterbalance negative experience with positive touch around the face and mouth. Stroking the face, working towards the mouth, kissing the face and mouth, and (if the child will tolerate it) letting the child chomp or suck on the parent's finger can all help the child understand that oral experience can be enjoyable. This will help to avoid later problems with hypersensitivity and teeth cleaning.

Gastro-oesophageal reflux

'Gastro-oesophageal reflux' is the term used when stomach contents come up into the oesophagus (gullet). Because stomach contents are acidic this can cause discomfort and pain. All young children will have some reflux and it will not cause problems. More severe reflux is particularly common in premature children and may also be seen in children with CP. Not all children who experience reflux will show overt vomiting. Other signs include crying and discomfort after feeds, arching, pulling the knees up to the tummy or sudden waking. Prolonged vomiting can compromise growth and weight gain. Children who have severe reflux may become reluctant to feed because they associate feeding with pain. It is therefore very important to limit reflux: some parents find that careful positioning after feeding, either in a semi-upright supported posture or in side-lying, may help reduce the effects of reflux. Small frequent feeds may be more comfortable than large feeds. Some children require medication to control reflux.

Introduction of semi-solid food

At around 4–6 months of age smooth purée is introduced to most children. In order to cope with the new texture the child must change the oral-motor pattern. When sucking, the tongue moves back and forth in the mouth. Initially a child will use the same pattern for solids and so food is pushed out of the mouth. The child consequently starts to use a different tongue action. The child also learns to time the mouth opening as the spoon approaches, and then uses the top lip to remove the food from the spoon. All these skills involve moving away from infantile reflexes and the development of voluntary control of the muscles involved in eating.

Most children with CP make the transition to a puréed diet easily. Others take time to develop appropriate oral-motor skills for this texture. If a child has struggled with breast- or bottle-feeding, it may be suggested that solids should be delayed until sucking has been mastered. However, unless there are specific medical reasons, the introduction of solids should not be delayed. Some children manage purée better than fluids, as the level of coordination required is different. The introduction of solids may also reduce gastro-oesophageal reflux.

Positioning

In typically developing children the transition to solids coincides with increased head control and the development of sitting skills. Oral-motor skills develop alongside other motor skills, particularly shoulder, neck and jaw stability. Consequently, children with delayed gross motor development will require additional postural support at mealtimes to facilitate oral-motor skills.

Support may be needed to help the child move from a semi-reclined position towards a more upright position. Some parents are able to achieve a good position with the child on the lap, but this becomes more difficult as the child grows and gains weight. In order to maintain flexion in the child's hips (and so prevent the child pushing back) it will be necessary for the parent to have one leg slightly higher than the other; to achieve a good trunk position for the child it may also be necessary for the parent to have additional arm support (Figure 13.4a).

Alternatives to sitting sideways on the lap include a wedge or V-shaped cushion against a table or wall, with the child facing the parent. Some car seats or child bouncers can achieve a similar position (Figure 13.4b).

A highchair may be a possibility, although extra support may be needed to prevent the child falling to the side. A lap strap may help the child to keep the hips flexed, so providing a stable base for sitting, and avoiding extensor spasms. Some children will be provided with specialized seating systems by their physiotherapist or occupational therapist for eating and drinking.

A general principle when positioning a child for feeding is to prevent the child pushing back into extension. When children arch their back their neck falls backwards: in this position it is more difficult to control food in the mouth, swallowing is more difficult, the airway is open and the risk of food or drink being aspirated is increased. Instead, the back of the neck should be elongated to facilitate oral-motor skills and increase swallow safety.

In addition to considering the mechanics of eating and drinking, an upright posture with face-to-face contact will help communication between parent and child at mealtimes.

Jaw support

Additional support for the child's jaw can help the development of the more mature tongue movements for eating solid foods. This can be provided by a parent from the side, or from the front. The fingers can be placed to support both the jaw and lips. It may take a child some time to tolerate this level of touch at mealtimes. As the child's skills develop, jaw support can be reduced (Figure 13.5).

Spoons

A small, shallow-bowled spoon will be most appropriate to help the child remove the food from the spoon though lip closure, without having to scrape off the foods against the child's gums or teeth. Applying gentle, firm pressure downwards on the tongue can help some children achieve better lip closure, and avoid forward tongue movement. A finger on the child's top lip may help to

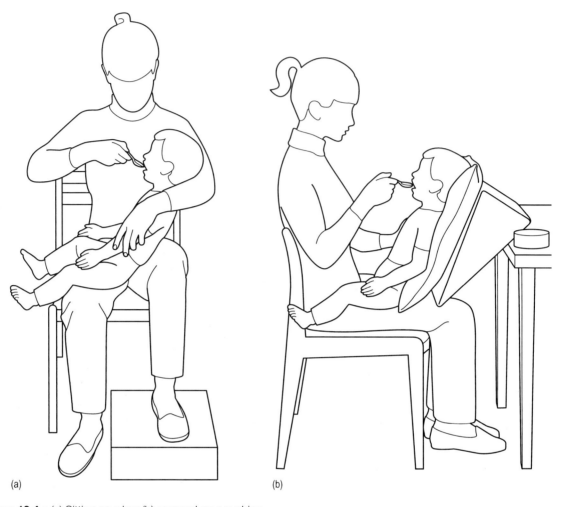

(a)

(b)

Figures 13.4 • (a) Sitting on a lap; (b) propped on a cushion.

bring the lip down to assist in removing the food from the spoon.

Some children with CP have a strong bite reflex, i.e. an uncontrolled strong jaw closing when anything is placed in the mouth, therefore a rubber or plastic child's spoon may be necessary. Bite reflexes may be inhibited though flexed positioning and desensitization programmes (see below).

Cup drinking

Children may be offered sips of fluid from a cup or spouted beaker from the age of 6 months. This is a skill that should be promoted in children with CP

as some children have difficulty moving on from reflex-driven sucking to the sipping action required for cup drinking. It is generally felt that prolonging the infantile suck may inhibit the development of more mature oral-motor skills. For children who have struggled with inefficient sucking, moving to sip-feeding using a cup may be more successful.

Initially, drinks may need thickening so they move more slowly, giving the child time to organize a safe swallow. This is particularly relevant if the child has some difficulty holding the fluid in the mouth by lifting the back of the tongue, and controlling the flow into the throat. For some children thickener can be reduced as drinking skills improve.

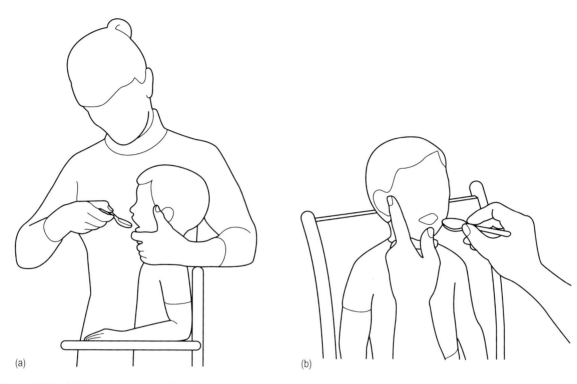

Figure 13.5 • (a) Jaw support from the side; (b) jaw support from the front.

For others, who continue to have poor oral control, it may be an ongoing requirement.

Progress in cup drinking depends largely on jaw stability and independent tongue movement. For children who are acquiring these skills slowly, external jaw support (with or without lip support) provided by the carer may be needed. This aspect of carer involvement should be considered when assessing a child's seating needs at mealtimes: the chair or standing frame and tray/table must allow the carer to provide appropriate support without compromising the carer's own posture and comfort. For this reason, review of seating systems to be used at mealtimes should be a joint undertaking, involving parents, physiotherapists, occupational therapists and speech and language therapists.

Developing chewing skills

Before typically developing children move on to the lumpier food textures, they have already engaged in a great deal of oral exploration. From the age of 4–5 months children tend to put everything into their mouths, and it is possible that this experience is necessary to allow the child to move on from purée and fluids, to more challenging textures that require differentiated tongue movements. A child with CP may not be able to pick up and transfer objects to the mouth, and consequently may be missing necessary sensory input. Parents should be aware of this potential need and help to provide the child with appropriate oral experience. It may be necessary to provide positive touch actively on the face and around the mouth through kissing and stroking, letting the child chomp on the carer's finger, supporting the child in bringing his or her own fingers to the mouth and holding teething toys for the child to chew on. This type of positive touch is particularly important if the child has had negative oral experience from reflux or invasive treatments such as ventilation or nasogastric tube use (Figure 13.6).

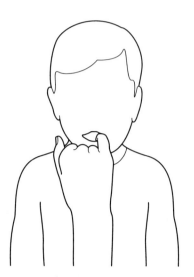

Figure 13.6 • Providing positive touch.

Lumpy purée is usually introduced to typically developing children at around 7 months of age. This stage of feeding may be problematic for a child with CP, particularly if there has been a history of gastro-oesophageal reflux: this can cause extreme hypersensitivity to texture and may result in gagging and a reluctance to feed. Also, more mature tongue movements are required for this texture. Children must learn to prepare the food so it is sufficiently smooth to swallow. Initially, children use a crude munching action that involves the jaw and tongue moving together to squash the lumps, before reverting to a suckle pattern to swallow the food. Gradually, the tongue movements become more refined and the food is moved around the mouth, using less jaw action and more controlled tongue movements. This enables children to move through the stages of soft-chew foods to foods of increasing firmness, moving towards the rotary chewing pattern that is required for chewy food such as meat.

Some children with CP who struggle with this texture may need to avoid the lumpy purée stage and instead move towards chewing through the introduction of bite-and-dissolve or bite-and-melt foods. Many popular snack foods are of this texture and so can be used for practice. Placing small pieces of food to the side of the child's mouth,

along the line of the jaw, can stimulate munching movements in the jaw and lateral (side-to-side) movements of the tongue.

For children who cannot cope with pieces of food in the mouth, that is, they continue to use a sucking pattern and so gag or cough on foods that are inadequately prepared for swallowing, an intermediate stage of chewing practice may be necessary. Pieces of chewable food can be placed in a pouch made of thin cotton using a moist handkerchief and then positioned along the jaw line within the mouth to stimulate chomping and lateral tongue movement, without having to swallow. A speech and language therapist who specializes in feeding difficulties can advise on the appropriateness of such techniques (Figure 13.7).

Once a child can cope with lumps, finger foods are typically introduced. Foods such as breadsticks, toast, thin sticks of cooked vegetables and lumps of cheese are offered to children to mouth. Again, a typically developing child tends to use a combination of chomping and sucking when making the transition from soft to chewable foods. A child with CP may also be able to progress through such textures, although may need help with holding the foods. However, some children do not make this transition as they do not have

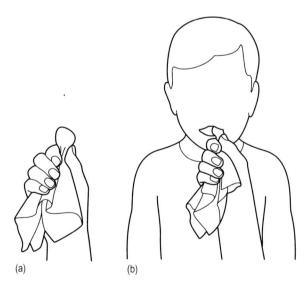

(a) (b)

Figures 13.7 • (a and b) Chewing practice, using a food pouch.

adequate oral-motor skills to deal with such textures safely: an inability to adapt to the challenge may result in choking and possible aspiration. A child with a bite reflex may be able to bite off pieces of food, but then produce only a sucking response so that the food is not adequately prepared for swallowing.

Postural management

Eating and drinking skills develop alongside changes in a child's gross motor skills; that is, as the child acquires head control and sitting balance, oral-motor skills also change. When the usual pattern of development is disturbed by CP it is often necessary to compensate through the use of seating and other postural management systems. Tensions can arise as a result of the need to develop both gross motor skills and oral-motor skills for eating and drinking. Parents may be advised that too much postural support can prevent a child developing head control or sitting balance. However, at mealtimes, if such postural support is lacking, it can have negative consequences for safe and efficient eating and drinking. A child who is struggling to maintain sitting balance will not be able to manage food within the mouth as effectively as the child who is given additional trunk support.

For efficient eating a young child should have a stable base, with the bottom on a supportive surface, with symmetrical hips flexed at 90° or less, feet on a flat surface (but not able to push back), sufficient trunk posture to ensure shoulder stability and independent head control. If a child with CP is not able to achieve these requirements independently, supportive seating (or an alternative such as a standing frame) should be provided, with hands-on support as necessary.

Nutrition

All children are monitored to check growth and weight gain. Historically it was expected that children with CP would remain small, but with developments in nutrition and dietetics it is now anticipated that most children should show adequate growth and weight gain. Although for the

health of both the child and for those who need to lift and handle the child, it is clearly undesirable that children with CP should be overweight, it cannot be considered ethical to restrict a child's growth in order that the child remains easy to lift. Keeping a child underweight will have a negative impact on the development of motor skills, the ability to fight infections and general well-being. Children with CP who are underweight may also have cold hands and feet, and may even sleep poorly.

Health visitors and doctors usually plot an individual child's height and weight on a growth chart. Obviously, not all children are the same weight and height, and so the centile lines on the growth charts represent the range that would be expected in the population. The 50th centile represents the weight where 50% of children of a particular age would be heavier, and 50% would be lighter. Weights and heights between the 9th and the 90th centile are considered to be within the average range. A child's growth and weight gain are related to size at birth and genetic factors in addition to maintaining an appropriate balance between nutritional intake and energy expenditure. The applicability of the standard growth charts to children with CP is not fully understood; however the majority of children would be expected to show a steady pattern of growth and weight gain, in proportion with each other, along centile lines within the average range. Specific weights at any one point in time are less important than the trend over time.

In children with CP there may be tension between feeding to maintain adequate growth and weight gain, and developing motor skills. From a developmental point of view it is desirable that a child should learn to sit, to self-feed and to move on from bite-and-dissolve foods to soft-chew and firmer foods. However, reducing the degree of postural support at mealtimes may result in less efficient feeding (as the child tries hard to maintain balance) and in turn this may lead to prolonged mealtimes or reduced food intake. Similarly, learning to self-feed may be more time-consuming, and so reduce intake. Studies of children with CP, compared with typically developing children, have demonstrated it can take up to 12 times longer to manipulate and swallow the same amount of purée, and up to 15 times longer to chew and swallow solid food (Gisel and Patrick 1988). As it is not realistic or desirable to extend mealtimes by such proportions this has significant implications for growth and weight in children with CP.

Self-feeding

As children develop they take an increasing part in feeding themselves. Between 6 and 9 months they learn to hold their own bottles and like to touch food and bring it to the mouth. They move on to a spouted cup and after 12 months control of the spoon gradually improves so that is not turned over as it approaches the mouth. Finger foods are held competently. Typically developing children become independent for spoon feeding by around 18 months. They can also drink independently from an open cup.

In order to help children with CP move through these stages, varying degrees of postural support may be needed. Some children will achieve independent feeding, but this may be dependent on appropriate seating (or standing frame). The height of the tray or table can make the difference between successful self-feeding and continued dependence. The table/tray should be high enough to provide a stable surface on which a child can rest the elbows when bringing a spoon to the mouth. For children who have difficulty grasping and manipulating the spoon, specific hand-over-hand assistance can be provided and then gradually withdrawn as motor control improves. Assisted eating for part of a meal or snack may help to develop functional skills, without compromising nutrition.

Some children achieve independence through the use of specialized equipment such as angled spoons, scoop plates and a NeaterEater. This type of equipment is typically provided by an occupational therapist (Figure 13.8).

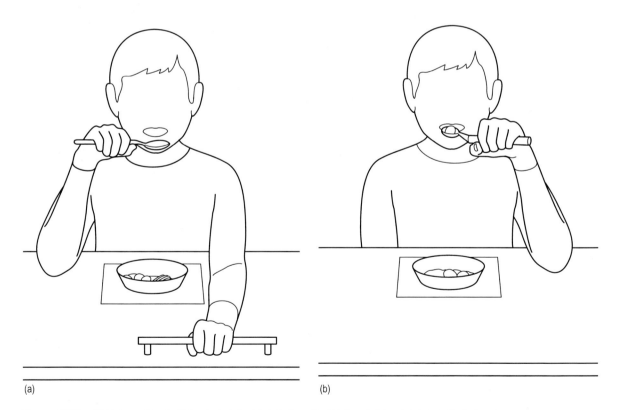

(a)   (b)

Figure 13.8 • (a) Using a hand rail for support and a mat under the bowl; (b) using an angled spoon.

Swallow safety

Most children with CP have a safe swallow, and feeding does not carry the risk of aspiration. However, a minority will have difficulties at the swallowing stage of eating and drinking. This is something that can change over time: children who have coped well can run into difficulties as they get older because of changes to the anatomy of the mouth and throat, or changes in postural ability. Signs of difficulty at the swallowing stage can include coughing, eyes watering, colour changes in the face, wet-sounding voice after eating or bubbly breathing during or after eating. Any such signs should be taken seriously, and a detailed assessment of swallow safety carried out by a speech and language therapist.

The therapist will carry out careful observation of eating and drinking (sometimes using a structured assessment; see Appendix 1). Listening to a child's swallow, using a stethoscope placed on the child's neck (cervical auscultation), can also provide information about the timing and efficiency of the swallow. Some children with particularly severe difficulties may require an X-ray swallow study (videofluoroscopy) to investigate swallow difficulty in greater detail. Such studies are carried out in hospital X-ray departments, usually by a specialist therapist. This requires a medical referral to a specialist service. Parents are usually involved in the study and are able to view the X-ray of their child's swallow, with the findings and implications for oral feeding being fully explained.

For many children any risk of food or drink going the wrong way, into the lungs, can be managed through careful positioning, with particular attention to the angle of the head and neck. Other strategies can include modifying food textures, such as purée rather than lumpy food, or thickened rather than thin, fast-moving fluids.

Supplementary/non-oral feeding

If a child is growing and gaining weight very slowly, and parents or medical staff are concerned about the child's nutritional status, a dietician may be able to provide support. Because of a slow rate of eating, a high-calorie diet may be recommended. Maximizing energy intake, whilst minimizing the effort required for feeding, through the use of calorie-laden foods may be sufficient to improve growth and weight gain. This may be achieved through simple measures such as adding butter, cream or cheese to foods, and selecting the highest-calorie desserts in the supermarket. Alternatively, supplements can be prescribed such as specially formulated drinks or desserts that are high-calorie and include additional nutrients. Again, dieticians can advise and request prescriptions via the child's general practitioner.

Despite the best efforts of parents, some children require non-oral feeding. This option may be considered in two main circumstances: (1) where oral feeding carries the risk of aspiration; or (2) when a child is unable to meet nutritional needs entirely through oral feeding. This may be a temporary or more permanent situation. Non-oral feeding may be suggested as an augmentative measure where the child continues to eat and drink as usual, but with additional tube feeds.

There are several options for non-oral feeding:

1. *Nasogastric tube* – a tube from the nose to the stomach. Very young infants may have a nasogastric tube until oral feeding is established. Older children may have a tube as a temporary measure during a severe illness. It is physically possible to eat and drink whilst a nasogastric tube is in place, but the tube can stimulate the gag reflex, leading to hypersensitivity, even when the tube is no longer present. Inserting the tube is very unpleasant for the child and it can contribute to aversive responses to oral stimuli, including food. It is not considered to be a good long-term option (Figure 13.9a).

2. *Gastrostomy.* This is inserted through the abdominal wall and into the stomach and so requires surgical placement. It has the advantages of being hidden under the child's clothing, and avoiding unpleasant stimulation of the nose and throat. It can also be removed, with rapid healing, if the tube is no longer required. It has the disadvantages of requiring surgery and, in some children, of increasing the risk of gastro-oesophageal reflux. Parents worry that the child may pull the tube out, and although this is very

rare, it would mean a trip to hospital for a tube change. In the past many children also had an operation to tighten the sphincter at the top of the stomach (a fundoplication) at the same time as a gastrostomy, but this is now a less common procedure (Figure 13.9b).

3. *Jejunostomy* – a tube inserted into the jejunum (below the stomach), usually though a gastrostomy. This is used to bypass the stomach if a child has very severe reflux or other stomach problems.

As children's feeding skills change over time, the possible indications for non-oral feeding may also change from infancy to adulthood. Some of the factors that may contribute to consideration of non-oral feeding include:

1. Poor suck–swallow–breathe coordination in infancy
2. Chronic lung disease (sometimes as a consequence of prematurity)
3. Prolonged reliance on nasogastric tube feeding
4. Difficulty meeting nutritional needs because of inefficient eating patterns
5. Epileptic seizures that interrupt time for oral feeding
6. Loss of infant reflexive feeding skills, with poor development of voluntary control
7. Swallowing difficulties leading to recurrent chest infections
8. Inability to meet energy needs to sustain growth and weight gain by the oral route alone
9. Prolonged mealtimes
10. Limited fluid intake, resulting in constipation and dehydration
11. Increasing number of feeders in school who are not as skilled as parents
12. Requirement to boost nutrition prior to bony surgery
13. Poor circulation
14. Compromised ability to recover from illnesses

In young children non-oral feeding may be a temporary measure, to be reversed as skills develop. In some children it is used only for fluids, for

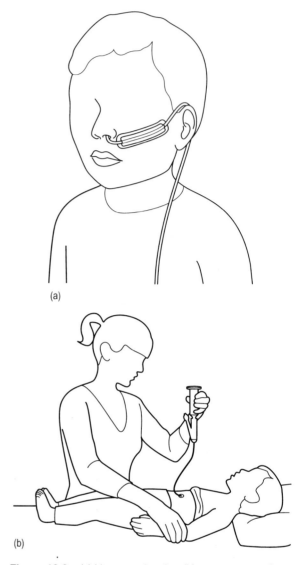

Figure 13.9 • (a) Nasogastric tube; (b) gastrostomy tube feeding.

medications or when a child is unwell. Some children are fed at home, but receive tube feeds at school. A small number of children with severe feeding difficulties are entirely tube-fed.

Most parents are understandably reluctant to consider non-oral feeding, particularly if their child has been feeding orally for some time. Research (Craig et al. 2003) into the emotional aspects of the decision-making process prior to gastrostomy suggests that parents' concerns include:

1. Loss of nurturing role
2. Lack of confidence in liquid feeds (compared with home-cooked food)
3. Loss of pleasure for the child
4. Loss of one of the normal experiences for the child/family
5. Surgery and anaesthetic risks
6. Fears about excessive weight gain, making the child more difficult to lift
7. Loss of hope about future progress, and fears that professionals are giving up
8. Negation of all past efforts to feed child

Although parents are very wary of gastrostomy, research also shows high levels of satisfaction postsurgery, with significant health benefits for the child, e.g. weight increase and fewer hospital admissions with chest infections (Sullivan et al. 2005) and improved quality of life for carers (Sullivan et al. 2004). In the past, gastrostomy was used as a last resort, often after years of struggling to meet a child's nutritional needs. In recent years it has been seen as more of a preventive measure to avoid failure to thrive, constipation and dehydration; to improve children's alertness, concentration and learning; and to provide nutritional back-up whilst working on oral-motor skills.

Constipation

Constipation is a common problem in CP. A range of factors are thought to contribute to the problem:

1. Poor fluid intake, often due to poor oral-motor control of fluids, leading to spillage or coughing and choking
2. Diet that is low in fibre
3. Inactivity, with long periods of time in one position
4. Disordered movement of the muscles of the gut

Some children with CP are prescribed medications that relieve constipation, but dietary management can play an important role. Fluid intake is often crucial. Offering thickened fluids may increase intake and reduce spillage. Foods with high water content, such as fruit purées (with added cream to increase the calorie content), mashed vegetarian jellies (animal-derived gelatine creates a rubbery texture that may be difficult to swallow) or mashed vegetables (with butter) may also help to increase both fluid and fibre. It has been suggested that live yoghurt or warmed drinks may stimulate the gut and assist bowel movement. One of the benefits of tube-feeding, often reported by parents, is a reduction in the discomfort of constipation.

Teeth cleaning

Dental health is important for all children. Most parents are aware of the need to limit sweet, sugary snacks and night-time bottles, and will introduce good oral hygiene routines from an early age. Children with CP and feeding difficulties may face additional threats to dental health: poor tongue control and drooling mean that the tongue is not actively moving around the mouth, helping to clear food debris and washing the teeth and gums with saliva. Mouth breathing, limited fluid intake and some medications can create dry conditions in the mouth that lead to acid build-up. Gastro-oesophageal reflux, if severe, may also contribute to acid conditions in the mouth.

Establishing good teeth-cleaning routines is important. Children who have experienced unpleasant oral stimuli, such as nasogastric tubes, ventilation, medication, gastro-oesophageal reflux or early feeding difficulties may be orally hypersensitive and therefore resistant to teeth-cleaning. Some children may not adjust readily to the sensation of a toothbrush in the mouth. Most children will overcome this if teeth-cleaning is approached in a sensitive fashion, with the gradual introduction of positive touch to the face and mouth. Once a child will accept a parent's finger in the mouth, a soft rubber finger toothbrush can be introduced to rub the gums. The child may then be able to progress to a rubber toothbrush trainer set, and then to a soft brush. An alternative might be to 'brush' the gums/teeth with a piece of moistened gauze or flannel, wrapped around the finger. It may be helpful to think of the mouth divided into four quarters – top left, bottom left, top right and bottom right – inserting a moistened finger/rubber toothbrush into the side of the child's mouth and then using gentle but firm strokes moving from the back to the front of each quarter. This may be the most easily tolerated method. Touch at the back of the mouth may stimulate gagging initially, therefore it may be necessary to work backwards very gradually.

Teeth-cleaning will stimulate increased saliva production and may therefore be best carried out in a side-lying position, where excess saliva can dribble out on to a towel if a child has been struggling to swallow the extra saliva.

All children should have regular checks from a dentist. Most districts in the UK will have a special needs dentist who will have expertise in the care of children with CP.

Saliva control

Drooling is normal in young children. Most children learn to control this as they mature, usually around 15–18 months, although some will drool until the age of 3–4 years in particular situations. The ability to control saliva develops alongside feeding and other motor skills. Head control in particular will play a part in how well a child can manage saliva.

Some children with CP are very slow to develop saliva control which can be distressing for families, and for the children themselves. It can contribute to dehydration due to loss of fluids, sore skin and wet clothing, and possible adverse comments from other children.

We swallow around once per minute when awake. This is an automatic act but is dependent on the ability to feel the build-up of saliva in the mouth, and good tongue movements to collect the saliva and push it to the back of the mouth for swallowing. Drooling is usually due to poor tongue movements and infrequent swallowing rather than poor lip closure or an overproduction of saliva (Senner et al. 2004).

There are five main approaches to the management of drooling in children: (1) oral-motor exercises; (2) medication; (3) surgery; (4) conservative management; and (5) intraoral devices.

Oral-motor exercises

A small number of children are able to achieve a degree of control of their saliva through tongue exercises. A speech and language therapist will be able to provide a programme of exercises to increase tongue control. Even if these exercises are carried out every day it may take several months to achieve any control, and this may only be when the child is concentrating. The degree of control will also depend on what the child is doing, e.g. the child may be able to stop drooling when sitting quietly, but may still drool when concentrating on school work. In order for a programme to work the following conditions are necessary:

1. Children must be aware of when they are drooling

2. Children must want to gain control and understand what is involved

3. The child and family must be prepared to practise the exercises every day

4. The child must be able to imitate a range of oral movements, including closing lips, sticking out tongue, moving tongue from side to side. Few children under the age of 4 years are able to do this

Medication

There are several medicines that are currently being used to control drooling. These are usually medicines which were originally developed to control travel sickness, but which have been found to be effective in reducing saliva production. Others are used in operations, before an anaesthetic to dry up saliva production. Some are administered through patches on the skin placed behind the ear or on the child's back; others are liquid medicines. Medication for drooling can have side-effects so should be discussed with a paediatrician or paediatric neurologist who has experience in this area before being prescribed.

Botox injections to the salivary glands are also being piloted in some areas of the UK. A referral to a specialist service would be required in order to consider such an intervention (Bothwell et al. 2002).

Other medications taken by the child may affect saliva production and management; for example, baclofen, prescribed to reduce muscle spasms, can increase drooling. Some epilepsy medications may also impact on drooling by either increasing or reducing saliva production.

Surgery

Surgery is usually only considered after medication (and oral-motor exercises, if appropriate) has been tried. Saliva is produced by three sets of salivary glands in the mouth. The submaxillary glands (the submandibular and sublingual glands) are responsible for the production of thick saliva, and the parotid glands produce watery saliva. This thin saliva is the one which is most likely to be drooled; therefore, it is often these glands that are targeted in surgery. There are several surgical procedures, which may involve cutting the nerve supplies to glands, removing glands or redirecting them so saliva is sent towards the throat, rather than into the front of the mouth.

Results of drooling surgery are variable. Some children gain long-term benefit; others have only a temporary improvement. Undesirable consequences can be a dry mouth, poor oral hygiene and some difficulties with chewing. Again this option will require discussion with the child's paediatrician/neurologist and a surgeon who specializes in this area.

Conservative management

For children who continue to drool, the following tips may be useful:

1. If the child is able to wipe his or her own chin, wearing a towelling sweatband on the wrist can be more appropriate than using tissues or a handkerchief

2. When wiping a child's chin, dabbing firmly rather than wiping across the mouth and chin will avoid stimulating further saliva production and may increase a child's awareness of the chin

3. A neckerchief in a soft, absorbent cotton may be more age-appropriate than a bib

4. Sweet drinks are thought to stimulate saliva production and so might be best avoided

5. Some children have found travel sickness acupressure wrist bands helpful, but only for short periods of time. These may be used for special occasions but are unlikely to be effective in the long term

Intraoral devices

A specialist dentist may consider making a dental plate for a child to wear for short periods of the day, and sometimes at night. The plate fits in a way that is similar to a temporary wire brace. It has ridges and bumps on it that are designed to encourage active tongue movement and may therefore be most suitable for children who can swallow when thinking about it, but who cannot manage to do this automatically. The intraoral device helps to stimulate the tongue to collect saliva and move it backwards for swallowing. This is a relatively new management option in the UK, although encouraging results have been seen in other countries (Johnson et al. 2004).

Summary

Feeding can be a key factor in the health of children with CP. Whilst CP can have a significant effect on the development of oral-motor skills for eating and drinking and saliva control, for many children mealtimes are a safe and enjoyable experience. Positioning, the use of special equipment and techniques and attention to dietary intake all have a role in minimizing the risk of poor nutrition, constipation and respiratory problems. For some children, faltering growth or swallowing difficulties require the introduction of augmentative feeding techniques, with advice and support from speech and language therapists, dieticians and doctors.

References

Bothwell JE, Clarke K, Dooley JM et al. Botulinum toxin A as a treatment for excessive drooling in children. Pediatr Neurol 2002; 27:18–22.

Craig GM, Scambler G, Spitz L. Why parents of children with neurodevelopmental disabilities requiring gastrostomy feeding need more support. Dev Med Child Neurol 2003; 45:183–188.

Gisel EG, Patrick J. Identification of children with CP unable to maintain a normal nutritional state. Lancet 1988; 1:283–286.

Johnson HM, Reid SM, Hazard CJ et al. Effects of the Innsbruck Sensory Motor Activator and Regulator in improving saliva control in children with CP. Dev Med Child Neurol 2004; 46:39–45.

Senner JE, Logemann J, Zecker S et al. Drooling, saliva production and swallowing in CP. Dev Med Child Neurol 2004; 46:801–806.

Sullivan PB, Juszczak E, Bachlet AME et al. Impact of gastrostomy tube feeding on the quality of life of carers of children with CP. Dev Med Child Neurol 2004; 46:796–800.

Sullivan PB, Juszczak E, Bachlet AME et al. Gastrostomy tube feeding in children with CP: a prospective, longitudinal study. Dev Med Child Neurol 2005; 47:77–85.

Further reading

Eating and drinking assessments

Evans Morris S, Dunn Klein M. Developmental pre-feeding checklist. In: Evans Morris S, Dunn Klein M (eds) Pre-feeding skills, 2nd edn. Therapy Skills Builders, Tucson, AZ, 2000.

Jelm JM. Oral-motor feeding rating scale. Psychological Corporation, San Antonio, TX, 1997.

Reilly S, Skuse D, Wolke D. Schedule for oral-motor assessment. Whurr, London, 2000.

Resources for professionals

Arvedson JC, Brodsky L. Pediatric swallowing and feeding: assessment and management. Whurr, London, 1993.

Arvedson JC, Lefton-Grief MA. Pediatric videofluoroscopic swallow studies: a professional manual with caregiver guidelines. Communication Skills Builders. Psychological Corporation, San Antonio, TX, 1998.

Evans Morris S, Dunn Klein M. Pre-feeding skills, 2nd edn. Therapy Skills Builders, Tucson, AZ, 2000.

Reilly S, Wisbeach A, Carr L. Approaches to managing feeding problems in children with neurological problems. In: Southall A, Schwartz A (eds) Feeding problems in children – a practical guide. Radcliffe Medical Press, Abingdon, 2000.

Scott A, Johnson H. A practical approach to the management of saliva, 2nd edn. Pro-Ed, Tucson, AZ, 2004.

Sullivan P, Rosenbloom L. Feeding the disabled child. MacKeith Press, Cambridge, 1996.

Winstock A. Eating and drinking difficulties in children. Speechmark Publishing, Bicester, 2005.

Wolf LS, Glass RP. Feeding and swallowing disorders in infancy: assessment and management. Therapy Skills Builders (Winslow Press), Tucson, AZ, 1992.

Useful website

Dysphagia website: New Visions (Suzanne Evans Morris): http://new-vis.com (with links).

Chapter Fourteen

14

Lifting and carrying

Julia Graham

CHAPTER CONTENTS

The typical child

Children of a young age with typical muscle tone are relatively easy to lift and carry. However, the number of times parents lift their baby, infant, toddler or child each day can result in a great deal of physical activity on their part.

For example, just think how many times a parent carries out the following tasks each day:

1. Lifting the child into and out of a cot or crib

2. Placing the child on a changing mat (usually at floor level)

3. Changing or dressing the child

4. Carrying the child up- and downstairs

5. Putting the child into and out of a highchair

6. Feeding the child

7. Bathing the child

8. Putting the child in and out of a buggy

9. Putting the child in and out of a car seat

10. Carrying a car seat

This activity is in addition to all the other physical work a parent has to do within the home, such as housework, shopping and looking after siblings. This activity also occurs at a time for mothers when their own body is still experiencing the after effects of the physiological changes that occur during pregnancy, making the mother more vulnerable to strain and injury.

As children grow, from as early as a few months of age, they become more active and begin to participate in the action of lifting, for example by reaching forward towards their carer. They anticipate the lift by stabilizing their upper-limb joints. They tuck their chins in and prepare for the movement they are about to experience. A parent or carer can carry a child knowing that the child will automatically hold on. As balance improves the child will adjust position, needing only minimal support. Thus the experience of handling is a dynamic one with the carer gradually reducing the amount of support and encouraging active participation of the child.

Figure 14.1 illustrates how one would usually carry a child with good balance.

Gradually the child assists in the movements more and more. At around 9–12 months the child may begin to creep or crawl towards the carer. The child begins to climb up the legs of the carer to a standing position, in anticipation of being picked up. Eventually the child does not need to be lifted as much, as the child begins to mobilize and makes his or her own way around the environment. The child begins to respond to the parental request to move from one place to another, for example to lie down on the changing mat, to come to the highchair

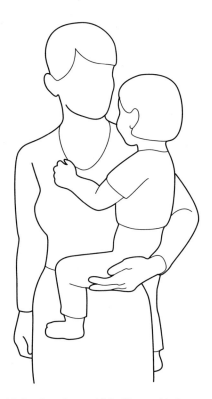

Figure 14.1 • Carrying a child with good balance.

at meal times, to climb into and out of a buggy or pushchair. Thus the need for parents or carers physically to lift their child becomes less and less as the child grows and develops gross and fine motor skills.

The child with cerebral palsy

A child with cerebral palsy (CP), however, presents a rather different scenario. When lifting the child the nature of the distribution of the CP and the effect the CP has on that child's muscle tone will influence how the child feels in the parent or carer's hands and how the child responds to the experience of movement.

A child with CP who has increased muscle tone will feel stiff to move and may not bend easily at the waist.

Equally difficult to move is a child who is floppy who may be difficult to grasp and hold; or a child who has fluctuating or changing muscle tone or experiences sudden uncontrolled movements.

Although the basic principles of lifting and carrying will remain the same wherever a carer is carrying the child, techniques of handling will need to be modified and changed according to the child's reactions in different situations and under different circumstances. It is, however, important that support is adjusted and withdrawn as the child progresses. This gives children the opportunity of adjusting their own posture, thus learning to maintain and regain balance, look around and interact with the environment.

Back care for parents and carers

It is important that, from the time your child is very small, you begin to lift and carry the child correctly, protecting both the child and yourself from unnecessary joint and muscle strain.

A child with CP will need your support as a parent and be dependent on your physical assistance for a much longer period of time (years) than a child who is able-bodied.

As your child grows, he or she will increase in both size and weight and this will increase the strain on you as a carer when physically lifting to transfer your child from one area to another.

If you can start to protect your back from the very beginning you will be more able to care for your child as the child, and you, get older.

Wherever possible as a parent or carer you need to encourage active or assisted movement from your child as this may avoid the need for you to lift the child's total body weight. Ask your child to help as much as possible. This type of approach will help to encourage the development of your child's independence skills and provide the child with a learning opportunity.

However, care must be taken with regard to your own posture when supporting your child and you are advised to seek the help of your therapist on the best way of doing this.

Back injury

A carer who is manually lifting a dependent child throughout the childhood and adolescent years, without any sort of mechanical assistance, can experience cumulative strain. This is a process by which damage occurs to the structures within the body, particularly the spine and upper limbs, over a prolonged period of time. It is caused by activities such as lifting, maintaining and sustaining poor body postures, repeated activity with little time for rest and recovery, overstretching and overtaxing body structures such as the muscles and joints.

The strength and stability of the spine depend on the integrity of the spinal discs and ligaments. These are the very structures which sustain cumulative injury due to the application of repetitive forces such as those imposed in a care situation.

Each time you carry out a physical lift incorrectly you may cause and accumulate damage to your body. Minimizing this activity by utilizing mechanical assistance and using correct lifting and carrying techniques will help protect your back for the future.

Risk assessments

Parents and carers may be aware that staff employed in health, social and education agencies, as well as those staff employed by the many other agencies with whom they may have dealings in the day-to-day care of their child, have to work within a framework of legislation regarding moving and lifting.

The legislative framework within Europe includes the Manual Handling Operations Regulations (1992). The legislation is in place to protect both staff and patients or clients (the children with whom we work).

The regulations require staff to carry out a risk assessment on any hazardous moving and handling task that has been identified in the management of the child in the course of their work.

A hazard is anything with the potential to cause harm.

A risk is the likelihood of that harm occurring and the severity of its consequences.

The aim of the risk assessment is to identify the level of risk involved to both the handler and, in this case, the child being handled, during the task. Once identified, the risk can be managed or reduced by introducing control measures such as handling equipment or training for those carrying out the task.

Risk assessments should be reviewed whenever there is a change to your child's condition, such as following surgery or growth.

Each child is a unique individual and it is therefore difficult to give specific guidance in a general text such as this. It is unwise to give advice on a weight that can be handled by a carer as each situation should be uniquely assessed in the following four areas: (1) task; (2) individual; (3) load; and (4) environment:

1. Each *task* carried out will present different issues. The task may be a straightforward transfer from bed to chair or it may be into or out of the bath, or into and out of a standing frame.

2. The *individual* is the person carrying out the handling. The skills and capabilities of parents and carers will vary greatly depending on their own circumstances. Individual handlers may be experienced, may be tired at the end of a long day, may have been unwell recently, or may have a back problem. All of these factors have the potential to affect their capability to handle.

3. The *load* may be a child with CP, each presenting differently, or the load may be an inanimate object such as a box or a piece of equipment.

4. Every *environment* will be different, but things to consider are space, clutter, lighting, noise and distractions.

The information given in this chapter presents very general advice on the main issues to be considered when lifting and carrying your child.

The therapists working with you should be able to advise and support you with regard to lifting and carrying issues and, if not expert themselves, should have the resources to discuss issues with a moving and handling advisor or a therapist who is a specialist in this field.

Carrying the young child who is predominantly extended

Bringing the child up to a sitting position from lying

Before sitting the child up, ensure that the child's weight is evenly distributed and that the child is lying as symmetrically as possible.

By rolling the child on to the side and semi-flexing the hips, then bringing arms forward, the child can be raised to a sitting posture through side-lying.

Figure 14.2 illustrates a way of bringing a child who is predominantly extended with arms flexed and retracted at the shoulders up to sitting. The carer's forearms can be used to keep the child's legs apart and turned out, thus leaving the hands free to control the child's shoulders, bringing these forwards and in. Handled in this way it will be easier for the child to bring the head and arms forwards and facilitate bending of the hips and legs.

When carrying a child who is predominantly extended by holding the child close to your body with hips and knees flexed, shoulders forward and hands in midline, as shown in Figure 14.3, carers are able to control the extensor tendency and maintain a good posture for both the child and themselves.

Care must be taken when holding a child on one hip as this introduces asymmetry to the carer's posture. It is recommended that carers alternate which side they use to carry the child as this will help maintain the symmetry of both the child and the carer's body posture.

Figure 14.4 shows a way of holding and carrying a child facing away from the carer. Carried in this way the child is encouraged to look at the environment, extending the head and spine in a controlled manner. The carer also maintains

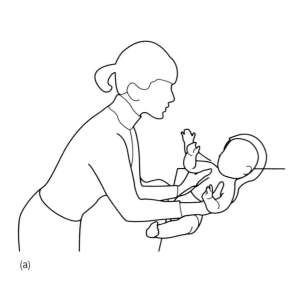

(a)

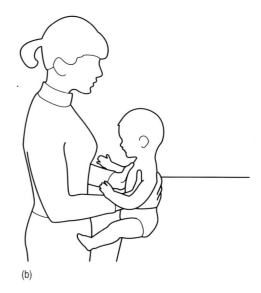

(b)

Figure 14.2 • (a, b) Bringing a child up to sitting who is predominantly extended.

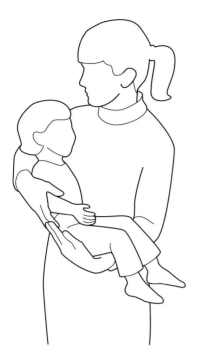

Figure 14.3 • Holding a child who is predominantly extended.

a symmetrical position, thus protecting the carer's back.

Carrying a young child with moderate to severe spasticity who is predominantly flexed

The young child who is predominantly flexed adopts a position in which the head is extended, chin is poked forwards and arms are turned in at the shoulders and flexed against the body. One or both hands may be fisted; hips and legs are turned in and partially extended.

One method of carrying such a child is demonstrated in Figure 14.5.

Figures 14.6 and 14.7 show how to carry an older child with moderate spasticity.

In this position you can keep the child's back extended and keep the legs separated and extended and turned out at the hips.

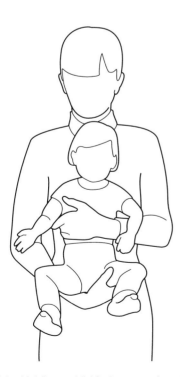

Figure 14.4 • Holding a child facing away from the carer.

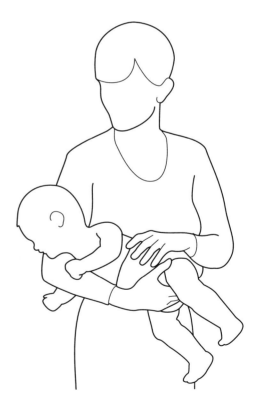

Figure 14.5 • Carrying a young child with spasticity who is predominantly flexed.

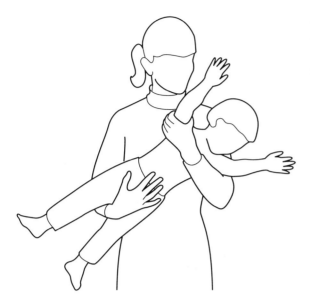

Figure 14.6 • Carrying an older child with moderate spasticity who is predominantly flexed.

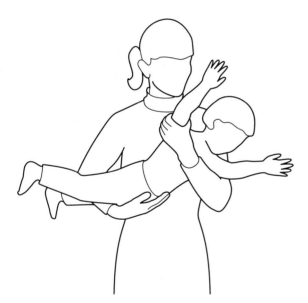

Figure 14.7 • Carrying an older child with moderate spasticity who is predominantly flexed.

Carrying the child with fluctuating muscle tone

Before lifting the child, 'gather' the child together by bending the legs and bringing the hands to midline. Bring the child up to sitting by either rolling the child on to the side or raising the child straight up, whichever is easier. Figure 14.8–14.11 illustrate suggested ways of carrying a child by

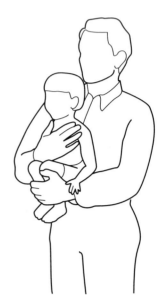

Figure 14.8 • Carrying a child with fluctuating muscle tone, giving pelvic support and shoulder girdle support if needed.

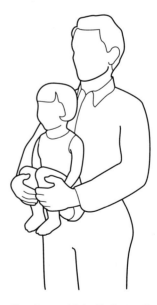

Figure 14.9 • Carrying a child with fluctuating muscle tone, giving pelvic support and shoulder girdle support if needed.

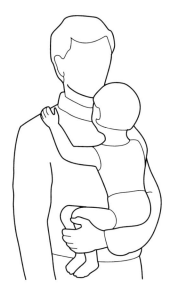

Figure 14.10 • Carrying a child with fluctuating muscle tone, giving pelvic support and shoulder girdle support if needed.

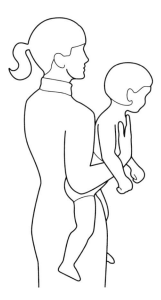

Figure 14.11 • Carrying a child with fluctuating muscle tone, giving pelvic support and shoulder girdle support if needed.

giving pelvic and, when necessary, shoulder girdle stability to enable the child to lift the head and shoulders, bringing arms forwards and extending the back to interact with the carer and the environment.

Carrying should always be kept to a minimum. Carers are often tempted to carry a child as it saves time or is done in response to a vocal demand for attention, but it must be remembered that whenever children are carried, they are deprived of an opportunity to move on their own and carers are increasing the strain on their own backs.

Equipment

Your therapist may have discussed with you the introduction of the use of handling equipment in the home. This can be difficult for parents and carers to accept as they may feel they have to carry out all the caring duties for their child on their own. However, using such equipment will help protect both you and your child so that you can enjoy family life together in the future. After all, if you suffer a back injury, who will look after your child?

You may be aware that, when at nursery, school or in respite care facilities, as a result of current legislation, your child may have been involved in a moving and handling assessment. During any transition from one activity to another or movement from one piece of equipment to another, the assessment should identify if there are any risks to your child or to the people handling your child. As a result of these assessments, in these environments your child may be using handling equipment. This may be a glide sheet (Figure 14.12), a handling belt (Figure 14.13), transfer board (Figure 14.14) or a hoist, to name a few examples.

Schools and therapy departments may possess hoisting equipment which will allow your child to access standing frames, treatment couches or hydrotherapy swimming pools.

Soft-play rooms and multisensory rooms with hoisting facilities may enable your child to continue to access and benefit from these activities as the child gets older, taller and heavier.

Despite the use of such equipment at school, you may not have started to use any of it at home but you may like to discuss this possibility with your therapist as it may help you in certain routines and would provide your child with more consistency in methods of being moved.

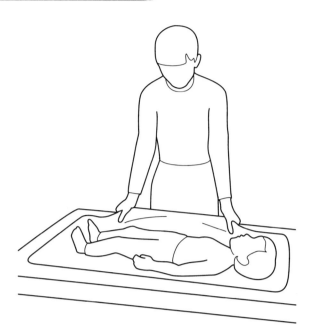

Figure 14.12 • A glide sheet.

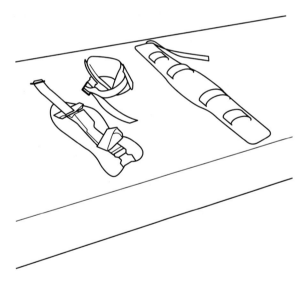

Figure 14.13 • Handling belts.

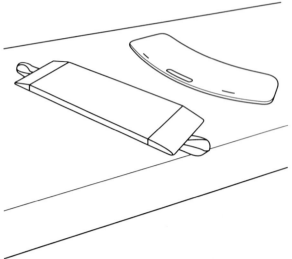

Figure 14.14 • Transfer boards.

Thus the child will be dependent on your help to move from one place to another.

If your child is likely to need hoisting equipment, adaptations to your home may be required. Prior to supply of the hoisting equipment your child should be fully assessed for the size and type of sling required, depending on the tasks for which it will be used.

Steps in hoisting a child from a bed to a chair

1. Where possible, raise the bed to a comfortable working height for the carers

2. Roll hoist sling in half lengthways

3. Supporting the child at the head, shoulders and pelvis as necessary, roll the child on to the side

4. Place the sling halfway under the child's body

5. Roll the child on to the other side

6. Unroll the sling from beneath the child's body so that it lies flat on the bed

7. Position the leg supports under the child's legs

8. Position the hoist near to the child

9. Lower the hoist down so that the loops of the sling can be easily attached to the hoist

10. Check that the sling is correctly positioned before raising the child off the bed

It is often an idea to plan ahead when considering the potential future need for hoisting equipment. Depending on the complexity of your child's disability, the child may not achieve the functional ability to take weight on the feet and carry out a standing transfer. Equally, over time the child may lose the skill of standing to transfer.

11. Taking care when moving the hoist and child, position the hoist over the child's chair

12. Carefully lower the child into the chair

13. Remove the loops of the sling from the hoist

14. Remove the sling from under the child

Below are the principal steps, shown pictorially, of hoisting a child from a bed to a chair.

Step 1

When hoisting a child from the bed to a chair, prepare the area and ensure you have all equipment needed to hand. Check the hoist is charged and in working order and before using the sling check that all stitching is intact. Roll the hoist sling lengthways away from you.

Step 2

Roll the child on to the side, placing the hoist sling as close to the child's body as possible (Figure 14.15). (If you are working alone, ensure that the bed guard is used on the opposite side of the bed. If you are working with a second carer, ensure the other person stands on the opposite side of the bed to you.)

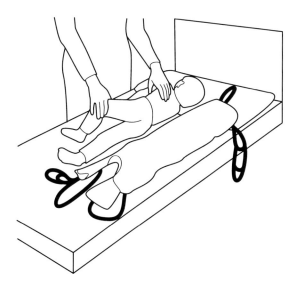

Figure 14.15 • Hoisting a child from a bed to a chair: step 2.

Step 3

Roll the child on to the hoist sling and on to the other side (Figure 14.16).

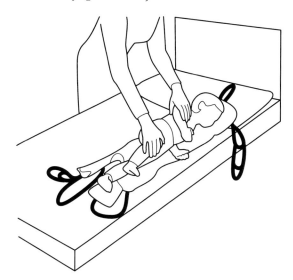

Figure 14.16 • Hoisting a child from a bed to a chair: step 3.

Step 4

Unroll the hoist sling from underneath the child (Figure 14.17).

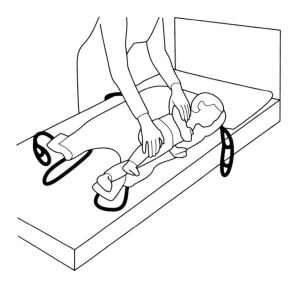

Figure 14.17 • Hoisting a child from a bed to a chair: step 4.

Step 5

Roll the child on to the back to ensure the child is flat on the positioned sling (Figure 14.18).

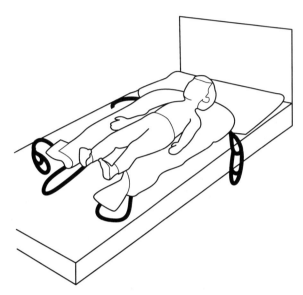

Figure 14.18 • Hoisting a child from a bed to a chair: step 5.

Step 6

Position the leg supports under the child's legs and attach the loops or hooks to the hoist (Figure 14.19).

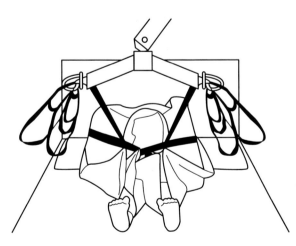

Figure 14.19 • Hoisting a child from a bed to a chair: step 6.

Step 7

Gradually begin to raise the child off the supporting surface, checking that the child is correctly positioned (Figure 14.20). If there are problems with the sling, lower the child to the bed and make the necessary adjustments before repeating the process.

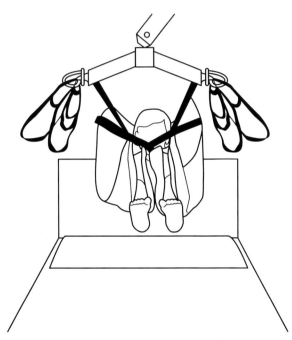

Figure 14.20 • Hoisting a child from a bed to a chair: step 7.

Step 8

Carefully manoeuvre the hoist into position in front of the child's chair. It is often easier to turn the hoist when standing from the side, with one hand on the boom and one on the upright frame. Once in position, gradually lower the child into the chair. Release the loops or hooks from the hoist and remove the sling from under the child.

Parents and carers may find hoisting equipment useful within the home to assist in the care of their child. All carers should be given training on how to use the equipment correctly and safely within the home environment and the child should be gradually introduced to and familiarized with the experience of being hoisted.

The training for carers should include:

1. How to adjust the environment in preparation for the handling

2. How to place the hoist sling under the child

3. How to connect the sling to the hoist

4. How to operate the hoist

5. How to move the child safely whilst in the hoist

6. What to do in an emergency

7. How to care for the hoist

Note: Using a hoist does not necessarily take away all the risks of moving a child. Carers should be aware of their own posture when using the hoist to ensure that they protect their own backs.

Lifting and moving tasks

One of the most difficult areas in which to handle your child is the bathroom. The bath is low and the child in the bath is wet and slippery when being handled. The posture of the parent is of paramount importance in this situation. If equipment has not been supplied to assist with this task, parents should ensure that they kneel down at the edge of the bath and do not stand in a stooped position to wash their child. Accessing the bath, shower or toilet can be very problematic. All children should be assessed within their own environment and provided with equipment to suit their individual needs.

Lifting a young child from the floor

Where it is not possible to use a raised or adjustable height-changing surface, correct handling and an awareness of posture can reduce the strain on carers for such transitions when the child has to be moved from a low level to a higher level in one movement.

Lifting a child on to and off a changing mat placed on the floor can be risky for carers' backs. Where possible the carer should kneel down close to the child. Roll the child on to the carer's forearm, placing a second hand under the child's pelvis, and raise the child, bringing the child close into the carer's body.

Carers should then step up into a half-kneeling position, adjusting their hold on the child if necessary. They can then rise to a standing position, having 'staged' the lift from the floor, being aware of their own posture as they do so. Figures 14.21–14.23 show the carer rising to a standing position holding the child.

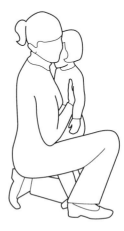

Figure 14.21 • Steps in raising a child up from the floor.

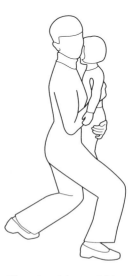

Figure 14.22 • Steps in raising a child up from the floor.

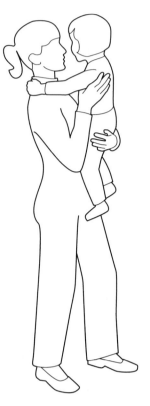

Figure 14.23 • Steps in raising a child up from the floor.

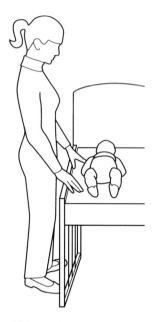

Figure 14.24 • Lifting a child out of a cot: step 1.

Step 2

Grasp the baby around the body (Figure 14.25).

Lifting a small child out of a cot

Lifting even a small child out of a cot can involve risks to carers' backs. To reduce those risks careful handling from an early stage should be encouraged. Manipulating the environment and adjusting your own posture using your body to assist in the lift can help to reduce the risks concerned.

Step 1

Prepare the environment. Lower the cot side. Prepare yourself: adjust your stance, place your feet in the direction of the movement. Keep your knees slightly relaxed and keep your spine in line (Figure 14.24).

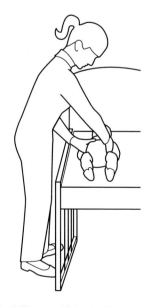

Figure 14.25 • Lifting a child out of a cot: step 2.

Step 3

Roll the baby towards you, on to your forearm (Figure 14.26).

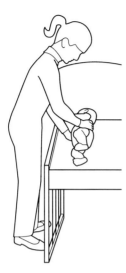

Figure 14.26 • Lifting a child out of a cot: step 3.

Step 4

Place the other hand under the pelvis of the child and lift up and towards your own body, keeping the child close (Figure 14.27).

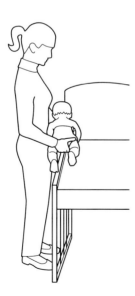

Figure 14.27 • Lifting a child out of a cot: step 4.

Step 5

Adjust your hold on the child, keeping the child close to your body (Figure 14.28).

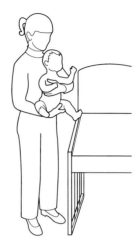

Figure 14.28 • Lifting a child out of a cot: step 5.

Lifting a child from a buggy or pushchair

When lifting a child from a buggy it is important to think about your posture as you perform the task.

Step 1

Lower your body to the level of the child. Kneel down alongside the buggy (Figure 14.29).

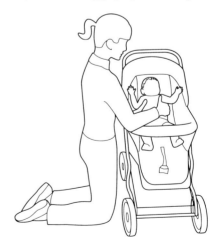

Figure 14.29 • Lifting a child out of a buggy: step 1.

Step 2

Lean the child forward over your forearm and place the other hand under the child's pelvis, gently easing the child out of the buggy (Figure 14.30).

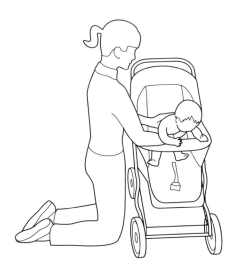

Figure 14.30 • Lifting a child out of a buggy: step 2.

Step 3

Bring the child close in to your body and adjust your hand hold as necessary (Figure 14.31).

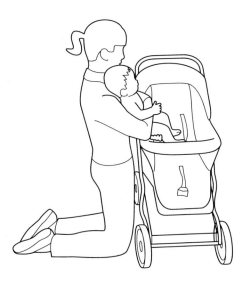

Figure 14.31 • Lifting a child out of a buggy: step 3.

Step 4

Raise one leg to assume a half-kneel standing position (Figure 14.32).

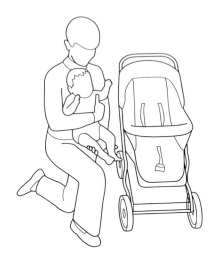

Figure 14.32 • Lifting a child out of a buggy: step 4.

Step 5

Rise to standing, transferring your weight from one foot to the other (Figure 14.33).

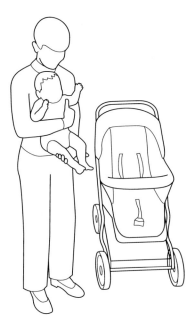

Figure 14.33 • Lifting a child out of a buggy: step 5.

Handling a child in special seating

If your child uses a special seating system, the close-fitting nature of the system usually means that putting a hoist sling around the child may prove difficult. There are now hoist slings available that are made of a fine silk-type fabric and these are much easier to slide into place. Placement of the hoist sling can involve a great deal of 'handling' of the child and carers should be aware of their own posture during the process. Some hoist slings can be left in situ but care is needed if your child has a delicate skin and this should be clarified with your therapist and the sling manufacturers in the first instance.

Before your child is supplied with hoisting equipment the manufacturers should be given a full assessment of their individual needs by a therapist or representative from the supply company. It is often useful to coordinate with school and respite care facilities when assessing for hoisting equipment so that the provision is compatible if possible.

Impact of sensory and cognitive deficits on lifting and carrying a child

When lifting your child, whether manually or by mechanical means, you must take into consideration how the child is going to react to the movement.

Children have a right to know what is about to happen to them and to be involved in decisions about such activities. It is important to involve a child in the discussion about why the child needs to be lifted or carried, and about how and when that lifting or carrying will take place. Wherever possible children should be given choices about who does the lifting and carrying and as much control over the process as they can cope with. If they have good upper-limb function, for example, they may be able to use the control buttons on a hoist during a transfer.

Children who have a sensory deficit such as a visual impairment may not be able to see you approach with equipment and may be startled when suddenly touched or handled. You will have to describe exactly what is going to happen and where you plan to move the child to so that the child can adjust and prepare themselves.

Children with a hearing impairment may not be adequately prepared unless you have given the appropriate visual cues or used the appropriate communication method.

Children who use augmentative communication aids on their wheelchairs may no longer have access to these when being lifted and may be unable to tell you that they are not yet ready for the move to take place. Discuss the activity with the child before taking away the communication aid so that they have an opportunity to tell you what they want and how they feel about it.

Children who have a learning disability may not understand what is expected or being asked of them. Try to adjust your language or use gestures to enable the child to understand what is about to happen.

A child who has problems with perceptual processing may find lifting and moving tasks difficult. If the child is unable to judge distances, depth and speed or does not know right from left, the child may have difficulty following directions or judging how far or how fast to move. Carers need to be aware of these issues for the child and adjust their preparation and handling of the manoeuvre.

How you approach the child and how you use your voice may affect the child's reaction to the lifting or carrying. Children with severe CP and increased muscle tone may startle if you speak loudly or suddenly. This may cause a further increase in their muscle tone, making them harder to move. Conversely children who have very low muscle tone may be more prepared for movement if their muscle tone is raised slightly by a more stimulating, lively approach.

The speed at which the movement occurs may also affect how the child responds to it. You will have to judge carefully how quickly or slowly you can carry out the task and give the child time to adjust to what is happening.

Carers must always be aware of children who may experience pain due to their disability and minimize this wherever possible.

The environment in which the lifting and moving takes place also has a great influence on the way in which the child reacts to the manoeuvre.

If children cannot focus on the task because there is so much going on around them, or there are sudden noises which may startle them, it may make the task much harder to perform. Their muscle tone and body posture will change in response to the environmental stimuli and this may make it more difficult to lift and move them. If there is something really interesting happening behind children, you will find them trying to get a better view by spiralling around in the hoist sling. This can be dangerous and you will need to manipulate the environment to reduce the risks during the procedure.

After every lifting situation carers should reflect on how well it went and how it might be improved in the future. Lifting, carrying and moving a child should not be a passive experience for the child, nor should it put the parent's or carer's back at risk of damage, now or later.

Acknowledgement

I wish to acknowledge the help of Helen Cullum with the photo shoots from which the illustrations in this chapter were based.

Chapter Fifteen

15

Toilet training

Anne J Wright • Rosie Kelly

Toilet training can be a difficult time for parents and children and the time it takes for a child to become clean and dry during the day will vary a great deal. The trick is to get a balance between praising a child for doing well and hiding your own disappointment when progress seems slow. We know that for some children with cerebral palsy (CP) toilet training is achieved within similar time-frames to children without CP. Studies have shown that for the child with a diplegic (lower-limb) motor disorder and no learning difficulties it is expected that toilet training is achieved by the age of 7 years (Roijen et al. 2001, Wright et al. 2002). For children with a four-limb motor disorder and learning difficulties toilet training may take a lot longer. Nevertheless, toilet training is an important developmental milestone in the life of a child, allowing independence and social acceptance.

Bowel continence is usually achieved before bladder continence and it is useful to have an understanding of these basic eliminatory functions in order to help with the training.

Basic bowel function

The bowel or gastrointestinal system is the system that handles food and fluid nutrients within the body. It is a single continuous system all the way from the mouth to the anus (bottom) and it is a tube-like structure that is able to push food along with a wave-like muscle action (peristalsis) (Figure 15.1). Food enters the gastrointestinal system via the mouth. It goes down into the stomach via the oesophagus. There is a useful natural reflex action

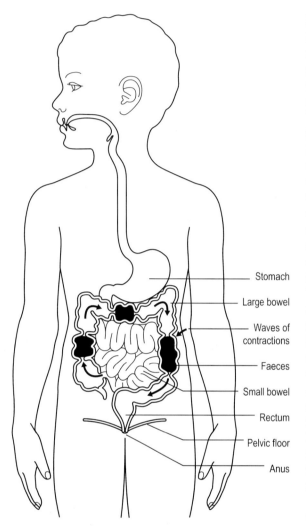

Figure 15.1 • The gastrointestinal system with formation of faeces in the large bowel.

Labels:
Stomach
Large bowel
Waves of contractions
Faeces
Small bowel
Rectum
Pelvic floor
Anus

large intestine as liquid slurry. The large intestine then extracts water from this whilst constantly peristalsing to move the forming faeces ('poo') along. By the time the faeces have reached the end of the large intestine they have solidified but are soft, and able to move along the intestine easily. The stool enters the rectum at the end of the large intestine. The rectal outlet is the anus and this is made up of two sphincters that act like taps. The upper one is the internal anal sphincter and this is under involuntary control (smooth muscle) whilst the lower one or external anal sphincter is under voluntary control and is made up of skeletal muscle which is part of the pelvic floor. This skeletal muscle may be affected by CP. When faeces enter the rectum, the rectum contracts and pushes the faeces down into the internal anal sphincter. The presence of faeces at the top of the internal anal sphincter is sensed by nerve endings which send messages via nerves in the spinal cord to the brain to let us know that we need to defecate. At this point an individual has two options: we can toilet and empty our bowels or, if inconvenient, we can exert a holding pattern by squeezing the voluntary external anal sphincter, which pushes the faeces back into the rectum, buying more time. However the rectum is not a storage organ but a short-stay holding centre and it will reflexly continue to squeeze the faeces back into the anus, constantly reminding us that we need to toilet.

During defecation the external sphincter is voluntarily relaxed and rectal contractions, along with relaxation of the internal anal sphincter, allow expulsion of faeces. If faeces are the correct consistency then it is not difficult to expel them and it does not hurt a child's bottom. Opening the bowels or defecating is a naturally slower process than urinating and, as most faeces are delivered to the rectum in 'lots', there is usually more than one 'poo' present, requiring a child to be patient and to sit and wait for the subsequent faeces to be expelled after the first. The 'lots' of 'poo' correspond to meals so that babies who milk-feed frequently tend to pass 'poo' frequently. As babies wean and their diets change to solid food, so the frequency diminishes with time so that opening bowels anywhere between three times daily and every other day can be normal.

by the stomach whereby when food enters it automatically causes the need for a bowel action down below to make room for more food to enter the system. This is called the gastrocolic reflex and this can be usefully used in bowel toilet training by placing the child on the potty about 15–20 minutes after meals.

After the stomach, food enters the small intestine where a series of digestive processes allow extraction of nutrients that enter the body. Following digestion in the small intestine what remains is largely waste and this transfers into the

Vital components that contribute to healthy bowels are normal faecal consistency allowing easy and non-painful expulsion of faeces, exercise and regular and complete bowel opening. These factors allow regular elimination of waste from the bowel in a healthy and timely manner. Fluid and fibre are important in achieving good consistency by preventing the faeces from becoming too dried out and therefore hard, and difficult for the bowel to eliminate. Exercise is useful because it aids the bowel in delivering faeces to the rectum.

Regular, complete bowel opening ensures regular elimination of waste and prevention of build-up. This is achieved with healthy toileting practice where children are willing to respond to messages from the bowel because the process is not unpleasant or miserable for them.

Basic bladder function

Urine is produced by the kidneys. The kidneys perform a very important excretory function in the body by continuously cleaning or washing the blood, removing toxins and controlling water and salt balance (homeostatic function). As a result of this they remove all the unneeded waste from our blood which they get rid of in water-based urine. Kidneys constantly produce urine in a drip-like fashion throughout the day and night. The urine is collected in pipes called ureters which transfer the drops of urine from the kidneys down into a balloon-like storage organ called the bladder. The bladder gets bigger as it fills with urine until it reaches its capacity, which is sensed via the nerves in the spinal cord, which go to the brain alerting of the need to pass urine. There is a tap-like sphincter at the bottom of the bladder made up of two components: this tap is constantly closed whilst the bladder is filling. This allows us to be dry. The upper portion of the tap is the internal urinary sphincter and this is under involuntary control consisting of smooth muscle. The lower portion is the external urinary sphincter which is under voluntary control and is made up of skeletal muscle. Skeletal muscle is affected by CP. Following toilet training urination (peeing) is voluntarily initiated by relaxing the external urinary

sphincter. The bladder muscle (detrusor) then contracts, squeezing urine out through the shorter outlet pipe called the urethra, expelling urine from the body in a continuous stream. Emptying urine from the bladder is generally a short process (seconds rather than minutes) and the bladder is always programmed to empty to completion before stopping (Figure 15.2).

A baby's bladder (30–60 ml) is obviously smaller than an adult's (average capacity 400 ml or greater) and the need to empty the bladder is influenced by the amount of fluid drunk as well as bladder

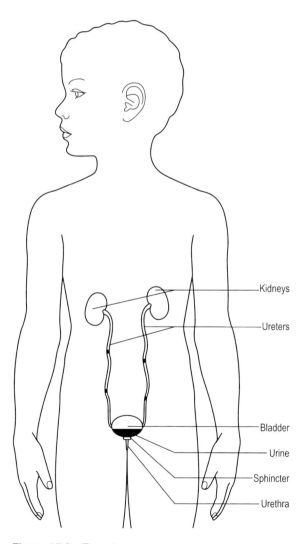

Figure 15.2 • The urinary system.

size. Babies will urinate frequently – anything up to 20 times per day. As the child gets older this frequency diminishes until, at the age of 5 years and above, the average child will urinate anywhere between five and seven times per day. Unlike the rectum, the bladder's main function is as a storage organ and it spends most of its time holding urine between short episodes of urinating. This system allows us to eliminate urine from our bodies in a timely and acceptable way. Urine is toxic to skin (as evidenced in nappy rash), so it is very important that the bladder system works efficiently.

Components of healthy bladder function include adequate fluid intake and responsive toileting. A healthy bowel can also be important for bladder function as constipation can disrupt normal bladder function and predispose to urinary tract infections (see section on constipation, below).

Achieving voluntary control over bowel and bladder

Recognition of the sensations from bowel and bladder indicating the need to defecate or pass urine as well as learning voluntary control over the bowel and bladder sphincters and the associated required action of toileting is the process that children achieve when they toilet train. This is a normal neurodevelopmental process involving maturation of the nervous system rather like learning to sit and talk. It is not something that children can be trained to do before their own nervous systems are ready and inappropriately early potty training attempts may be doomed to fail and create frustration and disillusionment in both child and parent. Like all developmental milestones, there is a large variation in the ages at which this will occur and developmental age is more important than chronological age. It is now generally accepted that potty training should not begin before 2–2½ years of age, although some children will train before this time and others a long time afterwards. More useful than stipulating age range is assessment of certain *readiness indicators*. These provide a useful checklist of the basic building blocks that indicate that toilet

training is likely to succeed. The more of these present, the better.

Toilet training readiness check

1. Your child is able to sit in a stable position either independently or with support for a few minutes

2. Your child has naturally stopped defecating at night time

3. Your child's faeces are solid and formed but not constipated

4. Your child is generally able to go at least 1 hour with a dry nappy

5. Your child recognizes the sensation of a wet or soiled nappy

6. Your child understands simple instructions

7. Your child is able to communicate his or her needs to you or another carer by means of words, sound, gesture, eye pointing or picture symbols

8. Your child understands what a potty or toilet is for

Sometimes it may be difficult to be sure about a readiness indicator. If you are unsure it would be worthwhile discussing the issue with an appropriate professional. Your physiotherapist can be consulted about seating issues and positioning, whilst a doctor or paediatrician can discuss whether there are any reasons why your child may not have normal sensation or offer help with faeces that are either too hard or too soft. It is worth modelling toileting behaviour for a child in order for the child to observe that it is a natural part of daily life and is part of social development. This can be done by pointing out the toileting behaviour of older brothers or sisters or indeed explaining your own. It helps to provide the vocabulary and words for a child to understand and to use and to start with this can be done by observing the child's own toileting when nappy changing. 'Oh, I see you've done a poo'. 'You have a nice wet nappy. That means you have done a pee'. Find appropriate means of communication and make sure that anyone who cares for your child will use the same labels and communication strategies as your child and yourself to prevent misunderstandings and frustration.

Getting started

If you feel your child is ready to start toilet training, having checked the above indicators, it is worth doing a bit of planning first.

A stable routine

Choose a period of time that will be stable from the point of view of the child's routine. If this involves other carers such as nursery and childminder, make sure that they are also able to participate and carry out the same programme. It can be confusing for a child to have different routines in different places. As far as possible try to accommodate the routine on an ongoing basis and not give it up on weekends and holidays. Some parents prefer to start training during warmer weather when their child can be lightly or partially dressed to facilitate easy removal of clothes.

A diary

Try keeping a diary for 1 week, recording when your child's nappy is wet or soiled. This will mean checking the nappy frequently for a few days but it may give you some idea of when to encourage the child to use the potty once the nappy comes off. This will increase your chances of success. Do not worry if there does not appear to be a regular pattern: you can begin by encouraging your child to try and 'pee' or 'poo' after meals.

The potty/toilet

Choose a suitable potty and make sure that one is always readily available and within view if possible. If your child is going to use the toilet straight away you will need to consider how easy it is to get to and if there are difficulties, such as only one toilet upstairs, it may well be worth providing an alternative such as a potty downstairs for ease of access.

It is very important that the potty/toilet seat is comfortable and that the child feels stable, safe and secure. Fear of falling off the potty will not help with toileting. Commercially available potties have a broad base and a wide lip with some back support. Some come with features such as a musical response that may reward and encourage children to perform. Domestic toilets are a standard one-size-fits-all and are often too big for children. Many children can be frightened of toilets, thinking of them as big white gurgling bowls that swallow down objects to an unknown destination. Equally they can present as cold and precarious. This will not be conducive to successful training. Using a toilet seat insert and a foot stool will help children to feel safer and more secure. Make sure that the environs are well lit and warm (Figure 15.3).

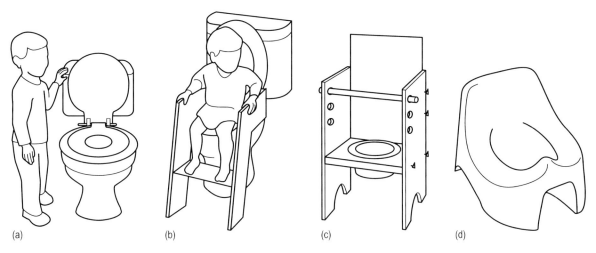

(a)   (b)   (c)   (d)

Figure 15.3 • Various potty adaptations for help with toilet training: (a) toilet seat insert; (b) foot support stool and hand rails; (c) potty chair with all-round support and safety rail; (d) potty with wide-based support and backrest.

Removing the nappy

You may want to start with your child still wearing a pull-up or nappy and remove it when the child is more reliably achieving toileting. If using modern disposables, these products are highly absorbable and the child will find it difficult to get the sensation of being wet after peeing. This can be helped by allowing children to wear ordinary cotton pants underneath the nappy or a piece of kitchen towel which will allow them to feel that they are wet. After a while it is useful to remove the nappy or pull-ups and have the child in pants. Accidents are bound to occur, so have some spare pairs of pants ready.

Getting going

Inform your child that you are going to start using the potty and start slowly by placing your child on the potty for a few minutes after the meal you have identified as being the most likely to produce a 'poo' and 'pee'. Encourage the child to remain seated for a few minutes but do not leave the child too long or insist the child has produced something. Make toilet training fun. It may help to allow the child to look at a picture book, recite nursery rhymes with you or play games such as blowing bubbles. This allows your child to feel more relaxed and more interested in going to the toilet. With time increase the frequency of pottying, praising any positive results in the potty/toilet but do not displaying any disappointment or negativity if the child either fails to produce anything or has an accident. A reasonable routine to aim for would be after meals and in between meals and on waking and before going to bed.

After a while your child will start indicating the need to toilet in anticipation of being placed on the potty. This is a very important step which should be praised and encouraged and, if your child needs help to access the toilet, this should be done as promptly as possible to reward the child's initiative and avoid accidents.

With time and consistency steady progress occurs for most children, although like any learning curve, ups and downs may occur.

Special considerations in children with cerebral palsy

Seating

During toileting the pelvic floor and sphincters have to relax in order to allow effective urination and defecation to occur. In order to maximize pelvic floor relaxation a stable seating position is required that provides truncal stability. Ideally the hips should be very slightly flexed and the thighs slightly apart. For some children this will be achieved with an ordinary potty and a toilet seat insert and stool. For others, however, much more support may be required and specialist toileting equipment may be appropriate. This may include potty chairs, support rails or other specialist adaptations (Figure 15.4). In this

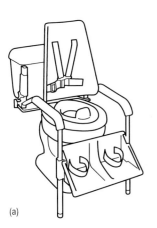
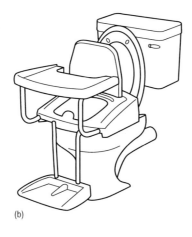

Figure 15.4 • (a, b) Various specialist toilet systems are available offering varying degrees of support.

(a)

(b)

case advice is best sought from your physiotherapist and occupational therapist who will be able to advise on seating support and specialist toilet equipment.

If possible, ask to try out the equipment first to see if it suits your child and if necessary the whole family. Check if it is a system that is removable for a toilet used by other members of the family. If your child experiences spasms try to move your child slowly and calmly into the toileting position, keeping the child's hips flexed and thighs apart. A pommel can be useful for keeping thighs apart. You may have to wait a while for your child to relax and achieve a good seating position, meaning that the child has to stay longer than a few minutes before having had a chance to toilet. Some

parents find it useful to sit on the back rim of the toilet and provide support and comfort for their child sitting in front of them until the child gains confidence to sit on the toilet alone (Figure 15.5a). Other parents have found it helpful to sit their child on a potty placed between the parent's legs on a chair (Figure 15.5b).

Equally some parents have found that sitting in front of their children on the toilet can provide adequate support. If straps and restraints are part of the equipment, be careful not to use them to keep the child on the toilet for too long and beware of edges or straps cutting into the child's body or legs. Do not let your child sit facing the back of the toilet (reverse sitting) as this position is easy to get the child into but difficult to get out

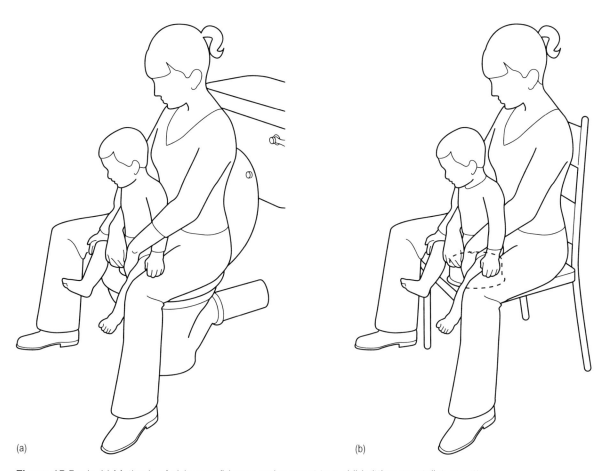

(a)

(b)

Figure 15.5 • (a, b) Methods of giving confidence and support to a child sitting on a toilet or potty.

of and the child risks falling backwards off the toilet. Never leave your child alone on the toilet.

Mobility

The ability of the child to access a toilet in a timely manner is essential for ensuring successful toilet training in the long term. To start with it is useful to use a potty which can be moved about the house. Once this is established, however, and the child needs to progress to using a toilet more consistently, it may be necessary to plan ahead for adaptations. Make sure your child can reach the bathroom safely and in time. If your child needs help walking or uses a wheelchair, make sure the bathroom or lavatory is large enough for the child and adult to turn around in or perform transfers from chair to toilet. You may find you need safety bars or hand rails round the toilet or even hoists as the child gets bigger. Portable commodes can be useful for night-time toileting or other situations when the main toilet cannot be easily accessed. Similar considerations will be needed at the child's nursery and primary school.

There are many different aids available and housing adaptations may be required. Advice is best sought from your occupational therapist who will visit your home to advise you and make any necessary referrals or recommendations.

Self-care skills

An inherent part of the toileting process is the self-care skills of removing and replacing clothes, wiping or cleaning after urination or defecation and hand washing. Some children find it difficult to manage tasks such as undoing buttons or pulling down trousers and it may help to have Velcro fastenings, poppers or trousers with a front flap. Figure 15.6 shows some positions which may help children pull their pants/trousers/skirt down and up again.

Cleaning, particularly after defecation, can be a considerable coordination challenge and it may help to use wet wipes rather than toilet paper to start with.

Reaching the taps and basin can also be difficult and it may be easier to have a bowl of water with a bar of soap in an accessible place or to use hand wipes.

Night times

Night-time dryness follows on after reliable daytime dryness but there can be a significant time gap between the two and most parents keep their child in night-time nappies until daytime toileting is mastered. Once your child has achieved

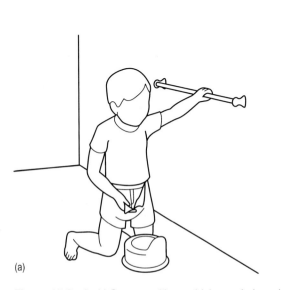

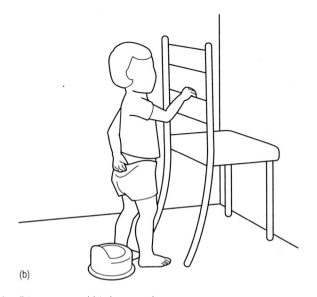

(a) (b)

Figure 15.6 • (a, b) Some positions which may help a child pull trousers or skirt down and up.

daytime dryness, night-time training can be started. You may find that your child is spontaneously dry at this time with dry nappies by morning. All that remains is for you to remove the nappy. For others, it is helpful to limit fluid intake 1–1½ hours before bed, when your child should have a last proper drink. It is very important for your child to have a 'pee' before bed and lots of children initially find this difficult to understand because they do not feel the need. Protective coverings for the bed protect the mattress and disposable or washable absorbent mats are also useful. It is important that the child is able to access the toilet at night if the child wakes up needing to pass urine and it may be that a potty or bucket by the side of the bed will do the trick.

Constipation

Avoiding constipation is an important prerequisite for healthy bowels and successful toilet training. Constipation occurs when faeces are retained in the large bowel for longer than normal. This results in the faeces being hard and difficult to pass. The result is infrequent passage (less often than every 3 days) of hard, rounded faeces which may hurt the child's bottom and may put them off opening their bowels in the future. Children do this by withholding the next time they have the urge to defecate and a vicious cycle can develop. The result is that faeces start to accumulate and back up. The large bowel does not like this state of affairs and will attempt to shift the faeces, with strong contractions that the child experiences as abdominal pain. If severe enough, softer liquid faecal matter (like slurry) from higher up in the colon will be pushed down past the hard blocked faeces and leak out of the anus. This can be confusing, as the soft faecal material may be mistaken for diarrhoea when in fact the child is severely constipated. Constipation can make anyone feel miserable, with poor appetite and abdominal pain. It can also affect bladder function by preventing complete emptying and predisposing to urinary tract infections in susceptible children.

Children with CP may be predisposed to constipation by virtue of the fact that food and fluid intake can be compromised by difficult feeding. Because of the motor disorder some may experience decreased mobility (and abdominal muscle use) and relaxation of the pelvic floor and external anal sphincter. Importantly, constipation may create unpleasant associations with toileting for the child which may sabotage toilet training attempts.

Conservative measures to encourage a healthy bowel habit include regular meals containing high-fibre foods and six to eight water-based drinks per day. It can be difficult encouraging children to eat high-fibre foods but raisins, fibre-containing cereals, brown bread, baked beans and baked potatoes are a start. In addition regular abdominal massage has been found to be useful with a gentle motion of the heel of the hand from the left of the umbilicus (belly button) down towards the lower mid-portion of the abdomen. If this does not do the trick and result in a regular, easily passed, soft formed stool then help and advice should be obtained from your doctor or paediatrician. It is important to do this earlier rather than later when the cycle of constipation may be very ingrained and prolonged treatment is more likely to be required. Your doctor will often prescribe laxatives to help. Laxatives are used for their local effect on the bowel in order to create a regular soft stool and they should be used on a regular basis in order to have best effect. The dose should be titrated in order to achieve the desired effect as too much will result in diarrhoea and abdominal pain and too little will result in ongoing constipation. There are two classes of laxative: softeners and stimulants. Softeners are used to make faeces softer and therefore easier for the bowel to push along. If softeners do not produce the desired effect on their own a stimulant may be required in addition. Examples of softener include lactulose and macrogol 3350 (Movicol) and stimulants include senna and bisacodyl.

Unsuccessful toilet training

Do not worry if toilet training does not seem to be going well. It may be that your child is simply not ready developmentally, and you should simply try again in a few months. It would be worthwhile discussing the issues with your health visitor or another professional to reassure you and to make plans for the future. If you have noticed any particular problems it is important to address these before trying again. If your child has not been able to toilet train despite fulfilling the readiness criteria and a concerted, consistent effort at training along the above lines, it is important to discuss this with an appropriate health professional. Your child may need to have bladder and bowel function more carefully assessed in the context of the child's motor disorder and associated development in order to pinpoint where the problem might lie.

Occasionally your child may benefit from a more intensive structured behavioural training programme (Azrin and Foxx 1974). Other strategies, such as using a body-worn buzzer alarm in the nappy or pants, may help your child to identify the sensations associated with a full bladder.

Some children with CP may have bladder dysfunction that prevents complete toilet training and requires diagnosis and treatment. In particular, a condition called bladder overactivity can result in your child passing urine frequently with very little warning (urgency) and urinary incontinence

results. This condition occurs in the ordinary population but is also reported in association with children with CP, when it is referred to as neurogenic bladder overactivity (Bauer 2002). Treatment usually involves bladder training and medication. Occasionally there is additional sphincter overactivity or an inability to relax the external urinary sphincter resulting in incomplete bladder emptying and treatment may involve clean intermittent catheterization as well. These conditions require specialist assessment and management and your general practitioner or paediatrician will be able to make an appropriate referral.

Either way it is very important to keep the issue of toilet training as a goal for you and your child as it is such an important part of long-term psychosocial esteem for the individual, with obvious implications for care issues. It can be forgotten among all the other pressing needs for your child and can present with other difficult issues if left too late. Keep on trying, but if you feel you are not achieving progress, do not hesitate to ask for help.

References

Azrin NH, Foxx RM. Toilet training in less than a day. Simon and Schuster, New York, 1974.

Bauer SB. Special considerations of the overactive bladder in children. Urology 2002; 60(Suppl. 5A):43–49.

Roijen LEG, Postema K, Limbeek YJ et al. Development of bladder control in children and adolescents with cerebral palsy. Dev Med Child Neurol 2001; 43:103–107.

Wright AJ, et al. The attainment of continence in cerebral palsy: a population based study. BPNA presentation 2002, Newcastle, UK.

Chapter Sixteen

16

Bathing

Revised by Eva Bower

Bathing a child with cerebral palsy (CP), encouraging the child to cooperate and perhaps eventually bathing independently often presents parents with problems, especially as the child grows heavier and longer. The difficulties faced, particularly when bathing the more severely involved child (levels IV and V on the Gross Motor Function Classification System (GMFCS): Palisano et al. 1997) arise as a result of the inability to sit. The more mildly affected child (levels I, II and III on the GMFCS), who can sit, is easier to manage. A child will not be able to learn to bath independently until sitting balance has been attained and the child no longer needs to rely on the hands and arms for support. This can be achieved by putting a child into a piece of equipment which enables supported sitting, leaving the hands free for use. In the typical child independent sitting, with little risk of overbalancing, is usually achieved by around 10 months.

To appreciate the difficulties a child with an unstable sitting base and inadequate sitting balance has to cope with when attempting to bath, one has only to think how much one relies on the ability to balance when taking a bath. For example, when lifting a leg to wash a foot, when adjusting one's position to wash one's back, and it becomes even more difficult if one has to bath using only one hand.

In this chapter some of the problems will be discussed and ways suggested that may make it easier to bath a child with CP. Suitable types of bathing aids, particularly seats, and ways of encouraging the older child to start bathing independently will also be considered.

Bath time is one of the daily routines that children enjoy. By 20 weeks of age the typical child will splash happily in the bath. Bathing often starts to lose its appeal when it means interrupting playtime or when children reach the stage of being responsible for bathing themselves.

Strategies which may help when bathing the young, small child

Bathing a child with CP is usually comparatively easy while the child is small so long as the base of the child's bath has an antislip surface for security. If the surface is slippery a small towel placed under the child will often be adequate or, if preferred, a small bathmat which sticks to the bottom of the bath.

The care and attention given to preparing oneself and the child before putting the child into or taking the child out of the bath are important. Some children are difficult to handle when lifting in and out of the bath. Some may throw their hands and arms backwards into extension. Others may have poor head control and low truncal tone and tend to slip through one's hands. Rather than lifting a child in and out of the bath in a semi-lying position it may be easier to hold the child if you flex the child first so that the hips are bent and the trunk and arms brought well forward (Figure 16.1).

If it is difficult to flex a child in the early months, as a short-term solution you might try washing as shown in Figure 16.2.

As the child grows bigger you might like to try washing as shown in Figures 16.3 and 16.4.

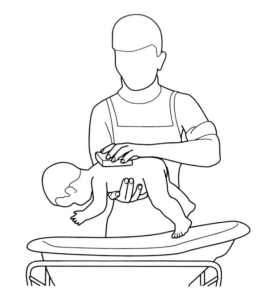

Figure 16.2 • Washing a small child who is difficult to flex.

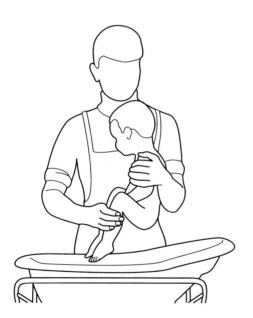

Figure 16.1 • Lifting a small child who extends in and out of a bath with the hips bent and the trunk and arms brought forward.

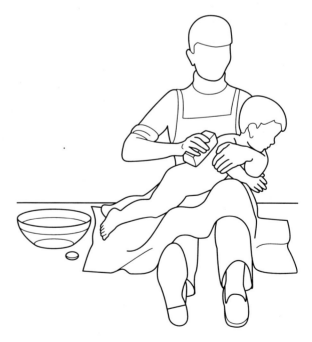

Figure 16.3 • Washing a child who flexes over the mother's knees.

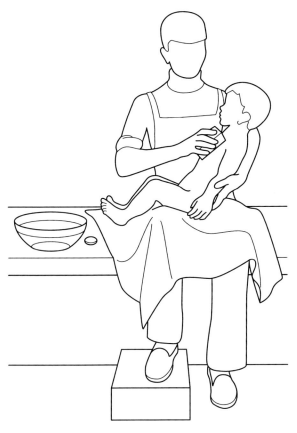

Figure 16.4 • Washing a child who extends on the mother's lap.

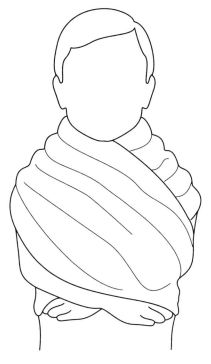

Figure 16.5 • Washing a child's face in a child who pushes the head back, using a towel wrapped firmly round the shoulders and chest to bring both arms forwards.

Some children push their heads back when they have their faces washed. This can sometimes be prevented by bringing both the child's arms forward and wrapping a towel firmly around the shoulders and across the chest (Figure 16.5).

Choosing a bath for the young, small child

The best type of child's bath is one that has a slight slope that supports the child's back. The bath stand should be firm and stable and the bath at a manageable height so that parents do not have to bend their back (Figure 16.6). If the child needs additional head support an absorbent foam pillow held in place with Velcro straps can be attached to the top end of the bath.

When the child grows out of the first bath parents often find it difficult to use a regular-sized bath. At this in-between stage it may be helpful to explore baths such as the one shown in Figure 16.7. Such a bath fits over most regular baths and is at a more convenient and manageable height. It can be filled directly from the bath taps and has a drain plug allowing the water to empty down the regular bath drain. This enables the parent to wrap a towel round the child whilst still in the bath before lifting the child out.

Another possibility is to bath a child in the base or tray of your shower if it has a non-slip floor. The problem with this is that it involves lowering the child to floor level and raising the child from floor level. For a child with poor head control and predominantly low tone it may be helpful to try out some of the versatile and easy-to-use swimming pool aids. Your physiotherapist or occupational therapist may be able to help you with this.

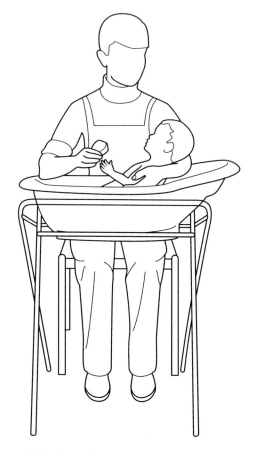

Figure 16.6 • A small child's bath with a sloping back placed at a convenient height for the mother to sit by it.

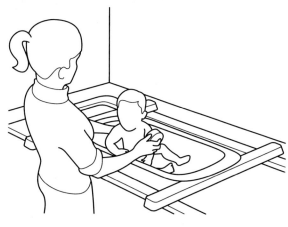

Figure 16.7 • A child's bath which fits into a regular bath so that the mother can kneel at the side of the bath.

Never leave your child unattended or alone in the bath and never leave your child unattended or alone in a bathing aid.

Interactive play with your child at bath time

For the parent your child's bath time may just be another daily routine but for your child it can be a good opportunity to learn through play. Where better to share the experience of interaction between a parent and a child than at bath time? This does mean setting aside extra time but it is likely to be time well spent for both.

Early communication is an important aspect of a child's development. At the stage when your child is still relatively immature in movement development yet relaxed and happy, bath time provides an excellent opportunity to lay down the foundation of what may develop into verbal communication. Encourage your child to look at your face whilst you speak. When your child responds by cooing and kicking keep the dialogue up between you, repeat the child's sounds and introduce new ones from time to time. Gently encourage and help your child to get two hands together and to look at them and also to splash them in the water. Get your child used to being moved by 'swishing' the child backwards and forwards in the bath. If your child enjoys it, do this with the child lying both on the back and front.

In many toy catalogues you will find a wide range of toys specially designed for a child to play with in the bath. Those which can be attached to the side of the bath and those with a suction base are particularly good.

Strategies which may help when bathing the growing, older child

Problems in handling may increase as a child grows older and bigger and is bathed in a standard-sized bath. Whereas a small child can be placed in a child's bath at a convenient height for a parent to manage, the normal-sized bath is deep and awkward in shape. The following are ideas that you might like to try at this stage.

Many children with mild or moderate involvement (levels I, II and III GMFCS) often feel rather insecure when sitting in a bath, even though they may have sitting balance. If your bath does not have a non-slip base a regular mat with suction cups that stick to the base of the bath should make a child feel more secure. Some children may feel happier if, in addition to the non-slip base, they sit inside two rubber rings (Figure 16.8). This provides lower trunk and pelvic support, leaving the child free to move the upper trunk and arms.

Another way of helping a child feel more confident and at the same time enabling play in the bath is by placing the child in a plastic laundry basket with a non-slip mat at the bottom (Figure 16.9).

Depending upon the child's amount of sitting balance, it may be helpful to use a suction hand rail threaded through the basket and attached to the side of the bath for the child to hold on to (Figure 16.10).

One mother whose child was more severely affected (level V GMFCS) found it easier to bath

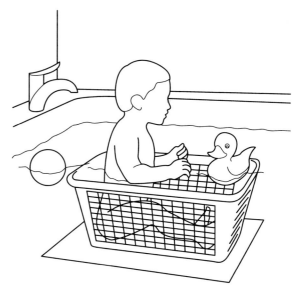

Figure 16.9 • Child sitting in a plastic laundry basket placed on a non-slip mat in the bath.

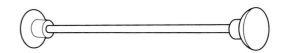

Figure 16.10 • Hand rail with suction caps for a child to hold on to.

her child if she put the child on the tummy on a half-inflated ball placed in the bath. This example is given to show how many parents can effectively manage their own child in everyday situations, especially if they have an understanding of the problems involved.

Choosing a bath seat

The first priority when choosing a bathing aid is to provide a child with a comfortable seat and a means of support that will enable a child to feel secure in the bath. Many of the seats can also be placed in a shower if the size and fixings fit. It is also important to make sure that the chosen bath seat makes it easy for you, the parent, to bath your child. This can be difficult as it is often not possible to take a bath seat home on temporary

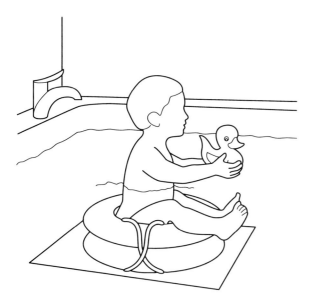

Figure 16.8 • Child sitting inside two rubber rings placed on a non-slip mat in the bath.

loan. It is in this sort of situation that support groups are useful as there will almost certainly be another parent who has faced a similar problem and may even have a similar bath seat to the one you have been recommended. The parent will be able to tell you if there has been any difficulty with:

1. Adjusting the seat or supports

2. Getting the child in and out of the seat

3. Washing the child all over, including the hair, back and bottom

Before purchasing a bath seat the following should be checked:

1. That the angle of the bath rest and the height of the seat are easily adjustable

2. That the material of the seat is comfortable and keeps its shape. Vinyl and plastic materials may be cold and slippery

3. The length of warranty and the availability of replacement parts

For the young child

With moderate sitting balance

For the young child who has good head and trunk control but only moderate sitting balance, a plastic moulded back support (Figure 16.11) and bath hand rails may be helpful. These can be adjusted to the width of a regular-sized bath and are attached by suction cups to the sides of the bath. The plastic moulded back support is attached to one of the rails and pivots to take up the natural angle of the child's back. The hand rails are placed in front for the child to hold on to as needed.

A slatted bath stool placed in the bath can also be used with the hand rail.

With inadequate sitting balance

A bath seat which fits across a standard bath has been found helpful for the child with limited ability to bend the hips. The seat may give the child an added feeling of security as the feet may rest on the bottom of the bath and the child can hold on to the metal bar surrounding the seat if and as required. The product usually has a plastic sling seat with holes for the legs to fit through and a plastic sling-type back rest (Figure 16.12).

A plastic corner seat fitted with a Velcro and buckle strap and a plastic abduction block may be another possibility for a child needing more support (Figure 16.13).

With no sitting balance

A bath chair may be suitable for children who have no sitting balance. The chair should be on castors so that it can be wheeled in and out of the shower if a suitable shower facility is available. Plastic and aluminium construction should control rusting and ease cleaning. A variable tilting mechanism is needed to accommodate children

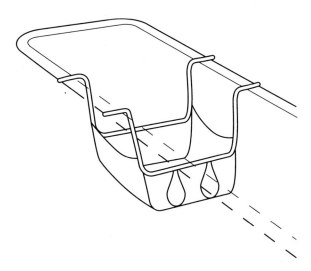

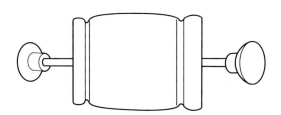

Figure 16.11 • For a younger child with moderate sitting balance but good head and trunk control, a plastic moulded back support with suction caps.

Figure 16.12 • For a younger child with inadequate sitting balance and difficulty flexing the hips, a seat that fits across the bath.

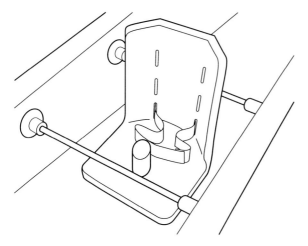

Figure 16.13 • For a younger child with inadequate sitting balance, a corner seat.

who push back into extension or those who fall forward into flexion. Adjustable head and foot rests, thoracic supports, abduction pommels and harnesses should be fitted as needed individually (Figure 16.14).

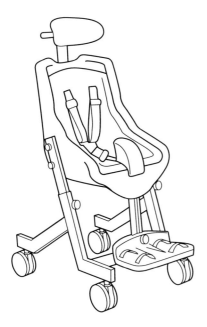

Figure 16.14 • For a younger child with no sitting balance, a bath chair.

For the older child

There are many bathing aids available for the older child. It will be necessary to assess the level of your child's sitting ability and then choose the most suitable. A useful assessment tool for this purpose is the Box Sitting Assessment Chart, which is part of the Chailey Heritage Clinical Services Levels of Abilities and is obtainable from Beggars Wood Road, North Chailey, East Sussex BN84JN, UK. A few examples of bathing aids for the older child are described below.

With adequate sitting balance

Figure 16.15 shows a bath support suitable for a child with good head and upper trunk control but needing support around the pelvis. It fits into a standard bath.

Figure 16.16 shows a similar bath support with a high, upright, plastic back rest suitable for a

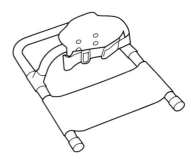

Figure 16.15 • Bath support for a larger child with adequate sitting balance, good head and upper trunk control needing pelvic support.

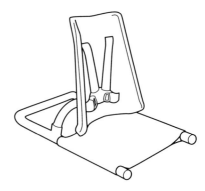

Figure 16.16 • Bath support for a larger child requiring trunk and some head control.

child requiring control for the trunk and possibly some head support. A harness supplies shoulder, chest and waist support.

With no sitting balance

Until a child is able to sit independently, a bath seat which holds the child in a semi-reclining position may be best. Figure 16.17 shows a reclining bath chair with a tilting back which can be used with belts for support. Figure 16.18 shows a similar reclining bath chair but with a more adjustable base.

Figure 16.19 shows a child lying in a powered bath lift. The child can be raised and lowered in the bath in this aid but still needs to be transferred manually on to this aid.

Unable to be put in sitting position

For the older child who cannot be placed in a sitting position the most suitable type of bathing aid may be a shallow bath made of thermoplastic material which is slip-resistant. This type of bath fits into a standard bath and is therefore at a more convenient height. It should be light and easy to move into and out of the bath, it should be filled with water from the bath taps and should have a large outlet for draining the water out so that the child can remain in the bath and then a towel can

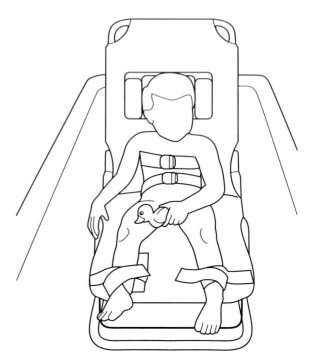

Figure 16.18 • Reclining bath seat, like Figure 16.17, but with a more adjustable base.

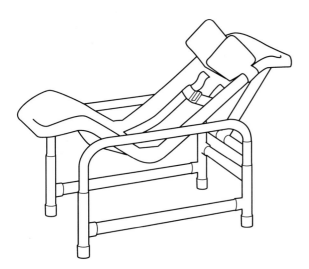

Figure 16.17 • For a larger child with no sitting balance, a reclining bath seat.

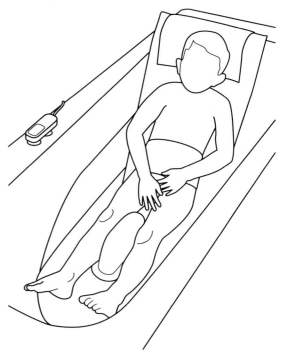

Figure 16.19 • A powered bath lift.

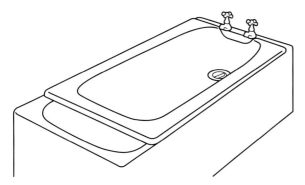

Figure 16.20 • For a large child unable to be put into a sitting position, a shallow bath.

be wrapped around the child before being lifted out. The effective length of the bath can be shortened by the insertion of a sloping back rest. As the width of the bath is similar to that of a standard bath there is sufficient room to roll the child on to the side, making washing easier (Figure 16.20).

A hand shower attached to the bath taps may also be helpful.

You may find that as your child gets heavier the only way you can manage is by giving the child a shower. It is recommended that you seek expert advice before embarking on major house adaptations, but a shower in an area with a sloping, non-slip floor for water drainage, and no steps into the area so that you can wheel your child directly into it using a chair made from suitable material for use in the shower is probably the best solution. A hand shower facilitates washing areas such as armpits.

Preventive back care for parents

One of the problems that often arises when bathing a child as the child grows longer and heavier is that it puts a strain on the parent's back which may predispose to problems in later life. To try to avoid this happening it is worth experimenting to see if kneeling on a cushion or sitting on a stool at the side of the bath reduces the strain on the back.

Bath time: a learning situation

I am, of course, not suggesting that you should do all the activities described every time you bath your child. I am conscious of the fact that bathing a child with CP can take a long time and therefore the time you spend playing may be limited; there is also the fact that other members of the family might want a bath too! No attempt is being made in this section to discuss which activities are suitable for a particular child either with a specific problem or at a particular stage of development. A variety of activities are suggested, some of which may be familiar to you, while others may be new. I leave you to choose those that are applicable to your child.

If your child is to feel safe and enjoy bath time the way to encourage confidence is to explain what you are doing before you do it. For example: 'I am going to wash this arm. Please help me by lifting it up as much as you can'. Touch and name the taps, explaining that one is for hot water and the other for cold. Show your child how to turn the water on and off. Let your child see you test the temperature of the water and explain why you do this. 'See the water running': demonstrate the difference between a light and heavy flow of water and let your child feel the difference. In this way you will not only make a game out of bath time but also create a valuable learning experience in a situation in which you will probably find it easier to secure your child's attention and cooperation.

Sensory awareness and motor learning at bath time

If you have a shower attachment to the bath taps a good way of helping your child develop an awareness of his or her body is by soaping the child all over and then directing a light spray of water at different parts of the body and encouraging your child to look, touch and if possible name the parts of the body sprayed. While your child is in the bath let your child feel the difference between a dry and wet sponge or flannel and encourage your child to squeeze the water out if possible. Drying your child with a slightly rougher towel, sometimes more firmly, sometimes more gently, can be made into a game and is another way of increasing awareness of the part dried.

Bath time is an excellent opportunity for letting your child practise hand function. Place floating toys and objects in the bath which are easy to handle. These could include household items such as empty plastic squeezy bottles, plastic yoghurt containers and corks. Encourage your child to notice the different ways in which they act in the water – some float whereas others sink. Practising filling and emptying and pouring water from one container to another is a way of helping your child to improve the timing and grading of movements and to develop eye–hand coordination further. There will be much less mess if these activities are undertaken in the bath rather than in the kitchen or living room.

Asking your child to give you the flannel, sponge and soap during washing and any toys before getting out of the bath are ways of practising grasping and releasing a variety of objects. It may also extend the vocabulary if the object is named.

Speech and movement

We often like to sing in the bath so if you find that your child likes to make a lot of noise while splashing about in the water, do encourage it. Speech may reinforce movement and control movement as it links intention with action. As your child develops communication and verbal speech skills, encourage your child to join in singing nursery rhymes with you that incorporate actions, such as 'This is the way we wash our face ... this is the way we wash our hands ... knees' and so on.

Working towards independence

Washing face and hands

It is especially important that, in preparation for going to playgroup and later to school, your child learns how to wash and dry his or her own face and hands if possible. Most typical children can wash and dry their own hands by about 24–30 months given the opportunity and a suitable facility.

Consider the steps involved:

1. Put plug in basin or operate plunger
2. Turn taps on
3. Pick up soap
4. Put soap on flannel
5. Wash face and hands
6. Rinse face and hands
7. Pick up towel
8. Dry face and hands
9. Replace towel
10. Let water out of basin

To achieve these tasks your child needs some mobility, stability and hand function. All of these will not necessarily be available to your child but you will appreciate that many of the movements needed to perform the tasks are also used in other daily activities. The central message in making progress in functional tasks is to break the task down into small stages or steps. Use as much carry-over of learning as you can from one task to another and, most of all, while stimulating and challenging your child to greater independence, never frustrate your child with a task beyond the child's capability. Remember: when children refuse to do a task, it is often because they *cannot* do it rather than because they do not want to do it.

Start teaching your child to wash his or her face and hands in sitting. For young children, as a standard basin is too high, give them a basin of water placed on a table in front of them (Figure 16.21). Later give the child a chair to stand on placed in front of the basin. At this stage the child can also try to manipulate the taps, which will involve reaching and grasping while maintaining a standing position (Figure 16.22).

Bathing

If a child reaches the stage of bathing independently the child may still be unable to get in and out of the bath alone without some means of support. Help may be given by a non-slip bath mat, a box or stool of the right height on which the child can sit before stepping in or out of the bath (Figure 16.23). Make sure there is something to hold on to: grab bars are useful for this purpose. At first ensure that the bath contains only a few centimetres of water and check the temperature of the water.

Some of the following items of equipment may help a child reach the stage of washing themselves:

1. A glove or mitten-type flannel

2. A mitt-type loofah

3. A wooden nail brush with indented sides which make it easier to grip, or a piece of webbing over the top of the brush through which the child can slip a hand

4. A long-handled brush

5. A liquid soap container

6. Soap and nail brush with suction caps

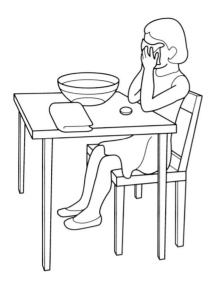

Figure 16.21 • Child washing own face and hands sitting at a table with a bowl of water.

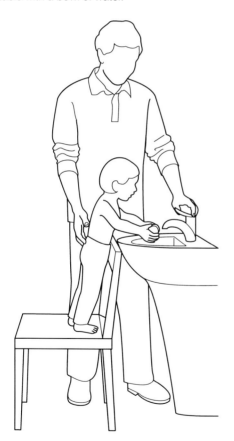

Figure 16.22 • Child washing own face and hands standing on a chair at a basin.

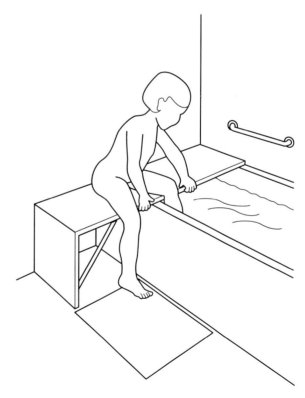

Figure 16.23 • Using a bathboard to get in and out of a bath.

7. If a shower spray is not a permanent fixture, a hand shower attached to the taps for rinsing

8. A large bath towel with a hole in the middle which can be slipped over the head, a terry towelling wrap or a towel with a tape which can be hung on a hook

9. A towel rail within easy reach and a stool or chair nearby for clothes

In this chapter I have tried to stress the importance of gaining your child's cooperation as early as possible and of working together with your child towards achieving the most independence allowed by the severity of the child's condition.

Reference

Palisano R, Rosenbaum P, Walter S et al. Development and validation of a gross motor function classification system for children with CP. Dev Med Child Neurol 1997; 39: 214–223.

Chapter Seventeen

Dressing

Revised by Eva Bower

In this chapter I shall discuss some of the problems that may arise when dressing or undressing a child with cerebral palsy (CP), ways of encouraging a child to cooperate and become as independent as possible with dressing and finally some ideas on more suitable clothing.

Before moving on to the more practical aspects of handling, or to put it another way positioning, holding and moving a child during dressing, I think it may be helpful to remind ourselves what complicated tasks dressing and undressing are. Not only does the child need to have sitting balance, good coordination between eyes and hands, the ability to reach, grasp and release, the ability to fix with one hand while moving the other but also the fine motor movement necessary to cope with buttons, zips and laces. The child needs to understand the difference between front and back, top and bottom, inside and outside and be able to distinguish between large and small openings on a variety of garments. The child must be able to plan movements in readiness for the tasks in hand. It is therefore not surprising that the majority of typical children are at least 5 years old before they are able to dress themselves without help.

A typical child usually starts to cooperate with dressing at about 12 months of age by holding out a foot for a shoe and an arm for a sleeve. At about 18 months, having achieved good sitting balance, and no longer needing to rely on the hands for support, the child will deliberately pull off shoes, socks, mittens and hat. Previously these items might have been snatched off unintentionally. Between 18 months and 2 years the child will start to cooperate more with both dressing and undressing and is usually able to take off all clothes by the age of 3 years. But the child will be at least 4 years before being able to put most of the clothes on. Between 4 and 5 years the child can dress and undress except for buttons, zips and laces. At 5 years the child usually learns to tie shoelaces and some time later begins to understand which holes to lace in and out of and in which direction. Although able to push feet into shoes quite early on it does not become apparent to a child which shoe fits on to which foot until later.

Dressing and undressing the child with cerebral palsy

General principles

1. Try to choose a position or positions for dressing and undressing your child which minimizes stiffness and unwanted movements, thus making it easier for both of you. Depending upon your child's characteristics these positions may be in lying, sitting, kneeling or standing.

2. Check to see that your child is lying, sitting, kneeling or standing as symmetrically as possible both before and during the activities. It is usually easier to dress the more affected side first and undress it last.

3. A priority when dressing any child is to make sure that all the clothes are within easy reach and where the child can see them if possible.

4. While your child is dependent upon you for dressing and undressing, make sure that your child is lying or sitting at a height which makes it as comfortable as possible for you.

5. Try to give your child lots of opportunities to help with both dressing and undressing, practising and using all the skills possessed, however limited. Always tell your child what you are going to do and what you want your child to do.

Positioning, holding and moving the child with cerebral palsy

Young children (under 8 months)

Most young children with CP are quite easy to dress and undress in the early stages as stiffness, unwanted movements and changing muscle tone do not usually appear until some months later.

If your young child does tend to bend or flop forwards, flexing rather a lot, it may be easier to dress or undress over your knees, as shown in Figure 17.1.

If your young child does tend to push backwards, extending rather a lot, it may be easier to dress and undress either over your knees, as shown in Figure 17.1, or on your lap, as shown in Figure 17.2.

Young children (under 1 year) with moderate stiffness

When some children with moderate stiffness reach the age of about 8–10 months there may be increasing resistance to certain movements such as parting the legs to put on a nappy or bringing the shoulders forwards and straightening the arms to put them through sleeves. Figure 17.3 shows a way of moving the legs to change a nappy and Figure 17.4 shows a way of moving the arms to put them through sleeves.

Figure 17.5 shows what is generally considered to be a more difficult way to dress a child in lying who has a tendency to turn the head to one side with an increase in bending or flexion of the arm on the skull side. Figure 17.6 shows that by rolling your child towards yourself you can encourage

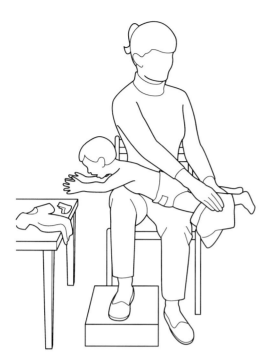

Figure 17.1 • Dressing or undressing a small child who flexes forwards.

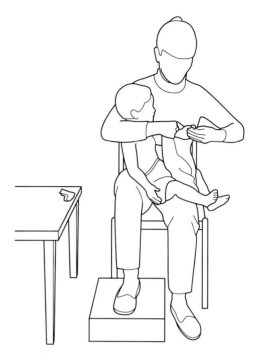

Figure 17.2 • Dressing or undressing a small child who extends backwards.

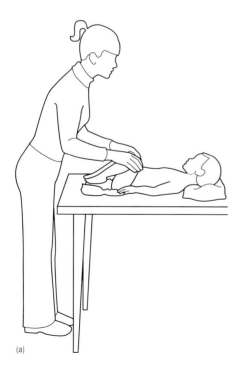

(a)

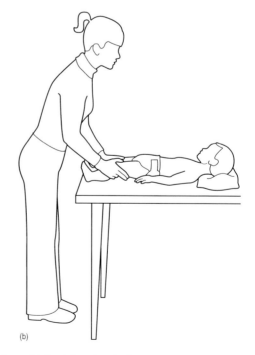

(b)

Figure 17.3 • (a) Bending a child's knees up and out to part the legs. (b) Straightening the legs down from the knees.

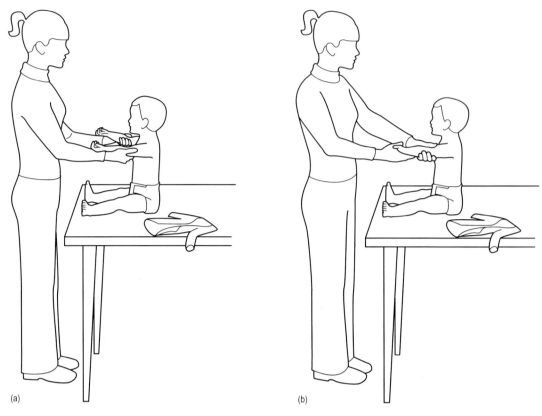

Figure 17.4 • (a) Turning a child's arms out and straightening them from the elbows. (b) Grasping a child's hand and keeping the elbow straight.

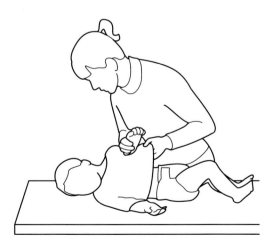

Figure 17.5 • A more difficult way to dress a child in lying (facing away from you).

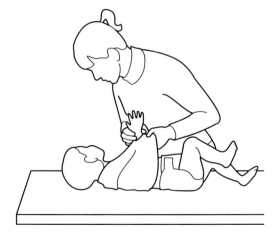

Figure 17.6 • An easier way to dress a child in lying (facing towards you).

participation, talk to your child and you can bring the child's shoulder forwards with the arm straight or in extension, which should be easier.

At this stage a child is still rather young to cooperate and problems sometimes arise because positioning, holding and moving may be too static, as shown in Figure 17.7. Figure 17.8 shows how, by introducing different positions and movements,

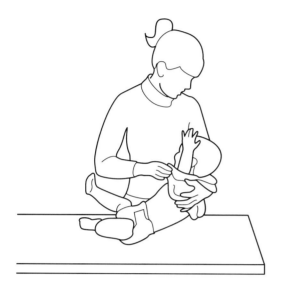

Figure 17.7 • A more difficult way to dress a child in sitting (child sliding about).

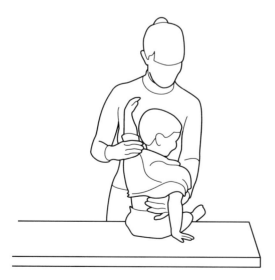

Figure 17.8 • An easier way to dress a child in sitting (child securely anchored).

you may, for example, encourage lifting up of the head and supporting or propping on the arm.

The young child who tends to push back into extension

With no sitting balance

If your child is dressed lying on the back the supporting surface should be inclined or tilted so that your child's head is slightly higher than the feet. This should make it easier for you, the parent, to bend or flex your child's head, bring the shoulders and arms forwards and bend your child's hips, knees and ankles.

Alternatively you could try dressing your child in side-lying, with the more affected side uppermost first for dressing, and the least affected side uppermost first for undressing.

With some sitting balance

If your child is dressed on your lap make sure that your child is in a good, stable, sitting position, hips bent or flexed and legs not too widely apart or abducted. By positioning your child in this way you should be able to turn your child's trunk or torso, making it easier for you to bring the shoulders forward and keep the hips bent or flexed, as shown in Figure 17.9.

The young child who sits with semi-extended hips, a rounded or flexed spine, chin poked forward, shoulders pulled forward and arms flexed by the sides

It should help you to dress your child more easily if once again you first check that your child is in a good, secure, sitting position. Then bend your child forwards at the hips and bring both arms forwards with straight elbows, palms facing up and turn the arms out at the elbows (Figure 17.10). By moving your child in this way you should find it easier to keep your child's back straight and head up and in turn this may help your child to straighten the back and lift the head.

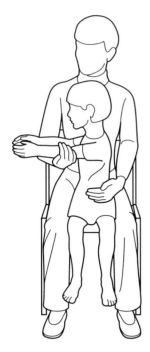

Figure 17.9 • Positioning a child who tends to push back into extension in sitting between your legs.

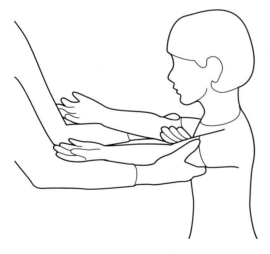

Figure 17.10 • Positioning a child who sits with a flexed spine and flexed arms.

The young child with unwanted movements and changing or fluctuating muscle tone

A child who later develops unwanted or involuntary movements and changing or fluctuating tone often has low truncal tone during the early months and if placed on the back lies with arms and legs in varying degrees of flexion, abduction and outward rotation. The child may also have a tendency to turn the head predominantly to one side, resulting in asymmetry of the trunk and pelvis. If your child is such a child, getting dressed lying on the back may become more difficult and dressing your child in side-lying or sitting on your lap may be easier. Probably the most comfortable position is for your child to lie on the tummy across your knees, if not too big, as shown in Figure 17.1, and especially so if your child is beginning to push the head and shoulders backwards and kick continuously.

The older child who can sit but has insufficient sitting balance

An older child who cannot sit and maintain balance when using both hands to dress may be helped by being given a point of stability using support at one of the following: hips, thighs, knees or feet. Where and how much stabilization is needed will depend upon the ability of the child to control the sitting position (Figure 17.11).

Sitting a child facing the back of a chair, as shown in Figure 17.12, is a good way of encouraging self-stabilization. By grasping the chair with one hand the child can lift and help to push the other arm through the sleeve. The box shown under the feet may provide another point of stability.

Sleeves, socks and shoes

Putting the older child's arms in and out of sleeves and putting on and taking off socks and shoes are two of the most common problems parents have to cope with – the former because of an increase in stiffness or flexor bending tone in the arms, the latter because of an increase in stiffness or extensor straightening tone in the legs. The following practical advice may help to overcome these difficulties.

Arms in and out of sleeves
Check to see that your child is sitting symmetrically, weight evenly distributed, hips flexed or bent and feet flat on the floor. It is very difficult

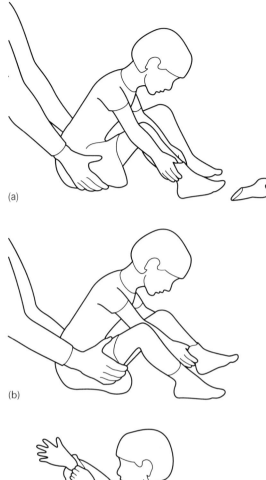

(a)

(b)

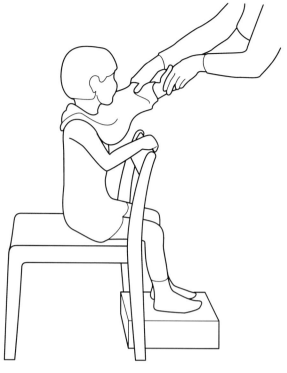

Figure 17.12 • Encouraging a child to self-stabilize sitting on a chair.

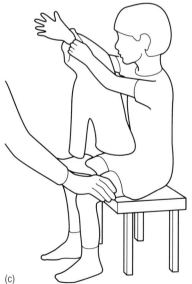

(c)

Figure 17.11 • (a) Supporting a child at the hips in sitting. (b) Supporting a child at the thighs in sitting. (c) Supporting a child at the knees in sitting on a seat.

to bring an arm forward while the shoulders and trunk remain back with the hips extended or straight. Do not take hold of an arm and pull as this will only result in an increase in flexor or bending tone. Straighten the arm first with outward rotation at the shoulder, being sure that the elbow is extended, then put the sleeve on. Do the same when taking the sleeve off (Figure 17.13).

Socks and shoes

Check sitting position as above. Do not try to put your child's feet into socks or shoes while the leg is extended and the foot plantarflexed or pointing downwards as this will result in an increase in extensor tone and toes will curl under. Flex the leg first, checking that the hip is outwardly rotated. It should then be easier to bring the foot up (Figure 17.14). When doing up shoes, always see that the foot is flat on a support.

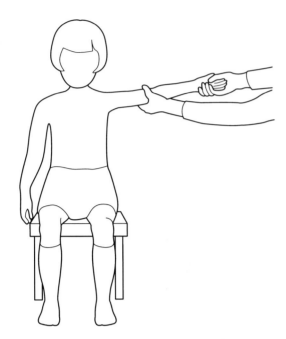

Figure 17.13 • Straightening the arm out before putting a sleeve through.

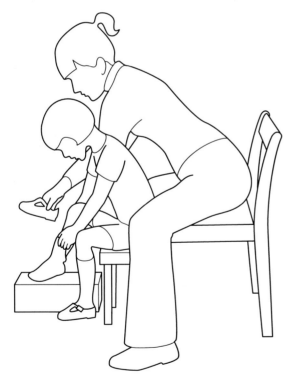

Figure 17.14 • Bending the knee up and out before putting a sock and shoe on.

Dressing and undressing the more severely affected child: level IV or V on the Gross Motor Function Classification System (Palisano et al. 1997)

Dressing and undressing a child with CP is never easy and becomes more difficult as the child grows older and heavier, especially if stiffness, unwanted movements or changes in tone increase at the same time as the child is growing and becoming heavier. As these children usually have little or no sitting balance they are often dressed or undressed lying either on a bed or a firm surface at a convenient height. As the stiffness, unwanted movements and changing muscle tone often increase when a child lies on the back it is worthwhile trying, at least partially, to dress or undress the child lying on the side. By rolling the child from side to side during dressing the child may not be in a position long enough to become stiff or to push back into extension (Figure 17.15). Side-lying should make it easier to put clothes over the head, put arms into sleeves, bend the hips and legs to put trousers on and do up clothes that fasten down the back. Figure 17.16 shows a changing table with adjustable height and Figure 17.17 a collapsible changing table attached to a wall.

Sitting on the floor/table/chair

Although in this chapter there are a number of illustrations showing a mother sitting behind her child, it is important that this positioning is only used while a child needs support when being dressed or perhaps when a child starts to dress independently. Then the fact that you are behind the child may give the child extra confidence. Try to be sure to leave a gap or space between your bodies as this may discourage the child from leaning backwards against you and also help the child move forwards from the hips.

Figure 17.18 shows a child in a nice position to appreciate what the mother is doing – the child's hands are in the same position as hers as the child completes the final stages of taking off a tee-shirt or in Figure 17.19 putting on socks. By keeping

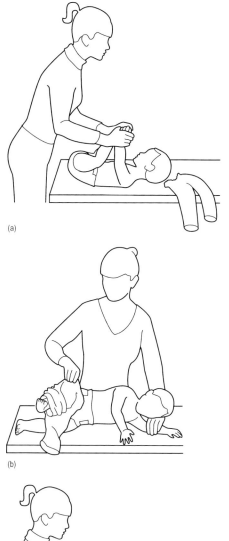

(a)

(b)

(c)

Figure 17.15 • (a) Rolling a child from side to side.
(b) Putting the trouser on to the uppermost leg first.
(c) Putting the trouser on to the second leg.

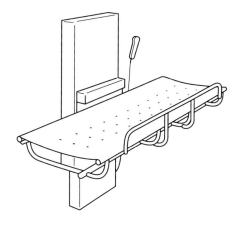

Figure 17.16 • A changing table with height adjustment.

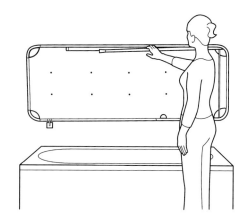

Figure 17.17 • A collapsible changing table.

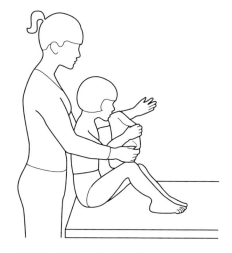

Figure 17.18 • Taking off a tee-shirt.

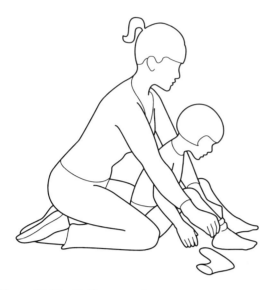

Figure 17.19 • Putting on socks.

the hips flexed and the trunk well forward, when the child lifts and brings the arms forward or lifts and bends a leg, there is less danger that the child will lose balance. As soon as your child can sit alone steadily, move to the side or to the front of the child.

Common problems and some suggestions

Early cooperation

You only have to watch a child being dressed or undressed to realize how most mothers chatter spontaneously to their children and how, even before a child can talk, the child babbles in response, going on later to demand immediate attention when wanting it. Many children with CP are unable to respond in this way and in time it often becomes easier for a mother not to bother to chatter to her child and to dress her child in silence. There will sometimes be occasions when, because of the extra time it takes to dress or undress your child, there will not be time to chatter but do try to make time whenever possible. It will be well worth the effort because if your child is always dressed in silence almost as if a doll,

your child may well become detached and passive and show little interest in what is going on.

Ways to encourage your child to dress or undress

Try not to miss opportunities of encouraging your child to be independent. When it becomes obvious that your child wants to try to help, give all the encouragement you can. At first it is likely that an enormous effort will be required on your child's part to achieve very little and your patience may run out before that of your child, but try not to interfere when your child does try unless, of course, the child gets into real difficulties. You can do this by watching carefully to see how much your child can manage independently and at which point your child needs some help. Only intervene then, but this needs time and patience on your part.

Skills needed

Before looking at ways in which you might encourage your child to dress or undress, let us look in greater detail at some of the abilities that are needed before dressing can become an intentional, purposeful and goal-related activity. The child will probably need to:

1. Sit unsupported and have good hip mobility

2. Look at what he or she is doing and be able to scan so that the eyes can guide the hands

3. Be able to adjust balance when moving the arms into different positions, for example lift an arm without falling backwards

4. Have sufficient stability or fixation at the shoulders so that skilled movements of the arms and hands can be performed, including moving towards and crossing the midline

5. Grasp, release and use fine finger movements regardless of the position of the arm, for example holding with one hand while pushing or pulling with the other

6. Understand the relationship between the openings on clothes and the parts of the body, for example, the difference between a large opening at the top for the head and smaller openings at the sides for the arms

7. Know the difference between up and down, over and under, back and front, inside and outside, left and right

8. Have the ability to sequence, for example know that socks go on before shoes, shirts before sweaters

9. Make an effort without an overflow of movements taking place in other parts of the body which affect the dressing process

On reading this list of skills you will soon appreciate that they include not only motor and movement achievements but also other aspects of development such as perception. Recognizing this, one would have to ask oneself what was preventing a child undertaking a particular activity, for example, putting on socks. Table 17.1 lists some of the questions one might consider and the function required to address each of the questions.

Some of the problems listed in Table 17.1 and others not listed may prevent the child from putting on socks so that it may be caused not just by one difficulty but by a number of difficulties interacting with each other. With such a diverse range of abilities necessary before a child is able to dress or undress, I am sure that you will realize that it would be a waste of time to concentrate, for example,

solely on a child's manipulative skills, without first having an understanding of the child's overall developmental level, including intellectual, physical (fine and gross motor), visual and perceptual abilities.

When a child starts to dress independently, each task should be broken down into small, easy stages. It is often easiest for the child to try to do the last part of the activity first. For example if the child is placed in a supported sitting position with the leg bent up and the sock placed over the foot, the child can then try to pull the sock up or off. It is necessary to watch carefully to see exactly how much the child manages to do alone and at which point the child needs some help. On the one hand try not to give your child more help than is needed but on the other hand do not allow your child to become frustrated.

Common motor problems

A few of the more common dressing problems are:

1. Having to hold and lift clothes, especially pulling them over the head, when some children will easily fall backwards

2. Opening clothes for which both hands will often be needed

Table 17.1 **Struggling to put on socks**

Question	Function required
1. Does the child understand what he or she has been asked to do?	Intellectual ability
2. Does the child have adequate balance to sit without the support of both hands or one hand?	Gross motor control
3. Can the child bend forwards sufficiently to reach the feet?	Gross motor movement
4. When the child bends one leg up, does the other extend so that the child falls backwards?	Gross motor control
5. Does the child have difficulty in using the appropriate movements for the task?	Motor planning ability
6. Does the child have the necessary manipulative skills and hand–eye coordination?	Fine motor control and movement plus visual focus and following ability
7. Is the child able to grasp with outstretched arms, maintaining the grasp while putting on socks?	Gross and fine movement control
8. Is the child able to cross midline?	Body awareness

3. Starting to put on a sock, which entails reaching down to a foot and pulling the sock over the heel

4. Starting to pull down pants

5. Putting the second arm into the sleeve of a coat

6. Doing up and undoing fasteners, especially those at the back

A child with hemiplegia or predominantly one-sided problems often displays associated grasping on the affected side when using the unaffected hand, making it difficult to use both hands together (Figure 17.20). Therefore when trying to take off socks it will sometimes be easier if the child self-supports with the affected hand, stopping this reaction (Figure 17.21). Then using the affected hand as a holding hand uses the unaffected hand to pull the sock off (Figure 17.22) or the shoe off (Figure 17.23).

Supplementing, timing and sequencing efforts

In many cases adaptations to seating, clothing or the use of splinting may be necessary to help function; it may also be necessary to provide spectacles

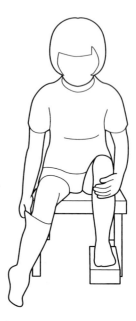

Figure 17.21 • Self-supporting with left affected side.

for a child who has difficulty in seeing what he or she is doing.

If you bear in mind that your child's functional level will be determined by developmental level not by chronological age, you will avoid asking or expecting your child to achieve something that is beyond the child's capabilities. There is nothing

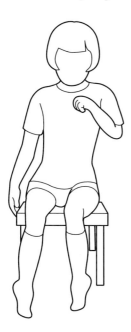

Figure 17.20 • Affected left side showing difficulty using both hands together.

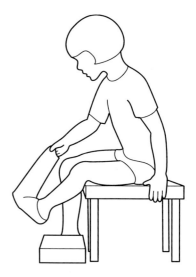

Figure 17.22 • Self-supporting with left affected side using right unaffected hand to pull off left sock.

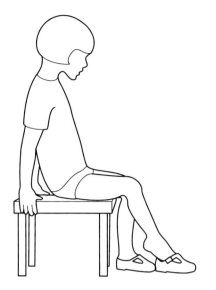

Figure 17.23 • Self-supporting with both hands using left foot to stabilize right foot while taking right shoe off.

more depressing for any of us than tackling a difficult task with no reward at the end.

When playing with your child it is a good idea to get your child to dress and undress a doll or teddy bear to understand the general principles of dressing. When encouraging your child to dress or undress, always do so at a time when you would normally be dressing or undressing the child, rather than practising it as an artificial exercise. All this will, of course, involve considerable input on your part as little can be achieved in a rush and your child will need time and a lot of repetition to master each new task.

Fortunately a child usually learns to undress before learning to dress, which has the advantage that undressing is usually done in the evening when hopefully there is less of a rush. If pressure on your time is a problem then the weekend may be a better time to start.

Training for gross and fine motor skills, which may include head and trunk control, sitting balance, hip mobility, grasp and release, has only one primary purpose, namely to enable your child to become functionally more independent in all activities of daily living.

Dressing is not only an essential functional activity in our society and climate but because it

requires the integration of a number of different skills it is a good situation in which to practise various skills. When working with your child remember the helpfulness of visually seeing what is to be done, vocalizing the intention of doing it and clear verbal instructions of how to do it. For example, you can help your child to relate to such phrases as 'Push your foot into your shoe' or 'Pull your arm out of your sleeve' by performing the movement on yourself first, then getting your child to perform the movement with as little assistance from you as possible and, if able to verbalize what he or she is doing, your child should be asked to say the words at the same time as performing the actions. As your child becomes more able both intellectually and physically, colours can be added to the phrases: 'Push your foot into your blue shoe'. This can be followed by: 'Pull your arm out of the top of your sleeve' and 'Push your right foot into your right blue shoe' and so on. In this way your child will not only be learning how to dress but also accumulating knowledge which can be used in other activities.

Some of the ways in which you can encourage children to master the basic movements of grasp, pull and push that they may use later when dressing and undressing are shown for the younger child in Figures 17.24–17.28 and for the older child in Figures 17.29–17.35.

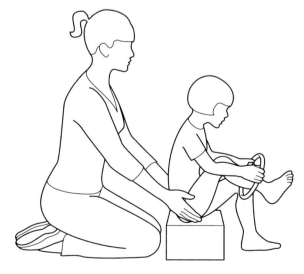

Figure 17.24 • Practising grasping, pulling and pushing with a quoit or hoop over the legs or trunk in supported sitting.

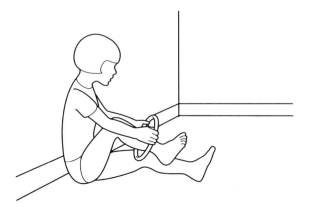

Figure 17.25 • Practising grasping, pulling and pushing with a quoit or hoop over the legs or trunk in supported sitting.

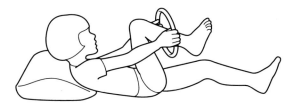

Figure 17.26 • Practising grasping, pulling and pushing with a quoit or hoop over the legs or trunk in lying.

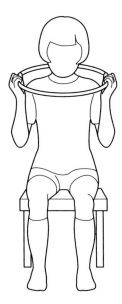

Figure 17.27 • Practising grasping, pulling and pushing with a quoit or hoop over the legs or trunk in unsupported sitting.

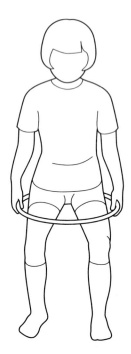

Figure 17.28 • Practising grasping, pulling and pushing with a quoit or hoop over the legs or trunk in standing.

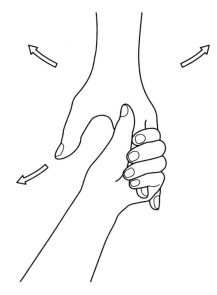

Figure 17.29 • By grasping your fingers, the child's arm can be moved in many directions while the child retains the grasp. This can be followed by the child moving your arm in many directions while you hold the towel. N.B.: Your finger is placed across the palm and out between the thumb and index finger.

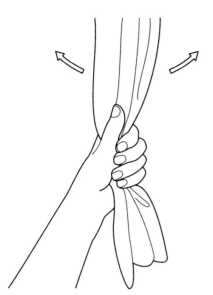

Figure 17.30 • By holding a towel, the child's arm can be moved in many directions while the child retains the grasp. This can be followed by the child moving your arm in many directions while you hold the towel. N.B.: The towel is placed across the palm and out between the thumb and index finger.

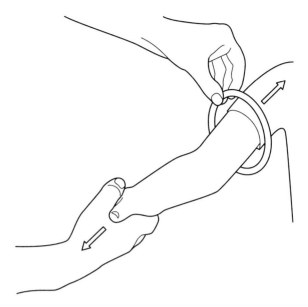

Figure 17.32 • Pull the child's arm through the quoit, taking the quoit up to the shoulder. Encourage the child to say 'push'.

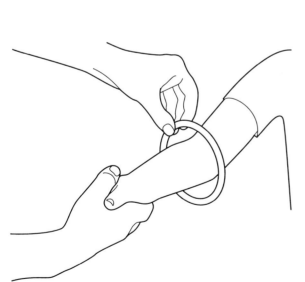

Figure 17.31 • Grasp the child's hand and the quoit.

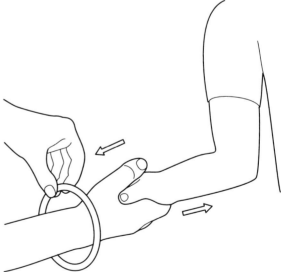

Figure 17.33 • Push the child's arm out of the quoit. Encourage the child to say 'pull'.

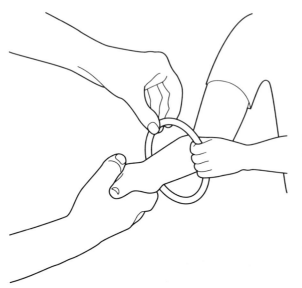

Figure 17.34 • The child holds the quoit and your hand and pulls and pushes the quoit with your help.

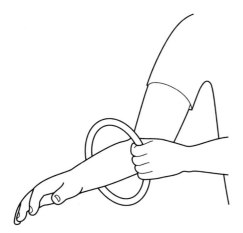

Figure 17.35 • The child holds the quoit independently and repeats the same movements.

Choosing a position for encouraging independent dressing

The position in which your child begins to dress will be determined by the ability to maintain a stable sitting base and balance when sitting. Positions that will make it easier for the child who has only moderate sitting balance when beginning to dress are shown in Figures 17.36–17.41. Ways

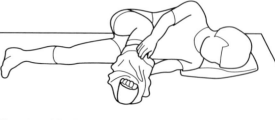

Figure 17.36 • Putting trousers on uppermost leg first in side-lying.

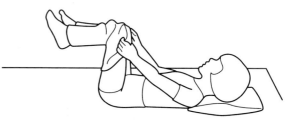

Figure 17.37 • Pulling trousers up to the thighs in lying.

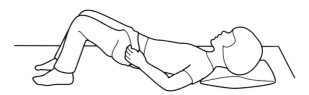

Figure 17.38 • Pulling trousers over the hips and pelvis by 'bridging'.

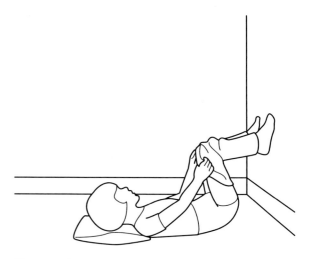

Figure 17.39 • Using a wall to lift the hips and pelvis to pull trousers on.

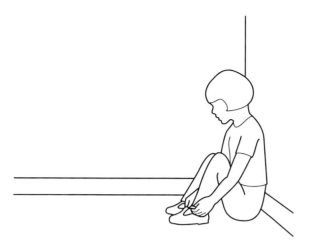

Figure 17.40 • Hips and knees bent to put on shoes leaning against a wall.

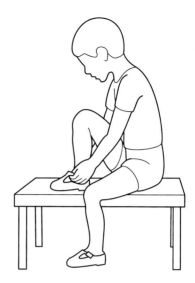

Figure 17.42 • Bending the right leg up and turning sideways to put on a shoe.

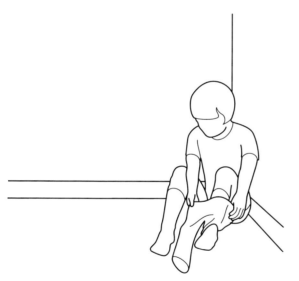

Figure 17.41 • Using a corner for support while pulling trousers on.

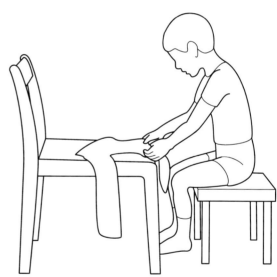

Figure 17.43 • Placing trousers into the correct position to put them on – back and top uppermost.

of giving a child who is mobile confidence when dressing are shown in Figures 17.42–17.49.

These are general points of advice and may need adapting to meet the specific problems of individual children.

Try not to continue to dress and undress your child out of habit or just because it is quicker. If children are going to be able to be independent, they must first be shown what to do and how to do it and then be encouraged to try for themselves, first with guidance and then on their own. If you think that your child should be doing more

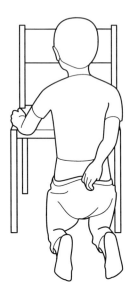

Figure 17.44 • Kneeling with a chair to pull up trousers.

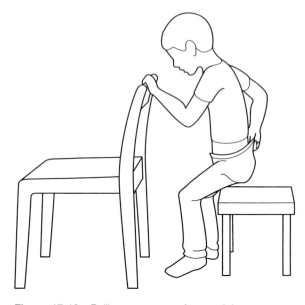

Figure 17.46 • Pulling up trousers from a sitting position.

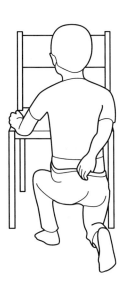

Figure 17.45 • Half-kneeling with a chair to pull up trousers.

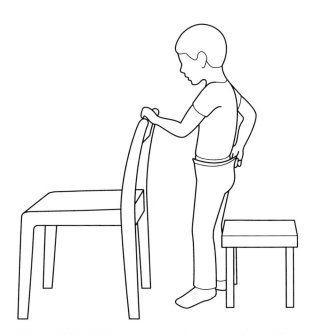

Figure 17.47 • Pulling up trousers from a standing position.

independently, leave your child to get on with it alone while you carry on with other jobs and you may be surprised on your return. Children can be crafty: I have known of a case where a mother was called to the front door to find on her return that her often bored and helpless child had self-dressed, something which no one had thought the child could do.

Clothing

As the choice of clothes is a very personal thing for parents when their child is young and for children themselves when older, clothing will be discussed in very general terms.

Materials

If possible choose clothes that include natural fibres such as cotton or wool. A blend of natural and synthetic fibres such as cotton 80% and polyester 20% or sweatshirt material is easily cared for and light and pleasant to wear. Other than for linings, it is better to avoid materials that have a slippery surface as they are liable to stick to the body.

For waterproof garments, although expensive, it is good to choose Gore-Tex or similar products as they are made of breathable fabrics and the garments are light and windproof. When choosing outer garments for winter wear, thermo-insulated materials or those with 100% polyester padding in the jackets are useful as they are warm and light and can be easily machine-washed.

Some young children with CP have sensitive skin and are apt to sweat a lot and as a result may become hypersensitive to certain fabrics.

Always check to see that the materials used for garments conform to safety regulations and are fully fireproof or fire-retardant.

Sleeves

All sleeves should be as loose as possible. Choose a shirt, cardigan, sweater or jacket with raglan or dolman sleeve as this provides the largest opening for the arm. This is helpful because it reduces the degree of accuracy or precise localization that the child has to use when putting the arm through it.

It is also helpful to have a wide opening at the bottom of the sleeve that is large enough to be able to slip your hand in and pull the child's arm through if necessary. If a cuff is tight the seam can be opened and edged with Velcro.

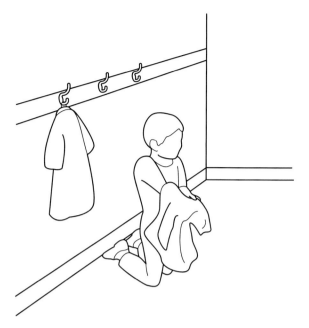

Figure 17.48 • Taking a coat or cape off in kneeling.

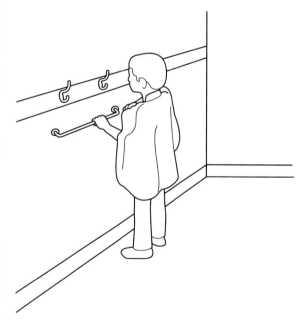

Figure 17.49 • Taking a cape off holding on to a rail.

Fastenings

One of the most difficult aspects of dressing or undressing for any child to cope with is fastenings.

Whereas it may be quite easy for a child to open and close fastenings on clothes laid out on a surface in front of the child, it is quite a different matter when the fastenings are on the clothes actually being worn by the child. This is particularly so if the child finds it difficult to look at what he or she is trying to do. Try out different fastenings with your child and then you can decide whether shank buttons, large press studs or even sewing up some button holes and sewing a strip of Velcro underneath is the answer. Velcro has the advantage of being most versatile and can be purchased in strips of varying lengths and widths. The secret of keeping Velcro in good condition is to brush it occasionally with a wire brush.

Some parents prefer buttons sewn on with elastic whereas others lift the buttons from the material by sewing a small button underneath. Large buttons or loop and button, zips and Velcro tape can also be used. Your aim is for your child to be independent and it is therefore worthwhile taking extra time and trouble choosing fasteners that your child can manage.

Suitable types of clothing

Body suits

A body suit is a warm and comfortable garment for a child made in either pure cotton or a mixture of 80% cotton and 20% polyester, sleeveless or with short sleeves, envelope neck and crutch popper openings. A reason for being enthusiastic about this garment is that it allows the young child the maximum freedom of movement and is good for any active movement session with your child.

Vests

The most suitable are those which have the largest openings for the head – the envelope cross-over opening for the younger child and a scoop neck with shoulder straps for the older child. If a wide shoulder strap is preferred, the seam can be opened and Velcro fastening used. Parents have recommended thermolactyl vests for use with children who feel the cold.

Pyjamas

For young children the most suitable night wear is probably stretch all-in-one sleep suits with popper fastenings. Usually they do not allow a generous amount of material for growing feet and it is advised to check regularly if shrinkage has occurred. The warning signs are if the material becomes taut, so that the child's foot remains in a plantarflexed (toes pointing to the ground) position. If this happens movement at the ankle may become restricted and the toes will start to bunch. For the older child, two-piece pyjamas with ribbed neck bands and cuffs at the bottom of sleeves and legs are suitable. If necessary, tops and bottoms can be held together by buttons and for the more severely disabled child a back panel may be found useful or, as an alternative to pyjamas, a loose night shirt.

Socks

Well-fitting socks are as important as well-fitting shoes and are an item of clothing it is better not to pass down through the family.

Socks should be bought with a high content of cotton as the feet of children with CP are often sweaty and this is especially so if the shoes do not allow sufficient air to circulate around the feet. Although socks are comparatively easy for a child to take off, putting them on can present quite a problem. Tubular socks with no heel shaping are therefore a good idea until the child becomes more proficient.

Tights are a useful garment. They are warm and have the advantage of being able to be pulled up to the waist with no fastening problems. Footless tights or long johns are a similar way of keeping the legs and pelvis warm without the problem of incorporating the foot and may be more acceptable for boys.

Shirts and jumpers

Children's tee-shirts with short or long sleeves, sweatshirts with or without hoods and jumpers should be bought generously and loosely cut. There are a large variety of neck openings from which to choose – roll, crew, scooped and with ribbed collars and cuffs – so that usually no special adaptations are needed. It is only as the child becomes older that difficulties may arise if a long-sleeved shirt is worn. Keeping a shirt tucked into trousers may present a problem. This can be remedied by buttoning the shirt on to the trousers or pants or by means of a tape sewn to the bottom of the shirt. If cuff buttons pose a problem, use two buttons connected by elastic. To save buttoning and unbuttoning the front of the shirt, edge each side of the front of the shirt with a strip of Velcro and sew up the buttonholes or sew on extra-large press studs.

Trousers, jog-suits

Boys' and girls' pull-on trousers, jog-pants with elastic tops or sweat pants are usually generously cut and are designed to stand up to hard wear.

One of the most useful garments on the market for children of all sizes is the jog-suit, either knitted or in cotton or polyester fabrics. Its great advantage is that the neck opening is simple, there are no fastenings to cope with and the trousers have elastic tops. It is a warm and comfortable garment for a child to wear and is to be recommended. Not recommended are the shiny nylon shell suits as they tend to be clingy, sweaty, sticky and not as warm or comfortable to wear.

Dresses

Shifts or pinafore dresses are most practical. They are simple to put on and have no fastenings. Some designs have buttons on the shoulders and these can be replaced with Velcro if you wish. In some cases it may be easier to dress a child if the pinafore dress has buttons on the shoulder and down one side.

Shifts and pinafore dresses can be made in a variety of materials and can be worn with a tee-shirt or jumper underneath.

For the older child who cannot dress independently a dress will be easier to put on if the fastener is down the back so that both arms can be put through the sleeves first.

Skirts

Skirts with elasticated waists and no fastenings which can be pulled up like a pair of trousers or pulled down over the head and shoulders can be usefully worn, often with a tee-shirt and tights.

Overalls

PVC and allied materials are best for overalls as they can be washed down without being taken off. If overalls are used at meal times, try to get those with deep pockets around the hem to catch any falling pieces of food. Back fasteners will be found the most satisfactory.

Bibs

Absorbent terry-towelling bibs with PVC backing provide the best protection for young children. These come either with simple ties at the back or in a poncho style which goes over the head and ties at the side. For the messy eater just starting to self-feed, overalls with long sleeves may be the answer. For the older child a bib with a moulded front to catch spills and an adjustable neck fastening which can be easily wiped clean and rinsed may be helpful.

Some mothers whose children dribble constantly have found that a piece of terry towelling or similar absorbent material placed under the child's top helps absorb excessive moisture. There are also available now scarves of absorbent material that are worth a try.

Capes and jackets

Capes with and without hoods, for both wet and fine weather, and ponchos come in a variety of materials and colours and as they have no sleeves are easier and quicker to put on. If required, a loop of elastic can be inserted for the shoulder and one for the arm to prevent them slipping off. The design of a poncho is so simple that it can easily be made. Padded jackets can be more difficult to put on and take off but fortunately there is a large range to choose from and it is advisable to try putting on and off a number before making a final decision.

For added warmth under a coat or instead of a cardigan another useful item is a sleeveless waistcoat or gilet which is again relatively easy to put on and take off. It can be knitted, made up of material or bought.

Mittens

Mittens are usually easier to get on and off than gloves. To try to prevent them from being lost attach a piece of elastic or tape to the waist.

Hats

As hats can be difficult to keep on, a hood with a band under the chin and a snap fastener or a combined hood and scarf are more serviceable. Many jackets and coats have detachable hoods which may be easier to manage.

Shoes

Before discussing some of the various types of shoes available, let us first look at the important role our feet play, both for balance and walking. To illustrate the point try the following:

Stand on one leg and feel the amount of movement in your foot and toes. Now stand with your weight on the inner side of your foot and try to balance on one leg. You will find that it is very difficult. Claw your toes and get someone to push you and you are very likely to fall backwards and lose your balance. Walk with your weight first on the inner, then on the outer edges of your feet and see the effect this has on your whole walking pattern and the posture of your body.

These are some of the problems your child may be experiencing when trying to walk.

If you have ever suffered from a pair of shoes that were the wrong size, I am sure you will remember the discomfort and blisters that you got as a result and how this affected the way you walked. I think this highlights the importance of checking that your child wears a well-fitting, supportive pair of shoes that can be easily modified if needed. Otherwise the ability to balance and the way in which your child stands and walks may deteriorate.

It is not possible to give specific advice regarding footwear as not only are the needs of any two children likely to be different but the types of shoes available are also likely to change.

Some children may need to have a pair of boots or shoes specially prescribed, providing an additional support to build up the shoe on the inner or outer side or alterations to the height of the heel. These adaptations may be carried out by an orthotist or sometimes by your local shoemaker or cobbler but it is always important to discuss the subject of footwear for your child with your therapist before going to buy shoes. Often your therapist will know which shop is the most helpful in your locality. Some shoes will be more suitable for your child than others, some are easier to adapt than others, and some are better made than others.

General comments regarding footwear

The first pair of shoes is just as important as subsequent pairs and even at an early age the right size is important. Each foot should be measured for length and width and the results compared to check if one foot is longer or wider than the other. Differences are more likely to be found in children with the hemiplegic, one-sided, type of CP where there may be a discrepancy in bony growth resulting from abnormalities in the soft tissues. It is also necessary to check how the child's weight is distributed both in and out of the shoes and that the shoes are easy to put on and take off.

A shoe that opens right down the front will make it easier to get the child's heel and foot well down into the shoe. If a child can walk, the child should be encouraged to do so in the shop before deciding upon which shoes to buy. If children cannot talk they will, nevertheless, soon let you know which pair of shoes they like best by the fuss they make when you try to take them off. Most children are proud of their shoes so if your child shows a preference for a certain colour, buy that colour if possible. This may be particularly important in a child who is capable of walking but reluctant to do so. Where a child has reached the stage of taking off and putting on shoes independently, while still in the shop, satisfy yourself that this can be done easily with the pair to be purchased. These days this is no longer such a problem as many shoes and boots have Velcro fastenings. Slip-on models, elastic-sided shoes, elastic laces and eyelets that can be adapted to make lacing easier are now widely available. It may seem obvious but do remember that the thickness of a sock or tights can also make a difference to the fit of a shoe.

Children in general and children with CP in particular are very hard on their shoes. A polyester resin, a rubber-like urethane which forms a glossy coat or an acrylic cement cap application which is evolved from dental and model plastic are different materials that can be purchased for protecting shoes. New products for reinforcing shoes are frequently being introduced, so watch out for them and ask your orthotist or therapist. Immediately your child's shoes show signs of wear ask your therapist to reinforce the toe caps or advise you how this can be done. Do not wait until a hole appears. Many mothers, as an added precaution, have a protective material put on a new pair of shoes before they are worn. Children's shoes are an expensive item so this is worth considering.

When special alterations have to be made to shoes it is helpful to check the way in which your child walks in them for the first 2–3 weeks to make sure that the alterations made have been beneficial, so that if necessary further changes can be made without delay.

If your child is unable to tell you that the shoes are uncomfortable check regularly to see if there are any areas of skin that look red or if there are any pressure sores on the feet. Keep an eye on the heels and soles of shoes to see if they are being worn evenly.

However attached your child may become to a pair of shoes, do not let the child wear them all the time at home. Shoes and feet need an airing.

The following are types of shoes that parents have found suitable for their children and can usually be purchased in good shoe shops.

For the younger child

Figure 17.50 shows a shoe which has a narrow heel and an arch support. Figure 17.51 shows a sports boot.

For the older child

1. Trainers which have soft, padded tongues and arch supports

2. Supportive sandals

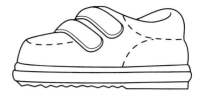

Figure 17.50 • A shoe with a narrow heel and an arch support.

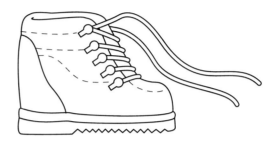

Figure 17.51 • A sports boot.

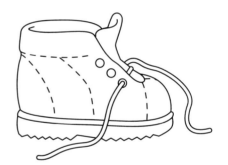

Figure 17.52 • A Pedro boot.

3. For the child who cannot keep shoes on, a pair of knitted socks with leather soles may be helpful

4. Wellington boots: these are now available made from PVC in all sizes and colours, short or long and with warm linings

5. Pedro boots are available in a variety of colours and sizes and are often recommended by therapists for stability (Figure 17.52). They are sometimes worn with ankle foot orthoses but this is not necessary as such orthoses provide their own stability and can be worn with trainers or plimsolls

A word of warning – although shoes are expensive, they are an article of clothing that should always have a high priority. Inexpensive shoes may not provide your child with the adequate support needed.

General points

Children with CP are often less mobile than typical children and as a consequence may well feel the cold more and need to wear extra clothing. This is particularly the case when sitting in a pushchair or wheelchair so it is especially necessary to wrap these children up well in rugs and/or specially designed sacks which cover the child's back, pelvis, legs and feet.

All children enjoy being told how nice they look and should be encouraged to take pride in their appearance. When old enough and within reasonable limits they should be allowed to choose the colour and type of clothes they prefer to wear.

Reference

Palisano R, Rosenbaum P, Walter S et al. Development and validation of a gross motor function classification system for children with CP. Dev Med Child Neurol 1997; 39:214–223.

Chapter Eighteen

18

Communication

Helen Cockerill

CHAPTER CONTENTS

How cerebral palsy can affect communication skills

Cerebral palsy (CP) is a disorder of posture and movement. Communication also involves move-

ment, from the early facial expressions and limb movements of a young child that are interpreted by carers as having meaning, to the intricate and complex oral-motor movements involved in the production of speech. Therefore, CP can have significant consequences for the development of communication between young children and their carers.

CP may also be associated with a range of additional impairments, including visual and hearing impairments, learning disabilities and epilepsy. These additional factors can also influence the development of communication.

In thinking about how to encourage communication in a child with CP it may be tempting to focus solely on speech. Many parents will ask the question 'Will my child speak?' – something that is not easy to answer in the early years (see Table 18.1). In this chapter we will consider a broad view of communication, that is, anything a child does that can be interpreted as having meaning and as giving a message about how the child feels and what the child wants. Typically developing children can express a great deal before they can speak and therefore we need to think about how such ability develops, how this might be affected by CP, and what can be done by parents and carers in the early years to maximize a child's communication potential. A brief overview of the major developmental milestones of speech and communication is given in Table 18.1.

Table 18.1 Major developmental milestones of speech and communication

Age	Behaviours
0–3 months	Cries, coos and gurgles, vowel sounds Startles to loud sounds Makes eye contact, responds to speech by looking at speaker's face Smiles
4–6 months	Responds to tone of voice Recognizes own name Participates in back-and-forth vocal play with adults Enjoys finger play, e.g. round and round the garden Interested in exploring objects Looks at what adults are doing and looking at Some consonant sounds in early babble, e.g. 'ba', 'da'
6–9 months	Stops and looks toward speaker when name is called Responds to 'no!' Tuneful babble with a range of sounds, e.g. 'bababababa', 'mamamama' Responds to 'where's mummy/daddy?' by looking around Reaches for desired objects Appears to recognize names of a few common objects Learning to press buttons to make noise-making toys operate
9–12 months	Points to request objects, checking back to adult's face Responds appropriately to some verbal requests, e.g. 'wave bye-bye' 'Talks' to people using phrase-like vocalizations (jargon) Uses a few words or word approximations Looks at objects pointed to by others Beginnings of functional play, e.g. brings hairbrush to head, telephone to ear
12–18 months	Communicates both to request and for social reasons Attract people's attention and then points, both to make demands and to show interest Understands simple commands, e.g. 'give it to me', 'come here' Understands several new words each week Produces a mix of jargon and recognizable words Names familiar objects, with some generalizations, e.g. 'daddy' for all men
18 months– 2 years	Engages in pretend play, e.g. feeding teddy Understands that pictures represent people and objects – can point to pictures of common objects in books on request Understands two-part commands, e.g. 'put the cup in the cupboard' Combining two to three words, e.g. 'mummy car' Speech becoming clear to unfamiliar people Starting to ask questions, and say 'no' or 'not' Uses a combination of spoken words, gestures and other non-verbal behaviours to communicate

(Continued)

Table 18.1 Continued

Age	Behaviours
2–2½ years	Vocabulary continuing to grow (around 500 words) Taking a few turns in conversations Acts out familiar routines in play, e.g. putting teddy to bed Plays alongside other children Gives a simple verbal commentary during play Picks out objects by function, e.g. 'which one can we eat?' Follows three-part commands, e.g. 'put mummy's shoes in the hall' Producing three-word sentences Asking 'what?' and 'where?' questions Starting to use grammar, e.g. plurals, pronouns and negatives
2½–3 years	Initiates and maintains simple conversations Increasingly participates in play with other children Asks and responds to 'who?/what?/where?' questions – starts to use 'why?' Understands many concept words, e.g. *in, on, big, wet*, and is learning colour words Vocabulary expands to an average of 700 words Talking about past events
3–4 years	Engages in pretend play with other children Understands sentences with five to six key words, including concepts, e.g. 'put the little horse by the big pig' Using increasingly complex sentences with grammatical features, including pronouns, verb tenses and possessives, but with some mistakes, e.g. 'I goed in grandad's big car' Tells stories about past events Can talk about the future, e.g. 'I going to seaside on holiday' Speech may contain some immaturities e.g. 'ambliance' for 'ambulance'
4–5 years	Engages in dramatic play with peers Can hold conversations with a variety of people on a range of topics Increasing understanding of sentences containing several concepts, e.g. 'which kitten has a white paw and black ears?' Understands early numbers Can give directions and reasons, e.g. 'the fire engine came because the cat was stuck up the tree' Using a vocabulary of several thousand words Attributes feelings to characters in stories Can follow explanations and is competent in using language as a medium for learning

Early interaction

From the moment of birth, parents look for meaning in their child's behaviour. Movements, facial expressions and sounds are interpreted as signalling that the child is hungry, tired, uncomfortable, excited or interested in people and events. Although such behaviours are probably not intentional in the early stages, they become more purposeful as the child develops the motor control to repeat specific movements, because of the response of the parents. For example, towards the end of the first year of life, if a child smacks the lips together and produces a 'ma' sound, parents may interpret this as an attempt to say 'mama'. Because of the delighted response of the parents, the child may repeat this sound and look for the same reaction.

During the first few months children are particularly interested in people. They 'invite' carers to talk to them by making eye contact and responding with interest to the special tone of voice and exaggerated facial expressions that we use when talking to young children. They can stop a 'conversation' by fussing or looking away, causing parents to make comments such as 'oh, you don't want to talk any more ... you've had enough for now'. There has been a great deal of research looking at this early interaction between young children and their carers, which has revealed the subtleties and complexities of the 'dance of communication', and how young children contribute just as much as the adults who are looking after them (Trevarthen and Aitken 2001).

CP can make this 'dance' more difficult. A young child who moves less or in different ways to typically developing children may provide fewer opportunities for parents to respond. Similarly, young children with low tone in their facial muscles may not give clear facial expressions that can be easily interpreted. An additional visual impairment may pose problems for parents seeking to establish contact with their child. Children with CP may respond slowly to their parents, distorting the timing of the interaction, and giving rise to misunderstandings. All these factors mean that early interaction skills may develop very slowly in young children with CP. What might be achieved in a few months in a typically developing child may happen over several years in children with severe CP and additional disabilities.

However, most parents of children with CP develop supersensitivities to the sometimes faint or idiosyncratic signals given by their children. They learn to leave longer pauses in order to give their children time to organize a response, and are alert to any possible signals that can be shaped into mutually satisfying communication exchanges. Close collaboration may be necessary between parents and others, including professionals, in order to interpret these early communication signals, for example, how children indicate

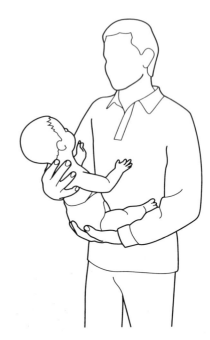

Figure 18.1 • Interaction between parent and child. 'Hello there – are you listening to Daddy?'

their likes and dislikes, how children show they are interested or wary, how children tell us that they have had enough. This is important for consistency: if everyone responds in a similar way to the things children do, they will learn that their behaviours can have an effect on those around – one of the fundamental principles in communication. Figure 18.1 illustrates interaction between father and child.

Object play

At around the age of 5 months, typically developing children shift their interests from people to the things they see around them. They still respond positively to people and being talked to, but are also keen to explore the world, hold objects and bring them to their mouths. Consequently, there is a shift in parents' language and they start to talk about whatever the child shows an interest in. Parents monitor where the child is looking, show the child objects that the child focuses on and talk to the child about them.

Children with delayed sitting balance and poor head control due to CP will need extra support to develop an interest in the world. Being in an upright, supported position will allow a child to look around and focus on objects and activities of interest, so providing parents with opportunities to talk about what is happening. Watching and following may take time, and parents will compensate for this by careful monitoring of their child's focus of attention and perhaps slowing down the rate at which they make comments. If a child cannot reach out to objects parents will need to present things in response to sustained eye gaze. This has implications as to how toys are positioned so that the child can readily focus on them.

Children with a visual impairment need additional support to explore the world. Objects should be presented slowly and extra time will be needed to help the child explore them in a way that makes sense. Figure 18.2 shows the father supporting the child and holding things where the child can see.

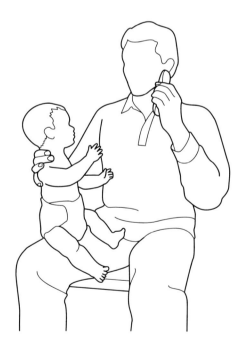

Figure 18.2 • Supporting the child and holding things where the child can see. 'Yes, that's Daddy's phone.'

Joint attention

The next stage in development comes when the child can shift attention between objects and people. This ability to look from an object to the person (who can talk about or give the object) occurs at around 9 months, and is referred to as joint attention. It is a very important part of communication development and language learning as it helps the child to match up spoken words used by carers with the objects and events those words refer to. At this stage, when something happens, young children often look to their parents as if seeking information on how to react. An example of this would be at about 10 months when children often start to become wary of strangers; they will look at their parents for guidance on how to react to the unfamiliar person. Again, this shifting of attention between objects and people may be delayed in children with CP, and affected by difficulties with independent head and eye movements. Children with CP will need extra time to make such shifts of attention if they are to achieve this important stage of communication that will lay the foundation for later skills.

Specific activities may need to be created to practise such joint attention skills; for example, showing a favourite toy to the child but waiting for the child to look at your face (gaze-switching) before handing it over. Some children have particular difficulty with voluntary eye movements and there may be a long delay between wanting to look and being able to turn the head and eyes in the right direction. These factors must be taken into account when helping a child to understand how powerful looking can be. Figure 18.3 illustrates joint attention: the child looks at the bowl, the mother asks if more food is wanted.

Gestures

Before speech emerges, typically developing children will be using a range of gestures: these include waving, pushing things away or shaking the head to reject, and pointing. Pointing can act

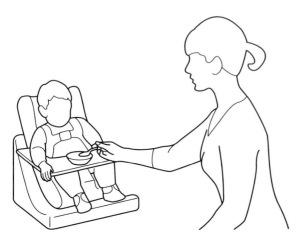

Figure 18.3 • Joint attention by parent and child. 'You're looking at your bowl. You want some more.'

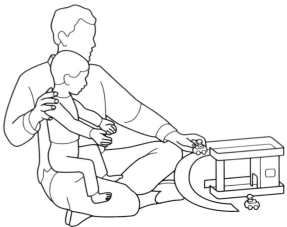

Figure 18.4 • Joint attention by parent and child. 'You're looking at the car on the top. It's ready to drive down the ramp'.

as a request well before children can ask for things by name. It also has a role in expressing an interest in objects and events which, in turn, prompts parents to talk about things, and thereby provide language learning opportunities. Pointing develops from joint attention gaze-switching but has the advantage of being easier to read; for example, a parent may or may not notice a child looking at a dog as it walks past the buggy and name it for the child, but if the child points and makes a sound the parent will almost inevitably respond by saying, 'yes, it's a dog … it says woof woof'.

A child with CP may not be able to point accurately, which can limit opportunities for language learning. Alternatives to pointing may include eye-pointing (looking from the object to the parent's face and then back to the object); looking and vocalizing; or looking and lifting an arm. All such methods can be used to indicate a difference between looking (for interest) and making a clear request.

As with other joint attention skills, specific opportunities for eye-pointing may need to be created. Sensitive parents can create activities where they wait for the child to direct play through eye-pointing. An example would be a toy garage with cars, helping the child to push the cars to the pumps or parking spaces in response to wherever

the child is looking. Figure 18.4 shows the child looking at the car and the father commenting on this.

In order to help a child develop an appreciation of the ability to express preferences and make decisions (important prespeech skills), choice-making opportunities must be created. These may include offering a choice of food at meal times, of toys when playing and of books at story time. Two or more objects can be placed in a position where the parent can see the child's face clearly, the objects can be named and then the child asked to look at the thing the child wants, for example: 'do you want jam or honey on your toast?'. It is important to give the child the thing that he or she has chosen, even if the choice is surprising, so that the child understands the power of communication (the choice can be reoffered a few moments later if the child has made a mistake). Sometimes children can be presented with a favourite toy and something of no interest in order to test whether they are making reliable choices.

If a child has an additional visual impairment choices can still be offered, but will need to be presented in more body-centred ways: placing two objects to each side of a child's face, or touching each hand, may be an alternative. Figure 18.5 shows the mother offering a choice to the child.

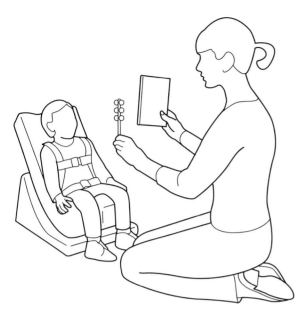

Figure 18.5 • Offering a choice. 'Do you want the book, or the bells?'

Speech

During the first year typically developing children progress from cooing and open vowel sounds to babbling (repetitive sequences of consonant and vowel sounds, e.g. 'bababa') and then to jargon (speech-like vocalizations with the intonation patterns of phrases, but no recognizable words). Progress in sound production is often closely linked to other motor skills, particularly head control, sitting balance and jaw stability. There is great variation in the age at which clear speech appears, but many children have a few words by 12–15 months, often around the same time as the child walks independently.

The emergence of speech is not simply a motor skill: it is also linked to a child's level of language understanding. Typically developing children are able to respond to simple instructions and questions such as 'where's daddy?' (the child will look around), 'give it to mummy' (when the mother holds out her hand), 'where's your spoon?' (during a meal). The child is probably also beginning to recognize and point to pictures in books, for example, 'where's the dog?'.

The exact incidence of speechlessness in CP is unknown, but many children are at risk of having no clear speech or limited natural speech that is only intelligible to familiar carers. The type and severity of CP influence the risk of speech and language problems. Children with hemiplegia or diplegia usually develop speech, although milestones may be delayed and perhaps dependent on the extent of any learning difficulties. Children with spastic quadriplegia often have significant physical disabilities and high rates of associated disorders, including severe learning disabilities, epilepsy or sensory impairments which, in combination with bulbar problems (control of the mouth and throat muscles), leads to marked communication and speech impairments. Children with ataxic CP may have a degree of dysarthria (inaccurate oral movements for speech production) or dyspraxia (inconsistent voluntary control of sequences of oral movements for speech). Athetoid or dyskinetic CP can result in involuntary movements and poor accuracy of the oral-motor movements for speech. However, it is not possible to predict which children are likely to have communication difficulties merely on the basis of a diagnostic label. This is partly due to difficulties of diagnosis and classification in CP (with many children being described as having a 'mixed' type), but also the complex interplay of cognitive, motor and sensory factors in the development of speech and language.

Children with CP may show limited vocalizations in infancy and babbling can be disordered, showing that speech production problems result from poor early motor control rather than a sudden failure to progress to words. It may be tempting to think that exercises for the tongue, lips and other parts of the speech production system will result in speech. Unfortunately this is not borne out by either research or clinical experience. The neurological control of speech is probably too complex to be influenced by massage or exercises aimed at the muscles involved. However, some attention can be given to maximizing a child's potential to develop natural speech. Postural support can help a child with breath support for speech, and provide head, neck and jaw stability, which in turn can increase control of oral-motor movements for speech production. Having inadequate support and struggling to maintain an upright posture can have a negative impact on breathing and the ability to produce voice. Many children experience variation in their speech due to the level of postural support, fatigue, general state of health, the communication situation and the emotional content of what they are trying to say.

Parents and carers will of course respond to any attempts to vocalize in order to encourage this aspect of communication. As with eye-pointing, it may be reasonable to expect a child to vocalize in order to make things happen. Too much pressure, though, can be counterproductive: for some children the more they try to produce a sound, the more body tension they experience, resulting in reduced ability to vocalize.

For a minority of children it may be appropriate to work directly on speech: this tends to be once the child has developed some intelligible speech, has an extensive vocabulary, is using full sentences and has achieved the maturity and intellectual level to think about *how* they are speaking as well as *what* they are saying. This is unlikely to be the case in the preschool years.

Although it may be appropriate for parents to *hope* that speech will develop, it may be realistic to consider that it may not, or that it may be very significantly delayed or disordered. Simply waiting to see if speech will appear may mean that time that could be spent encouraging effective nonverbal skills is lost. By developing other methods of communication some of the frustration that can occur due to limited speech may be avoided, at an age when children are learning about language and communication in its widest sense.

Speech and language therapy assessment

Children who are slow to develop communication skills may be referred to speech and language therapy. This can be instigated by the child's general practitioner or paediatrician, or by the parents themselves. The role of the speech and language therapist is to assess and work in partnership with parents (and schools) to develop a child's communication skills. The focus of therapy will be on effective communication in its widest sense, rather than simply speech development. In order to provide advice that is specific to the individual child the therapist may carry out assessments of varying degrees of formality. There is a range of tests that have been standardized, that is, we know how children typically perform at specific ages, taking into account the variation we would expect in the population. However, these tests have all been standardized on typically developing children who do not have physical, sensory or intellectual impairments. They often depend on physical responses such as pointing to pictures, handling toys or speaking; consequently it may seem unfair to administer them to children with CP. Adapting them for children who eye-point or who need additional supports such as signing will mean that strict scoring criteria cannot be applied, and any comparisons with typically developing children should be interpreted with caution. Despite their limitations, tests may have a role in helping to establish a profile of a child's communication strengths and difficulties, allow tracking of a child's progress over time and provide guidance on areas of development to target in therapy. Table 18.2 gives examples of some of the tests commonly used by speech and language therapists in the UK.

Augmenting natural speech

For many children with CP who are slow to develop speech we might consider a range of strategies and methods to expand their communication skills beyond the preverbal stage. Parents are understandably concerned that such a step may have a negative effect on speech development. The recent interest in child signing has shown that the early introduction of signing does not stop typically developing children developing speech, and research from other disabled populations, such as children with Down's syndrome, suggests that signing can speed up speech development, in addition to avoiding some of the frustration that can arise from delayed speech. There is a lack of research in this area in CP, but the evidence we have does not suggest that augmentative

Table 18.2 Speech and communication assessments

Test	Functions covered
Receptive-Expressive Emergent Language Scales (Bzoch K, League R 1991: Pro-Ed Inc/nferNelson)	Language understanding and expression Birth–7 years
MacArthur Communicative Development Inventories (Fenson L, Dale P, Reznick J et al. 1993: Singular)	Parental questionnaire covering early gestures, vocabulary and grammar (understanding and expression) Words and gestures: 8–16 months Words and phrases: 16–30 months
Reynell Developmental Language Scales (Reynell J, Hartley L 1985, revised by Edwards S, Fletcher P, Garman M et al. 1997: nferNelson)	Language understanding and expression 15 months–7.6 years The earlier edition is standardized for children using eye-pointing
Pre-School Language Scale 3 (UK) (Zimmerman IL, Steiner V, Exatt R: UK adaptation Boucher J, Lewis V 1997: nferNelson)	Language understanding and expression Birth–6 years
British Picture Vocabulary Scale, 2nd edition (Dunn LM, Dunn LM, Whetton C et al. 1997: nferNelson)	Understanding of single words 3–15 years
Clinical Evaluation of Language Fundamentals – Preschool UK (Wiig EH, Secord W, Semel E 2000: The Psychological Corporation)	Broad range of receptive and expressive skills 3–6.11 years
Renfrew Action Picture Test (Renfrew C 1997: Speechmark)	Expressive skills 3–8 years
Test for Reception of Grammar: version 2 (Bishop D 2003: The Psychological Corporation)	Understanding of grammatical contrasts 4 years to adult
Pre-Verbal Communication Schedule (Kiernan C, Reid B 1987: nferNelson)	Measures the communication skills of children who cannot speak or who have a few words/signs/symbols
Pragmatics Profile of Communication Skills in Children (Dewart H, Summers S 1995: nferNelson)	Flexible parental interview assessing communication in a range of situations Birth–4 years
Early Communication Assessment (Coupe O'Kane J, Goldbart J 1998 Communication Before Speech, 2nd edn)	Preintentional and early intentional communication Children and adults with severe, profound and multiple learning disabilities
Social Networks: a communication inventory for individuals with complex needs and their communication partners (Blackstone S, Hunt Berg M 2003: Augmentative Communication Inc.)	Explore an individual's communication strategies with a range of communication partners Children and adults
Paediatric Oral Skills Package (Brindley C, Cave D, Crane S et al. 1996: Whurr)	Detailed assessment of oral skills for feeding and speech Birth–adult

(Continued)

Table 18.2 Continued

Test	Functions covered
The Apraxia Profile (Hickman LA 1997: The Psychological Corporation)	Assessment of automatic and voluntary oral movements 2–12 years
Verbal Motor Production Assessment for Children (Hayden D, Square P 1999: The Psychological Corporation)	Oral-motor skills for speech 3–12 years
Children's Speech Intelligibility Measure (Wilcox & Morris 1997: The Psychological Corporation)	Intelligibility of speech 3–10 years

and alternative communication (AAC: signing, pictures, symbols and computers) will prevent speech. On the contrary, there is some evidence that augmentative forms of communication will facilitate speech development (Schlosser 2003). It may also be the case that signing or pointing to a picture or word whilst speaking will increase the comprehensibility of dysarthric speech. If and when intelligible speech develops, any forms of augmentative communication can be discarded if no longer necessary.

Although AAC is increasingly used in schools by children with CP, it is less popular with many families. This may be because it is seen as 'unnatural' and involves changing well-established patterns of non-verbal communication that have developed over the early years. It may also be due, in part, to the level of attunement that families and children achieve. Subtle or idiosyncratic communication signals may be recognized by families but not by less familiar communication partners. Speech may be intelligible to parents and siblings, but not to people outside the immediate family.

An increasingly common concept in the management of children with CP is that of a circle of communication partners (Figure 18.6). This idea was developed as a way of understanding how a child may communicate in different ways with different people.

People in the child's first circle, that is, the child's family, may understand the child's speech, but those in the third and fifth circles (acquaintances and unfamiliar partners) may not. Consequently

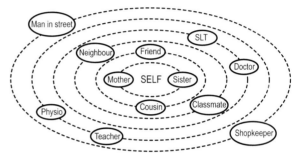

Figure 18.6 • Circle of communication partners (based on Blackstone 1991). SLT, speech and language therapist.

AAC may not be so necessary within the home, but would have a vital part to play in enabling a child to participate in school and community activities. Approached in this way the decision to implement AAC is seen not as a polarized choice between speech and non-speech methods, but as a way of equipping a child for both family and community life. The fourth circle (professionals) may be regular and familiar partners for intensive periods in a child's life but are rarely long-term partners. They may have priorities such as enabling the child to access the curriculum in school where the child will need to demonstrate knowledge, talk about the past and future and learn to read.

The circle of communication partners concept highlights the need for flexibility with regard to a child's communication needs and prompts us to think about multimodal communication, that is, a combination of natural speech, gesture and sign, pictures and symbols and electronic communication aids. At different stages in the child's life, in response to the demands of the situation, and the skills of the various communication partners, aspects of multimodal communication will be more or less important. If a child needs AAC in school it is not helpful if parents devalue or make negative comments about this form of communication.

Some of the possible AAC systems are described below. The decision as to which systems are appropriate for an individual child is likely to be a team one, involving parents and speech and language therapists, teachers and other professionals involved in the early years (for an overview of AAC methods and teaching strategies, see Von Tetzchner and Martinsen 2000). Parents have a central role in the decision to introduce AAC and in implementing strategies and so should be regarded by professionals as collaborators in the development of each child's communication skills (Granlund et al. 2001).

The overall purpose of introducing AAC to a child with limited natural speech is to reduce the gap between what the child understands and how that child is able to express ideas. Exactly how much a child with CP understands can be difficult to establish with accuracy, but is likely to reflect the child's general cognitive level. However, it is necessary to match comprehension and expressive skills

in order to avoid frustration, and also to avoid the sense of failure that can result if a child is required to use AAC systems that are too complex.

Unaided communication: signing

For children who are able to make hand shapes, and who are starting to use natural gestures, signing may be an effective communication method. Even for children who cannot produce accurate finger movements, gross approximations to signs may be of some benefit: for example, bringing the hands together could indicate a child wants 'more' food or play, whereas moving the hands swiftly apart can indicate the child wants to 'finish' (Figure 18.7). Putting a hand to the forehead may make a child's attempt to say the word 'hot' more likely to be understood.

In order to learn signs children will need adults producing signs alongside speech repeatedly, much like any child will need to hear words many times before starting to say them. It may take weeks, months or years before children will learn the specific meaning of a sign and before they attempt to imitate it and go on to use the sign for functional communication. Parents will need training in how to use and adapt signs in

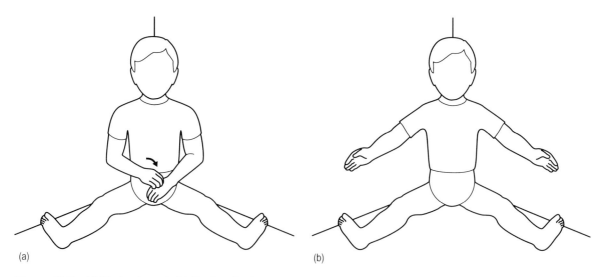

(a) (b)

Figure 18.7 • (a) Signing 'more'. (b) Signing 'finished'.

ways that make them more appropriate for their own child; for example, for a child with a visual impairment, taking the child's hands and moving them to form the sign for 'up' can help the child to anticipate the movement and perhaps participate in the change of position when being picked up. This is an example of how AAC can be used to facilitate a child's understanding of language, that is, as an input system, rather than necessarily expecting children to use AAC to express their own wishes. A child may require repeated exposure to AAC as input, before moving on to AAC as output. This mimics the normal developmental process of hearing and learning the meanings of words before being able to use them.

Aided communication

Objects

Another way of supporting a child's understanding of what is about to happen is to present objects consistently alongside speech. An example might be giving a child a spoon before offering food. Because the spoon is an integral part of the meal time it can come to represent that activity, that is, it is an 'object of reference'. This can be particularly useful for children who are not thought to have reliable understanding of spoken messages. Children who are passive may be able to take a more active role in daily activities if given such input; children who become distressed by changes of activity may be calmer and more receptive if they can anticipate events. Care should be taken when selecting objects of reference to ensure they are connected to that activity in an obvious way; for example, a toy car used to represent a car journey may not have an immediate meaning for a profoundly disabled child, whereas a piece of the strap from the car seat may have a closer association (Park 1997). Figure 18.8 illustrates a seat belt being shown to the child to indicate a car journey.

Children who show anticipation of events on seeing objects of reference may be able to move on to pictures, depending on their vision, and their ability to understand that two-dimensional pictures can represent three-dimensional objects or events.

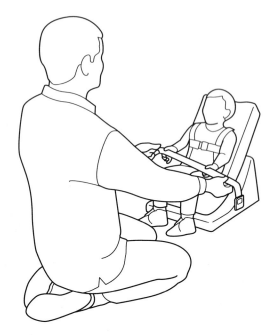

Figure 18.8 • Using objects to aid anticipation of events. 'Here's your seat belt. It's time to go in the car'.

Pictures

Once children are able to use non-verbal communication to indicate choices using real objects it may be appropriate to introduce pictures for expressive communication. By replacing real objects with pictures the child will develop the skills to 'talk' about things that are not actually present, in the way that a typically developing child uses spoken words. Like signing, pictures can be effective in giving communication partners clues if the child's speech is difficult to understand, or they may serve as an alternative form of communication if the child does not have speech, but has specific ideas the child wishes to communicate.

Pictures may also have a role in supporting language understanding. A child may not understand 'we're going to the hospital today', but may recognize a picture of the hospital if it is a place that the child has visited several times before.

Pictures can vary in complexity. Initially a child may need to see a photograph of the actual person, place or object being talked about. The next stage would be recognizing that a line drawing (colour or black and white) can represent a person, place, object or activity. This level of abstraction makes it possible to represent concepts that are difficult to photograph, for example, 'fast' and 'more'. Line drawings can also increase applicability of objects and events: 'cuddle' can be used for a cuddle with mum or dad, granny or a doll.

Several vocabularies of line drawings have been developed for children with limited speech. These are usually described as symbol systems and have the advantage of consistency, that is, the same symbols will be used in the nursery, the school and the therapy clinic. Most have computer software packages so that parents and professionals without drawing skills can create communication materials (see websites and addresses at the end of the chapter for further information on different systems and sources of information).

A good way to introduce pictures is to make personalized scrapbooks and photograph albums. These can include photos of people who are important to the child. Leaflets, tickets and photos from special outings and events can be collected: these could then be used when discussing what has happened. This will enable the child to 'talk' about past events, something which may not be possible for a child with limited speech. If a child has speech that is not easily intelligible, people who were not present at the event under discussion may be helped to understand what the child is trying to say with the aid of the pictures. Packaging from favourite foods can be used to indicate preferences and to make choices. Reduced versions of the covers from videos or storybooks can be a more efficient way of presenting choices rather than having to take all the videos or books off the shelf to find out which one the child wants. Figure 18.9 shows a chart offering the child a number of choices for places to go.

Experimentation may be required in order to discover how best to present picture materials for an individual child. The size and layout of pictures on a page will need to match a child's visual and motor skills. Some children will be able to point directly to pictures, others will have inaccurate fist-pointing or may rely on eye-pointing. Previous experience of eye-pointing to objects can transfer

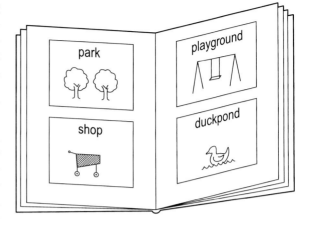

Figure 18.9 • A chart offering a choice of places to go.

to using pictures for communication (see sections on joint attention and gestures above). Positioning will also need careful consideration as the parent should be able to see both the child and the pictures the child is selecting.

If a child has limited speech but does have the ability to indicate 'yes' and 'no' to questions, it may appear that asking questions may be a more efficient way of communicating. Although this can undoubtedly be quick and effective in many instances, it also has its limitations: the child must wait for the carers to ask the right question, and initiating a new topic will be difficult. Introducing pictures is probably best seen as an initial step in the process of expanding communication: once the child understands how powerful pictures can be in conveying specific messages, more extensive personalized communication systems can be developed. Vocabulary for curriculum topics, specific activities, interests and a wide range of communication situations can be developed, enabling the child to initiate and conduct conversations across various settings. This process of expansion of a picture-based system is likely to take place over many years if the system is to meet the child's changing needs.

Printed words always accompany picture symbols, and so can be a useful part of developing early literacy skills. Parents may question the value of pictures or symbols: why not simply teach a child who has limited speech to read?

Most children are highly competent language users before they develop literacy skills. Literate adults who are skilled readers can forget what it is like to be unable to read until they travel to a foreign country and are suddenly dependent on pictures and visual signs if they cannot read the language. In developmental terms, pictures can be read and understood several years before text can be deciphered.

Technology

The past 20 years have seen the development of communication technology. Many children with CP and limited natural speech now use communication aids with speech output. These are usually described as voice output communication aids or VOCAs. Some children use specialist software packages on standard laptop computers; others use dedicated communication aids, which are computer-based electronic devices that do not have all the other functions offered by a PC. Communication aids can allow children to express themselves in some situations where a communication chart or book may be inadequate, for example on the phone, or when talking to other children who do not understand symbols. However, learning to use communication technology effectively will take time and requires specific teaching/therapy.

To hold a conversation via a communication aid requires two basic skills: (1) selecting a message; and (2) operating the communication device. In order to select a message a child must be able to recognize a range of pictures or symbols on the screen or membrane keyboard of the VOCA and be able to remember which one or ones will call up the appropriate message. Understanding the meanings of pictures, and remembering where messages are stored, involves a great deal of learning and is therefore dependent on a child's cognitive skills and on specific teaching.

As with communication charts and books, some children will be able to access the pictures directly (by pointing to a precise location on the touch screen or keyboard), but many children will not be able to achieve this degree of accuracy and so will operate the device via switches or a joystick.

If the child is to operate switches efficiently it will be necessary to identify a motor action or actions that the child can produce reliably and with minimum effort, even when tired or unwell. In order to select pictures from a display on a screen the child will need to learn 'scanning and selecting', that is, using one switch to move a cursor around the grid of pictures in the screen, and using a second switch to select the desired picture when it is highlighted. An alternative method, if a child can only reliably activate a single switch, is to have automatic scanning, that is the cursor moving around the screen at a predetermined rate, with the child activating the switch at the correct time to select the desired picture. Scanning and selecting is a skill that can be difficult to learn. Recent research with typically developing children suggests that this skill is rarely acquired before the age of 4–5 years. If a child has significant physical disability or an additional learning disability, it can take years to develop competence. For some children the accessing of communication technology will remain extremely effortful, and they may find low-tech communication charts more effective. Figure 18.10 shows a switch-operated VOCA.

In the early stages of AAC introduction it may be necessary to practise the two skills of symbol learning and accessing separately. A range of

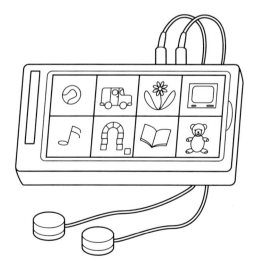

Figure 18.10 • Switch-operated voice output communication aid.

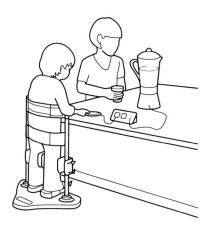

Figure 18.11 • A child operating a blender via a switch and adapter.

simple technology can be used to help develop a child's accessing skills. Switch-activated toys can foster understanding of cause and effect, that is, the child presses the switch and is rewarded by the battery-operated car moving. Special adapters can be used so that fans, food mixers, tape recorders and other electrical devices can be switch-operated. These are often more rewarding than switch toys, particularly if they involve the participation of other children; for example, operating the music for a game of musical chairs, making milkshakes in a blender at a tea party and operating a foot spa. Figure 18.11 shows a child operating a blender with a switch.

Simple VOCAs that have only one prerecorded message can also increase a non-verbal child's participation in games, singing or storytelling activities. By pressing the switch within a structured activity the child can experience the potential effectiveness of voice output at a basic level. Figure 18.12 shows a mother saying the first line of a refrain from a song book and the child responding via the VOCA with the second line.

Summary

All children with CP have ways of communicating with their carers. Some children will remain at the level of emerging communication and so be dependent on skilled interpretation of their

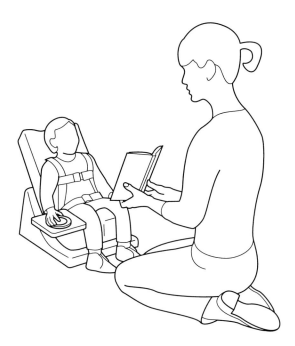

Figure 18.12 • Pressing a switch to speak a message. *Mum*: 'And the wolf said…'. *Child*: 'I'll huff and I'll puff, and I'll blow your house down.'

behaviours by parents and other familiar people. Children with severe learning disabilities may not progress beyond the early stage of preverbal communication. Some children will achieve full independent communication through speech. Others will have specific difficulties with intelligible speech and will require AAC to support natural speech. The majority of parents adapt their communication styles to match the needs of their child, and achieve mutually rewarding interaction. Many parents need support from professionals such as speech and language therapists to extend their child's communication skills if speech is limited, particularly as the child comes into contact with less familiar people, and is required to function within the school context. By working though some of the stages outlined above, parents can help a child to develop effective communication skills. The rate and extent of communication development will be influenced by each child's motor, cognitive and sensory impairments, and also the child's personality and opportunities for communication within the home. Many children with CP require AAC in order to demonstrate what they understand and wish to communicate. A multimodal approach to communication may need to be actively pursued. If and when children develop sufficient natural speech to match their communication needs, AAC systems can be abandoned. If speech intelligibility with all communication partners is not achieved, AAC can offer ongoing support for self-expression.

References

Blackstone S. Interaction with the partners of AAC consumers: part 1 – interaction. Augment Commun News 1991; 4:1–3.

Granlund M, Björck-Åkesson E, Olsson C et al. Working with families to introduce augmentative and alternative communication systems. In: Cockerill H, Carroll-Few L (eds) Communicating without speech: practical augmentative and alternative communication. MacKeith Press, Cambridge, 2001.

Park K. How do objects become objects of reference? Br J Special Ed 1997; 24:108–114.

Schlosser RW. Effects of AAC on natural speech development. In: Schlosser RW (ed.) The efficacy of augmentative and alternative communication: towards evidence-based practice. Academic Press, London, 2003.

Trevarthen C, Aitken KJ. Infant intersubjectivity: research, theory and clinical applications. J Child Psychol Psychiatry 2001; 42:3–48.

Von Tetzchner S, Martinsen H. Introduction to augmentative and alternative communication, 2nd edn. Whurr, Chichester, 2000.

Further information

1 Voice (support group for children and families using AAC), PO Box 559, Halifax HX1 2XL. Tel: 0845 330 7862. www.1voice.info.

ACE Centre, 92 Windmill Road, Headington, Oxford OX3 7DR. Tel: 01865 759800. www.ace-centre.org.uk.

ACE Centre – North, Units 11 and 12, Gateshead Business Park, Delph New Road, Delph, Saddleworth OL3 5DF. Tel: 01457 829444. www.ace-north.org.uk.

AFASIC (Association for all Speech Impaired Children), 2nd Floor, 50–52 Great Sutton Street, London EC1V 0DJ. Tel: 020 7490 9410. www.afasic.org.uk.

ASLTIP (Association of Speech and Language Therapists in Independent Practice), Coleheath Bottom, Speen, Princes Risborough, Buckinghamshire HP27 0SZ. Tel: 0870 241 3357. www.helpwithtalking.com.

CALL Centre, Patersons Land, Holyrood Road, Edinburgh EH8 8AQ. Tel: 0131 651 6236. www.callcentrescotland.org.uk.

Communication Matters (UK Chapter of the International Society for Augmentative and Alternative Communication), c/o ACE Centre, 92 Windmill Road, Headington, Oxford OX3 7DR. Tel: 0870 606 5463. Fax: 0131 555 3279. www.communicationmatters.org.uk.

Royal College of Speech and Language Therapists (RCSLT), 2 White Hart Yard, London SE1 1NX. Tel: 020 7378 1200. Fax: 020 7403 7254. www.rcslt.org.uk.

SCOPE (for people with CP), 6 Market Road, London N7 9PW. Helpline: 0808 800 3333. www.scope.org.uk.

Chapter Nineteen

19

Hand function and fine motor activities

Dido Green

Development of skilled use of the hands

The hand provides a mechanism for developing children to access information about their environment and to control their immediate world. The vast combination of movements of the hands and fingers support increasingly complex actions to achieve dexterity. For example, the ability to rotate the wrist and maintain grasp while keeping the elbow and shoulder stable, but not stiff or rigid, allows the child to hold and manipulate objects such as shaking a rattle to practise circular movements, providing early practice for later drawing and writing.

The hand does not work in isolation, but is dependent on a number of postural and cognitive processes to move beyond simple reflexes to voluntary actions for engagement with objects and people. Increasing strength of the arms and hands enhances the development of several postural functions such as pulling to stand and weight shift. The process of acquiring movement skill is associated with experience, practice and feedback (Shumway-Cook and Woolacott 1995). These principles of motor learning are important when considering the initial motivation to use one's hands for a variety of purposes, including communication and emotional expression, as well as the manipulation of objects. Fitts and Posner (1967) defined three main phases of motor learning:

1. Cognitive – determination of what is to be done

2. Associative – refinement of strategy

3. Autonomic – skill is largely automated

Competence in fine manipulative skills emerges from an interaction of the individual with the task and the environment, interlinked with intellectual development. The internal drive to plan and evaluate movements is supported by having an understanding of the task and the consequences of actions, until eventually premovement planning becomes automatic (Fitts and Posner 1967). A number of factors are important when considering the development of hand skills. High amongst these are the enjoyment of the sensory experience and exposure to numerous opportunities to interact

actively with the environment, for example, waving the hands to obtain a consistent response from adults. Sufficient time is required for practice, especially through play with opportunities to gain feedback from the consequences of movement.

Stages in the development of typical hand use

The main stages of the development of hand function are described in Table 19.1. This shows the interaction between postural control, skilled upper limb (arm and hand) functions and sensory perceptual abilities.

Trunk and head control

Strength and stability of the muscles around the shoulder and upper trunk are essential for reaching

Table 19.1 Typical development of hand function over the first year

Age (months)	Posture	Reaching and grasping	Fine motor skill
4–5	Trunk and head lifted off surface	Leans on forearms and hands for support Swipes at objects whilst lying on back	Grasp reflex reduced. Hands begin to open. Begins to shape hand to an object's size and shape
6–7	Stable trunk with independent arm and leg movements	Hands and arms used to prop and assist postural stability	Visual regard and tracking for early eye–hand control (spatial-temporal accuracy). Palmar grasp with thumb out of palm. Raking actions of fingers
7–9	Independent sitting, weight shift and emergent trunk rotation	Reaches with one arm while bearing most of body weight through the other extended arm and wrist. Both hands hold objects. Forearm rotation for control of release	Transfers objects from one hand to another Holds objects with thumb opposed to object/fingers (radial palmar) and wrist extended
10–12	Shoulder stability and head control	More precise control of grasp and release	Objects held between thumb and fingertips (radial digital grasp). Places shapes into smaller containers. Prewriting skills

and grasping, contributing to hand–eye coordination and object manipulation. The young child will lean on the hands and forearms to lift the trunk and head off a surface when lying on the tummy. The child gains strength to sustain arm extension and shift their weight from side to side. Once the child has more stable trunk control, the child can reach out with one arm while supporting the body weight through the other arm with the hand open. The ability to take weight through an extended arm and wrist strengthens the muscles of the shoulder as well as the arm and wrist (Figure 19.1). Wrist stability is also important for providing a stable but mobile base for fingers to move and manipulate objects within the palm. The muscles of the hand are designed to hold items most effectively with the wrist in line with the forearm or slightly extended.

Adequate shoulder and wrist stability is also important for a child to help with propping in sitting or standing and pulling to stand and to have confidence to experiment with shifting weight around a central point (Figure 19.2).

The ability to maintain a stable trunk frees the head and arms for independent movements. The young child needs to keep the body still when turning the head to watch and listen to objects as they move across the child's line of vision/hearing without losing balance. Experiments have suggested that when young children have their head and body stabilized, reaching can be achieved

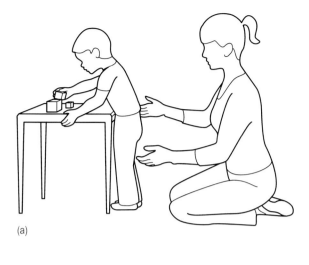

(a)

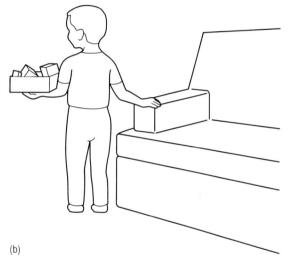

(b)

Figure 19.2 • A small table or sofa provides a good base to encourage early independence. Use extra cushions as required. (a) Learning to stand up and support oneself with minimal help. (b) Weight-bearing on an extended arm rotated outwards by reaching away from the body.

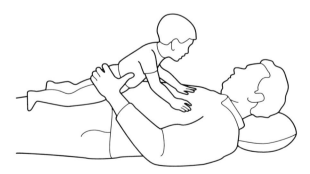

Figure 19.1 • Preparation for reach and grasp. Child takes weight on extended arms and wrists to strengthen muscles of the shoulder. Father helps the child to self-support by stabilizing the child's pelvis.

earlier (Shumway-Cook and Woollacott 1995) (Figure 19.3).

What are sometimes described as 'postural background movements' or 'counterpoising mechanisms' refer to subtle shifts in weight distribution of the trunk for movement efficiency (Levitt 2004). Larger weight shifts such as rocking from side to side contribute to early rolling and trunk

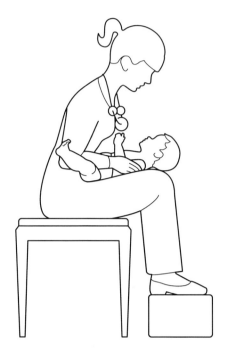

Figure 19.3 • Supporting the child to assist reaching and encourage visual and auditory awareness.

rotation. This enables the two sides of the body to work together in harmony rather than as one unit. An important outcome of these early movements is the ability to dissociate actions – that is, to separate some body movements from others. The child can then alternate arm and leg movements in reciprocal crawling and/or creeping or reach for a toy with one arm whilst the other sustains the body weight. These skills contribute to later bimanual (two-handed) control.

Reaching

Reaching towards objects is interrelated with visual and auditory responses. As it is not always easy to determine when a child is listening and tracking sounds, the development of hand–eye control is more often measured, although some of these principles may equally apply to hand–sound actions. The newborn child is only able to regard objects momentarily. Later, the child will move the eyes in all directions without head movement to sustain regard on small objects within reach or gaze at more distant objects such as a picture on a wall.

There are differences of opinion as to the extent that reflexes contribute to early voluntary control of reaching movements. Some theories suggest that reaching results from the blocking or incorporation of primitive reflexes into voluntary movements. Others argue that reflexes provide the foundation for complex movements or that hand–eye coordination emerges concurrently with the maturation of reflexes rather than as a modification (Schmidt and Lee 2005). Research has suggested that young neonates can reach forward towards objects providing their heads and trunks are stabilized, suggesting an innate ability to coordinate pre-reaching actions, independent of reflex integration. Despite these differences of opinion, there is evidence that experience is important for improvement in accuracy and skill.

Successful reaching emerges alongside important developmental changes such as postural control, freedom of head and arms to perform separate movements and improved eye movements. At this stage there is a transition from visually triggered – when visual location of the target initiates the movement – to visually guided movements allowing precise adjustments for greater accuracy when reaching (Paillard 1982, Goodale et al. 1996). Visual feedback from movement experience is essential for visually guided skills to develop. Children will continue to be reliant on external visual or auditory feedback to guide reaching movements and grip strength for lifting objects until 8 or 9 years old (Forssberg 1998).

Grasping and releasing

The ability to shape the hand to an object's size and shape (hand orientation) begins to occur at the onset of successful reaching (Keogh and Sugden 1985). More refined grasps emerge later. Children show a range of grips, sometimes deemed inappropriate or ineffective by adult observers, as they move through childhood. Table 19.2 gives details of the ages at which children typically attain manual skills.

The child experiments with shaping the hand and balancing the grip force with the texture,

Table 19.2 Typical attainment of manual skills

Age (months)	Fine motor skill
5–36	Prewriting
10–24	Formboard
11–36	Block construction
18–30	Paper activities (page-turning/folding)
8–31	Pegboard
29–36	Stringing beads
20–48	Fastenings
36–48	Pencil/scissor control

shape and weight of the object through visual information and also through sensory receptors in the skin, joints and muscles. Grip force has to be adjusted to the object's surface tension to prevent slippage or damage to fragile objects (Forssberg 1998). The younger child will err on the side of caution and open the hands wider and grip harder with a delay in overcoming the inertia of a static object. By 1 year of age, hand shape is adjusted more precisely to the object's spatial dimensions, with the visual system remaining crucial for programming the timing of reaching, lifting and manipulation of the object (Forssberg 1998). Children continue to show delays in adjusting to changes in the sensory characteristics of objects, such as an unexpected increase in the weight of an object when a mug is filled with liquid, until more adult grip responses emerge at around 9 or 10 years of age (Eliasson et al. 1995).

As important as the ability to hold items is the ability to let go of them. Initial release of objects is involuntary. The child begins to finger items in preparation for transferring these from hand to hand (Erhardt 1994). It is not until the child is able to rotate the forearm to turn the palm up (supinate) that the child can control letting go and transferring objects. More precise control of release, with the wrist extended, may be achieved by the end of the first year as the child places shapes into smaller containers (Figure 19.4) (Erhardt 1994, HELP 1985).

Grasps are described according to the position of the hand in relation to the object. More refined grips develop as the child differentiates movements of individual fingers.

By 12 months many children will have achieved a fine pincer grasp, although they may opt to use a range of different grips throughout play (Figure 19.5):

1. Reflexive grasp (Figure 19.5a), in which the child squeezes an object into the palm of the hand in response to contact, often with wrist flexion (bent). Once a voluntary grasp is achieved the child can work towards opposing the thumb to fingers.

2. Radial–palmar grasp (Figure 19.5b), in which the object is held more towards the thumb rather than the little fingers with a neutral wrist position.

3. Inferior-scissor grasp (Figure 19.5c), in which the object is held between a tucked-in thumb and fingers.

4. Key or scissor grasp (Figure 19.5d: lateral pincer), in which the thumb holds the item against the side of a curled index finger.

5. Chuck grasp (tripod) (Figure 19.5e), in which the item is held between the thumb and first and second finger pads.

6. Fine pincer grasp (Figure 19.5f), in which the child holds a small item between the thumb and fingertips.

In-hand manipulation, raking, translating and rotating

The ability to distinguish each finger and move each one independently emerges over the first year. The ability to isolate the index finger for touch pointing and then imperative pointing (pointing to request something) is an important aspect of both hand skills and early communication. The manipulation of objects within the hand begins as a child tries to rake small objects towards the palm. The skill to move small items from the palm to the fingertips emerges later and is related to the ability to open the hand for controlled release. The child will continue to develop skills throughout early childhood in transferring items from thumb to different

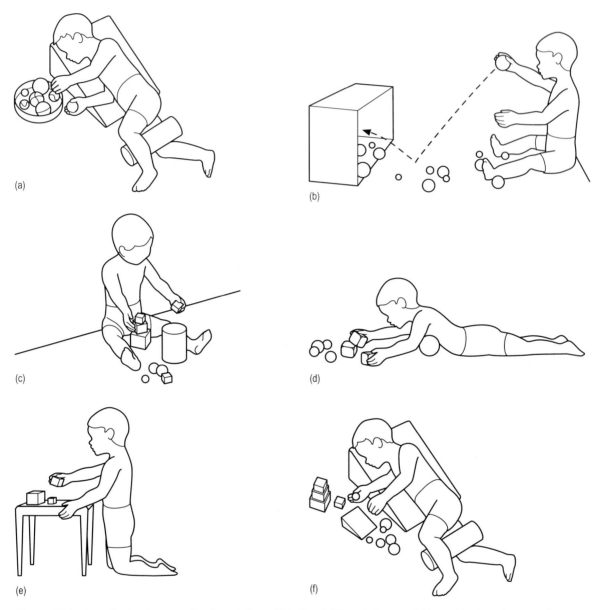

Figure 19.4 • Learning basic perception from balls and blocks of different sizes, weights and textures to promote adjustment of hand grasp. (a) Provide balls to retrieve and feel. (b) Introduce more balls with different textures and weights. (c) Drop balls into a container for sound and to develop precision of release. (d) Introduce different shapes and textures. (e) Introduce more blocks to build towers and encourage weight-bearing with arm reach. (f) Use different shapes such as ramps to roll balls down and towers to knock down to promote hand–eye coordination.

fingers and controlling rotational movements within the hand for more refined skills such as turning buttons to fit through buttonholes and placing coins through differently angled slots (Figure 19.6). Manipulative skills may also be classified by the comparative actions of the thumb and digits: simple, reciprocal or sequential patterns (Sugden and Utley 1995).

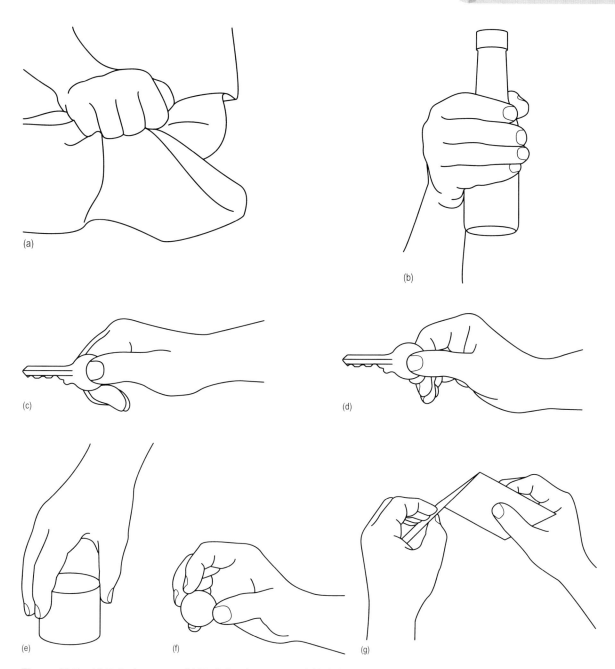

Figure 19.5 • (a) Reflexive grasp. (b) Radial–palmar grasp. (c) Inferior-scissor grasp. (d) Key or scissor grasp (lateral pincer). (e) Chuck grasp (tripod). (f) Fine pincer grasp. (g) Using both hands with varying grasps.

Perceptual–motor integration

Matching sensory cues with meaningful perceptual information is integral for planning skilled movements. Early attempts to imitate actions are seen when the child mimics facial expressions and arm movements to communicate. Perceptual–motor matching develops in the first year as the

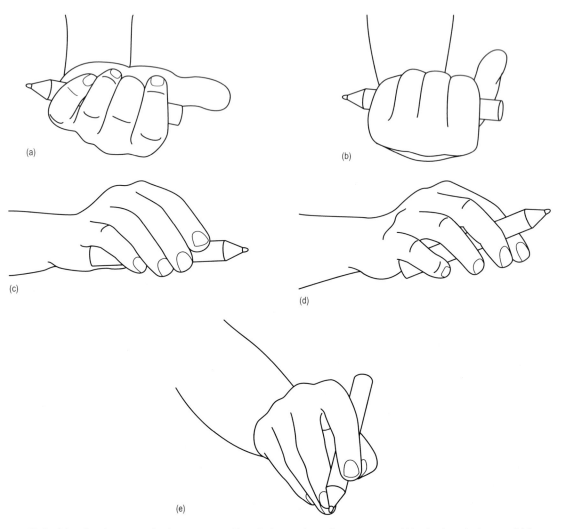

(a)

(b)

(c)

(d)

(e)

Figure 19.6 • The development of using a crayon. Translating and rotating a crayon within the hand when scribbling provides additional visual feedback of hand position. (a–c) Translation from palm to fingertips. (d, e) In-hand manipulation of a crayon.

child watches adults write and draw and then attempts to place marks on paper. Awareness of size, shape and form enables the child to marry improved manipulative skills with an understanding of objects and environments so that, at 3 years, a child can not only copy a line, cross and circle, but starts to be aware of the impact that graphic symbols may have in communication (Callaghan 1999). Further development of one- and two-handed skills continues over the next few years.

Notable in all aspects of upper-limb movement skills as they develop through the course of childhood is the spontaneous initiation of a great variety of upper-limb postures.

Identification of atypical use of the hands

There are no hard and fast rules that apply in determining what is typical, let alone atypical.

The range in ages by which a hand posture is obtained and used functionally is quite broad but more important is the ability to achieve a variety of hand positions spontaneously and voluntarily. A child with cerebral palsy (CP) may have varying degrees of neurological involvement contributing to impaired hand function. This may be due to inadequate muscle recruitment, impaired sensation and stereotypic posturing affecting coordination of reaching and grasping and/or poor understanding of how to use tools and manipulate toys. When one side of the body is weaker or less reliable than the other, children may adopt one-handed or alternative strategies using their less involved upper extremity or teeth or body, further contributing to learnt non-use of the weaker, more impaired hand.

During the first year, observations of hand development will be quite general and relate more to postural control and ability to support body weight on the forearms and hands. Towards the latter half of the first year, it may be apparent that the child has difficulty sustaining eye contact on an object to reach towards it or hand postures may look clumsy with the wrist bent and hand clenched, the fingers acting as one unit rather than emergent individual and isolated finger movements. A lack of variety of spontaneous and fluid (not fidgety) upper-limb movements, especially those that result in changes in posture or loss of balance, may be of concern. Incoordination when reaching and grasping may also indicate poor motor control. The arms may have too little resistance to stretch and appear weak (possibly hypotonic) or conversely feel stiff with too much resistance to stretch (hypertonic), contributing to difficulties reaching towards and manipulating objects. By the end of the first year, if the child does not hold and release objects such as cubes, toy cars or rattles with ease, or hand positions remain limited to fisting around the object with the thumb stuck into the palm of the hand, or there is a prolonged grasp of an object before lifting it off a supporting surface, it is usual to consult a medical practitioner who may refer the child to a physiotherapist or occupational therapist specializing in child development.

Assessments

A number of assessments are available to determine the extent to which the child's development may be behind or deviant from that which would be expected at their chronological age. Most do not address hand skills until the child is over 1 year of age, when the basic hand skills are expected to be more established. Therapists will also document any resistance to stretching and the range of movement at the shoulder, elbow and wrist and atypical and persistent postures such as a constantly flexed wrist or thumb tucked into the hand. From 1 year onwards, tests are available which investigate the extent to which any motor problems influence speed, strength and sensory perceptual skills and the impact of these on the performance of daily activities. Assessment of basic motor actions in relation to perceptual reasoning and task understanding is also included. Once complex and functional hand use is more established, other assessments are available which look at performance in tasks involving manual dexterity or upper-limb function, for example, throwing and catching balls. Table 19.3 sets out some of the most frequently used tests of upper-limb functions of the younger child.

Few of these tests will be feasible for use if a child has more significant motor problems, learning difficulties or a sensory impairment. It has also been suggested that the relationship between advanced movement skills and knowledge about objects is somewhat different in children with visual impairment from sighted children (Bigelow 1992). The use of developmental scales such as the Denver curriculum (Frankenburg et al. 1992) may provide better indicators of any discrepancies in skill attainments.

As well as performing fine motor tasks such as holding a spoon, pencil control and ball skills, the quality of movement and atypical posturing may be of concern. A few specific assessments allow for measuring the quality of movements, such as the Quality of Upper Extremities Skill Test (DeMatteo et al. 1992) and the Melbourne Assessment of Unilateral Upper Limb Function (Randall et al. 1999). More recently developed

Table 19.3 Published assessments of upper-limb skills

Test	Age	Key upper-limb skill measured
Alberta infant motor scale (Piper and Darrah 1994)	Birth to 18 months	Shoulder stability and arm movements for weight-bearing when lying and kneeling Reaching from extended arm support Crawling and pull to stand
Erhardt scales (Erhardt 1994)	Birth through childhood	Describes hand positions Identifies risk factors such as stiffness and deformity
Posture and fine motor assessment of infants (Case-Smith 1992)	2–6 months	Posture and hand skills Helps set targets for monitoring progress
Peabody developmental motor scales (Folio and Fewell 2000)	Birth to 6 years 11 months	Grasping Hand use Hand–eye coordination, manual dexterity, e.g. stacking cubes and puzzles
Bayley scales of child development (Bayley 1993)	1–42 months	Mental scale explores perceptual reasoning Motor scale tests body control, fine and gross motor skills
Miller assessment for preschoolers (Miller 1992)	2.9–5.6 years	Fundamental cognitive functions in addition to sensory and motor skills for the identification of mild, moderate or severe developmental delay Child needs to understand language

tools such as the Manual Ability Classification System (Amer et al. 2005) and the Assisting Hand Assessment (Krumlinde-Sundholm et al. 2006) provide reliable methods of classifying the extent of difficulty using two hands and the effect this has on function as well as monitoring progress.

In addition to problems maintaining trunk stability for reaching and grasping actions, the child with CP will often have difficulties manipulating objects and using hands and arms for emotional expression and more precise communication. Parents are usually best at identifying problems in movement and skill development and any concerns should be mentioned to key medical professionals.

Promoting hand skills

The early development of hand skills, especially hand–eye coordination, provides a foundation for later independence in a number of daily living tasks. Children with CP may need to rely on their hands to hold walkers, assist transfers and mobility or communicate needs, either directly or by accessing augmentative communication devices. The ability to flip or turn the pages of a book and point to choices may transform the communication skills of a child.

Providing the child with additional opportunities to practise and rehearse movements is essential. Conventional interventions emphasize engagement in activities by simplifying the postural demands and manipulative requirements of objects. First and foremost is the need to provide enjoyable sensory experiences of touch. Many children who have had early experience of negative touch, for example needles and plasters, may show some hypersensitivity to tactile (touch) sensations and may express discomfort or withdraw from a comforting stroke or cuddle.

Sensory enjoyment

The following suggestions may help the child find tactile contact less aversive.

Active use of hands

1. Encourage children to rub their hands on their face, arms and legs by holding the arm firmly but not tightly just above the wrist. If the child has difficulty opening the fingers, use a firm and constant grasp across the joints of the wrist and fingers to assist opening the hand against a firm surface, avoiding contact with the highly sensitive palm (Figure 19.7a).

2. Assist a stroking action to encourage rhythmic and hence predictable tactile experience so the child feels more in control and comforted by the contact (Figure 19.7b).

Avoid unpredictable touch imposed by others

1. This is more tickly and may be uncomfortable for some children. If the child seems hypersensitive to touch, avoid contacting the head or body from behind. For example, do not ruffle the hair, however affectionately.

2. Allow time to accommodate to changes in body contact and inadvertent touch using firm and consistent contact whenever possible.

Keep a more constant physical contact

1. When stretching limbs, try to keep more constant contact by having one hand remain still on the child's arm or leg whilst the other slowly and smoothly moves the limb, giving sufficient time for the child to feel comfortable with the tactile contact.

Provide a variety of pleasurable tactile experiences

Do not follow tactile experiences with invasive medical procedures such as suctioning or placement of the child in positions that require difficult postural adjustments.

1. Place different items and textures between the palms, beginning with firm toys that hold their shape and then those that have a different texture or are malleable.

2. Change the texture of familiar objects by covering them with different surfaces such as a wash cloth or cellophane over a block.

3. Help the child experience different surfaces such as: (a) wet and dry; (b) warm and cold; or (c) sticky and smooth.

4. Avoid more slimy textures until confident that the child is happier with a range of tactile experiences.

5. Once the child is comfortable with touch or with assisted exploration of different textures,

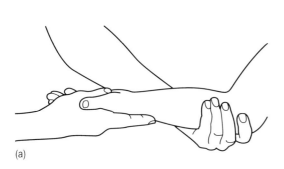

(a)

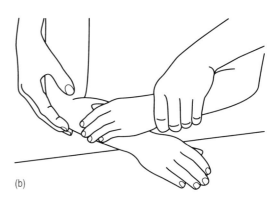

(b)

Figure 19.7 • Assisted grips for self-stroking and forearm rotation. (a) Gently rotate the forearm whilst providing pressure through wrist and elbow. (b) Assist self-stroking by holding across back of hand.

engage the child in interactive play such as blowing kisses, tickling and hide and seek.

6. During personal care and daily activities encourage the child's participation in the task, for example hand-over-hand holding of a brush. Draw attention to the hands and also to the feet during washing and bathing. For the child who is unable to hold soap, making a mitt out of a flannel cloth is a useful way of encouraging children to wash themselves with less random, unpredictable and tickly contact from the carer.

Visual regard leading to visually guided reaching

The position of the child is imperative to minimize the effort required to keep the head and body stable. A number of strategies may be used to help the child fixate and respond to visual or auditory stimuli:

1. Place smaller children on your lap with a small wedge under your feet to provide an incline to the legs and help direct the child's vision to your face.

2. Keep the child's head in midline and provide some support to the back of the shoulders, which will free the child's arms to reach towards your face or a bright pendant or bell around your neck (Figure 19.8).

3. A cupped headrest or shawl placed across the back may help support the head and keep the shoulders forward making it easier to move the arms.

4. Place the child in the cot in a semi-reclined position using a wedge or blanket strapped to the sides of the cot. Some support or wedge under the bottom may also be necessary to stop the child sliding down the cot. This may help the child reach towards a toy or hanging mobile (Figure 19.9).

A child should not be put in a hammock unless an adult is nearby to supervise.

5. Bright, shiny and noisy objects, such as a rattle covered with aluminium foil, may encourage the child to locate by vision and or sound.

6. Move objects slowly in an arc in front of the child's vision to develop head control. Some children may rely on head turning to operate switches later.

7. Once the child can follow the rattle with the eyes, take the arc a bit further to develop head turning, reducing the support to the head.

The association of sounds and images with motor actions will be helpful in developing an understanding of the environment and assist with learning how to use or respond to these stimuli independently. Remember to allow sufficient time, which might be longer than with some children, for the child to focus, fixate and follow movement, sounds or sights.

1. Encourage the child to look at familiar objects.

2. Shiny and noisy objects may attract the most attention, such as looking at shiny objects on shelves, stopping in front of a ticking clock, rain on a window pane or reflections in a mirror.

3. When too heavy to carry, the child's trunk can be supported on the tummy whilst lying across your lap looking at objects (Figure 19.10).

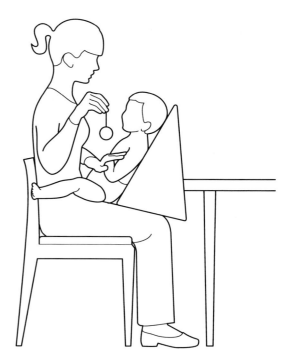

Figure 19.8 • The child sits astride the mother's lap with a wedged cushion for comfort and support. The mother prevents the child pushing back by holding the arms forward across the child's chest. She may support the child's head in midline and help the child focus on her face or follow the ball without moving the head.

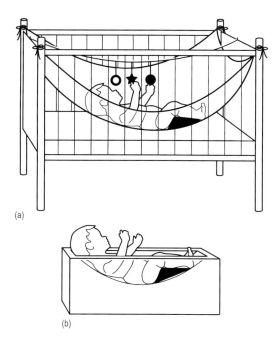

Figure 19.9 • (a) Blanket strapped to sides of cot for a semi-reclined position. (b) Foam section cut out to provide a hammock shape.

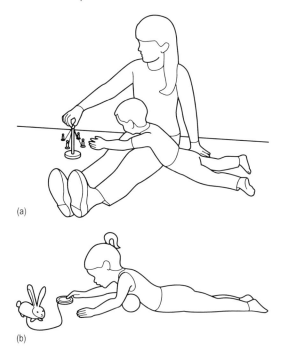

Figure 19.10 • (a) Child's tummy supported across mother's lap. (b) Use of a roll to help a child operate a switch for a toy.

4. Pets may provide an excellent resource to focus visual and auditory attention, and also smell and touch.

5. Draw the child's attention to typical home objects and noises such as the doorbell or telephone ringing, bathtub bubbles, water dripping from a tap, clicking on and off an electric light switch, kettles whistling and other similar events.

6. Encourage the child to look from one stimulus or object to another, alternating different sounds or images to attract attention and develop eye and head control.

7. Use your own face to attract your child's attention, talking, smiling and nodding your head to encourage the child to look up at you during breast- or bottle-feeding.

8. Later encourage the child to track objects from side to side and up and down as well as near to far to develop eye movements further for targeting and reaching objects.

9. Wear bright or funny hats, use hand puppets or wave bright scarves to provide animation to help the child follow moving objects (Figure 19.11).

10. Swiping at bubbles can be a fun means of refining reaching skills. You could place a drop or two of food dye into bubble mix to add colour contrast.

Once the child is able to sustain visual attention on interesting objects the child can practise coordinating hand–eye movements.

1. Place mobiles across cribs or set above the play area on the floor to provide feedback on range and effort of swiping actions and early reaching, to encourage greater precision for targeted actions such as hitting switches to operate toys and communication devices. Remember to get down to the child's eye-view to check what will actually be seen.

2. Provide extra support if necessary to keep the head in a midline position and bring the shoulders and arms forward.
   (a) C-shaped cushions with some dycem (non-slip mat) placed underneath the trunk can be used for some children.
   (b) Padded-out laundry baskets can be used to position the child as well as being useful to attach objects to promote reaching.

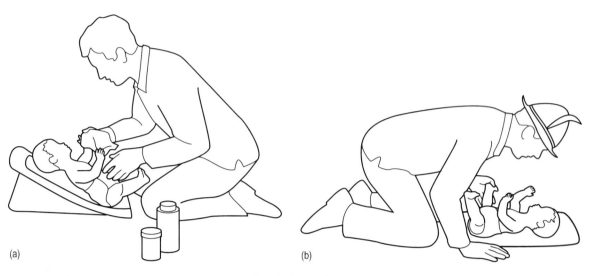

(a)　　　　　　　　　　　　　　　　　　　　(b)

Figure 19.11 • (a, b) Encourage hand–eye coordination during routine activities.

Many toy gyms and activity triangles are available commercially which have been tested for safety and durability.

1. Look at a number of catalogues or shops before making a final choice to ensure that the size of the frame and the weight, colour and sound of items are suitable for your child.

2. Additional items can be added to some commercial frames but, if fabricating your own, place items that are within the child's visual and reaching range, with or without assistance to guide arm movements, so that arm movements make an object move in a fairly consistent way.

3. Bright or noisy objects can be added to commercially available mobiles with clothes pegs or stitching.

4. Home-made mobiles can be made with more traditional lampshade frames or clothes hangers.

5. Avoid objects which have a spiral, rotary effect that lasts beyond the relative immediate action of the child as this may confuse the visual-motor perceptual organization and strobe effect toys may precipitate epileptic fits in some children.

6. Place items around the home such as shiny bracelets wrapped in coloured cellophane or tin foil, strips of crêpe paper, decorations left over from festivals. But remember, items within reach may be grabbed and placed in the child's mouth. Therefore attach a large ball at the base of a string containing the smaller items so that, when the child swipes at the ball the bright, shiny or noisy items move but cannot be grabbed and placed in the mouth.

7. Primary colours are easiest for many children to focus on, but for those with a visual impairment, black and white contrast may provide better visual stimulation.

8. For the child who has difficulty reaching forward to swipe at objects within range, attaching bracelets with bells or shiny surfaces to the child's wrists or ankles may help the child organize self-directed movements and associate these with sights and sounds.

Children who have difficulty organizing head and eye movements with reaching and targeting may also have difficulty discovering where their body parts are. Different positions can be used to help children look at and grasp their hands and feet and thus begin to learn about their own boundaries and relationship to their environment. Figures 19.12–19.15 illustrate some techniques to position the child to support symmetrical and stable postures for play and learning about body parts.

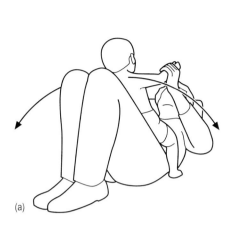
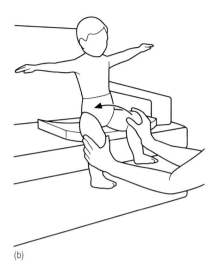

Figure 19.12 • A child needs good trunk control, pelvic stability and balance before being able to use both hands for skilled activities in sitting. (a) The child sits across the father holding his hands. To encourage an improvement in head and trunk control, the father moves his legs sideways, encouraging the child to make the necessary postural adjustments. Later the father may progress to just holding one hand if the child becomes more competent. If the child's arms feel heavy the father can stretch them out above his head with the shoulders outwardly rotated (turned out). (b) Place a square of foam on the base of a sofa, or use a roll or ball, to encourage balance reactions. Tip the child slowly from one side and wait a second before moving the child back to midline to encourage the child to accommodate to the postural change.

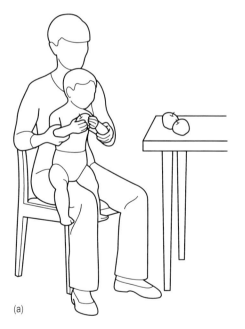
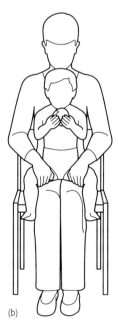

Figure 19.13 • Different positions to help the child who flexes (bends) to grasp an apple and take it to the mouth. (a) Sitting across the mother's knee the child is helped to grasp an apple from the table with extended (stretched) arms. As the child takes the apple to the mouth the mother stops the child's arms from pressing down and turning in by supporting under the elbows to keep the child's arms away from the body. (b) If a child has a tendency to extend the hips and legs and push back when lifting the arms, try controlling the legs as shown.

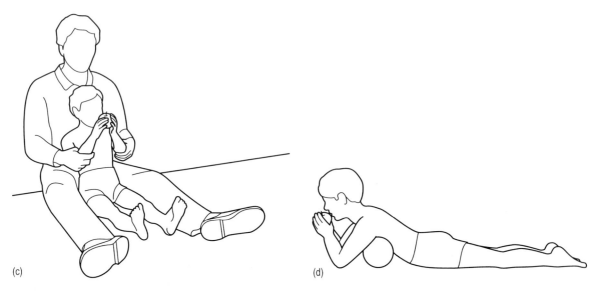

Figure 19.13 • (c, d) Two positions which may be used with a child who needs more postural support.

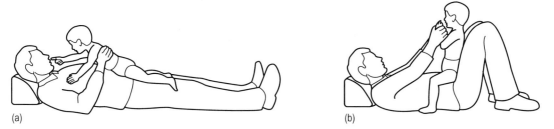

Figure 19.14 • Different positions for the child with increased tone. (a) Laying the child on the father's trunk supporting the child under the armpits so that the child is able to take weight on one open hand and reach forward with the other hand. (b) Sitting the child across the father's trunk and guiding the child's hands towards the child's face. Encourage the child to touch and name nose, eyes, mouth and ears. If the child has poor trunk control and slips backwards, place a wedged cushion between the child's back and the father's knees to bring the child's trunk forwards so that the child's body weight is going through the bottom and legs.

Stimulating toys that encourage location of images and sounds, such as those that reflect light, click, rattle or play a tune, are commercially available in most countries. Most such toys do not need to be purchased through specialist companies.

1. Rattles, teething rings or other objects that a child may place in the mouth, gaining important additional sensory information about texture and shape of the object, should be the correct size for the child to hold but not so small that there is a danger of swallowing, nor too brittle with parts that may snap.

2. Toys with two handles or those that can be lifted easily by slipping a hand under a lever for early cause and effect will encourage early hand skills.

3. Toys and objects that respond when poked, patted, pressed, banged and pulled or pulled apart can all be used to promote the child's hand–eye coordination and early fine motor skills.

4. Switches can be linked to battery-operated toys to promote targeting.

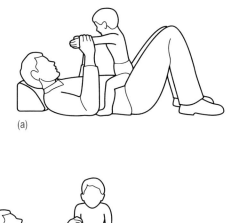

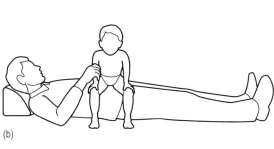

(a)

(b)

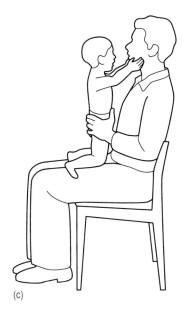

(c)

Figure 19.15 • Different positions for the child with fluctuating tone and involuntary movements who needs a stable base for improving body awareness and use of the hands. (a) The child grasps the father's thumbs as he pulls the child towards himself, keeping the child's arms straight. The father can try to give a quick backwards movement and then pull the child forwards again to try to give the child a feeling of grasping while at the same time trying to increase the tone in the trunk (making it firm). Try also to encourage the child to push against the father's hands. This may give the child a feeling for reaching forwards in a controlled way. (b) The father holds the child firmly just below the shoulder. The child should place the hands on the knees and be encouraged to move slowly forwards to put the hands on, in front of and beside the feet and then return to the sitting position with the hands on the knees. The father should gradually remove the arm support if possible. (c) The father provides steady, firm pressure through the pelvis and hips to encourage the child to maintain the extension of the trunk when lifting the arms up.

5. Items such as saucepans and lids with large spoons continue to be universal favourites for the young child.

Hand skills

Good seating and positional systems are imperative when poor postural control and atypical movement postures affect the reaching, grasping, releasing and more dextrous hand skills, especially if the arms are needed to prop and maintain an upright posture.

1. Strengthen the muscles around the shoulder by encouraging the child to lean on the elbows or on the hands in various positions such as lying prone, sitting and standing (Levitt 2004).

2. Place a small half-roll under the hands to help cupping and develop musculature of the thumb and little finger.

3. Encourage rocking actions over the arms with a roll under the tummy as a foundation for reaching away from the body.

Voluntary grasp of objects can be promoted in a variety of playful settings. A good game to play to help the child reach forwards is to place a favourite toy just out of reach on a soft piece of cloth (Figure 19.16), encouraging the child to grasp or rake the cloth to pull the toy towards him or her (Levitt 2004).

Help the child plan and sequence reaching and targeting by accompanying movements with action songs.

Being able to open and close the hand is a prerequisite for manipulating objects within the hand. The child who is hypersensitive to touch, as discussed earlier, may automatically clench the fist against tactile stimuli. Similarly, some children

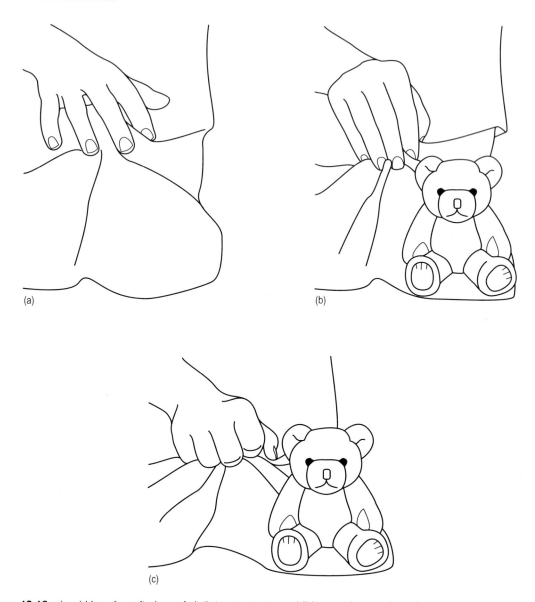

(a)

(b)

(c)

Figure 19.16 • (a–c) Use of a soft piece of cloth to encourage a child to reach and rake to bring a toy closer.

who retain the grasp reflex will automatically fist around an object that touches their palm. A desensitization programme should be instigated if necessary following consultation with a therapist. Weight-bearing through one open hand whilst encountering different sensory experiences in the other hand exposes the child's sensory-perceptual system to a range of tactile sensations to promote active exploration of objects.

In cases when the thumb stays tucked into the palm, some therapists may recommend a thumb strap, providing this does not cover the palm, to keep the thumb out of the palm for periods during the day to allow the highly sensitive palm to

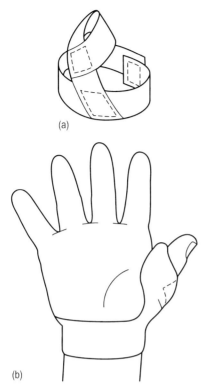

Figure 19.17 • (a) Simple thumb strap to keep thumb extended and abducted. (b) Thumb strap applied to hand.

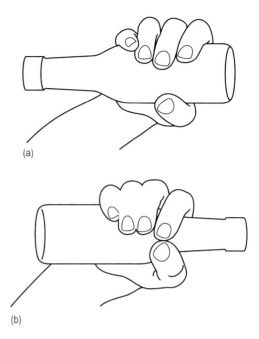

Figure 19.18 • (a) Contoured bottle with wide end at the thumb to encourage thumb opposition. (b) Contoured bottle with wide end at the little fingers to shift grip force towards the thumb and encourage opening-up of the hand.

experience different sensations, notably weight-bearing on different textures. A well-designed thumb strap can also help the child maintain a degree of wrist extension that will assist the ability to oppose the thumb to the fingertips (Figure 19.17).

As the child develops strength and control of hand muscles (the thenar and hyperthenar pads in the palm) the child begins to hold objects towards the thumb side (radial) rather than the outer, little-finger side (ulnar) of the hand.

1. To promote this, small cones or contoured bottles with the small end placed on the ulnar (outside) of the hand will encourage the thumb to oppose the fingers (Figure 19.18a).

2. If the child maintains a clenched fist with wrist flexed and bent outwards, place the cone with the wide edge towards the little finger to help the child shift the force of grip towards the thumb and help to open up the hand (Figure 19.18b).

3. Use opportunities during the day, such as at mealtimes or when bathing, to encourage the child to reach and grasp items.

4. Offer toys with different textures, shapes, sizes and moulds (density).

5. When the child can grasp an object, promote a radial–palmar grasp by providing the child with objects that can be held with one hand:
   (a) Use 2.5-cm (1-inch) cubes or blocks in posting games to encourage the child to grasp with the index and middle fingers against the thumb.

6. These same items can also be used to encourage the child to use two hands for bimanual tasks such as banging two cubes or saucepan lids together. The duration of noisy games may need to be restricted according to the tolerance of other family members.

7. When the child has developed the ability to bring two hands together, encourage the child to hold a container steady with one hand and to drop items in with the other.

The ability of the two arms to work together cooperatively will be important for performing bimanual tasks such as holding one side of a jacket still to place a button through a buttonhole.

As visual fixation and fine motor skills develop:

1. Place smaller (edible) objects within or just outside reach.
   (a) For example, place a raisin, piece of cereal, rice or pasta on the child's tray or bowl and encourage the child to rake this into the palm.

2. When encouraging the child to grasp objects, do not be upset if the child drops them, as releasing items is as important as holding them for skilled use.

3. Gradually reduce the size of the opening of the container to force the child to use the thumb and fingertips to rake up the small item against the fingertips (Figure 19.19).

Fine motor skills are also influenced by sensory discrimination and the need to manipulate items without vision.

1. To promote sensory awareness, hide items in containers filled with a little water, pasta/rice or sand. Let the child empty the container to find the object, later reaching in to find the hidden item by touch.

2. If the home environment is not suitable for outside sand and water play (Figure 19.20a), use the bath or an inflatable children's splash pool to contain the mess.

   Never leave a child unsupervised in any pool.

3. Use containers, such as boxes, cans, waste baskets or purses filled with different items and mixed textures (Figure 19.20b).

More dextrous hand skills are achieved with the wrist held in slight extension.

1. Position toys above the child's wrist level to encourage wrist extension.

2. Place textured pictures or switches on a vertical surface such as a wall or easel for the child to feel with the fingers which should encourage wrist extension.

3. Use an angled surface such as a slant board when drawing or finger painting to promote a better hand posture.

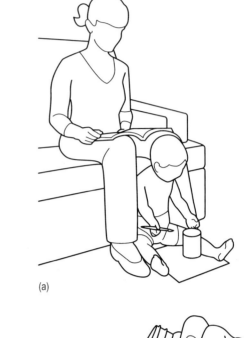

(a)

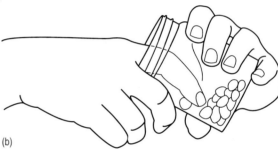

(b)

Figure 19.19 • (a) The child is supported at the shoulders and the pelvis by the mother's legs and feet whilst playing on the floor. (b) Reduce the size of container openings once the child is able to rake and release small items with the fingertips.

4. Similarly, encourage the child to press down when rolling pastry or playing with dough to take weight through the hands with the wrist and fingers extended.

5. For the child who requires more postural support, place the child over a prone wedge, roll or large ball to promote the ability to self-support through open hands.

6. When positioning the child on the tummy or when leaning forward, provide opportunities for the child to bear the weight of the body through the arms, rotated outwards on to extended wrists and hands to help strengthen the musculature

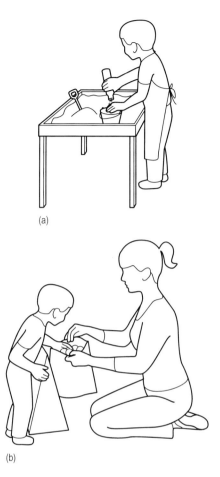

(a)

(b)

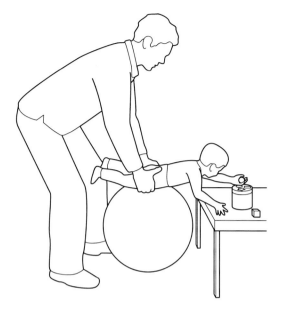

Figure 19.21 • For the child who requires additional postural support place the child over a large ball, wedge or roll to encourage the weight to be taken through an extended arm and open hand.

Figure 19.20 • Sensory discrimination. (a) Use a sandpit set at waist height so that the child is supported and encouraged to bend forwards from the hips with a straight back. (b) Hold a bag containing objects such as a comb, brush, spoon and apple hidden amongst foam balls. The child should be encouraged to identify the object without seeing it.

around the palmar arches for good effective grip strength and object manipulation (Figure 19.21).

The ability to release objects voluntarily has repeatedly been mentioned as equally important to holding on to an item.

1. Providing the child is not overly sensitive and contact to the palm does not provoke a grasp reflex, encourage the child to squeeze wet sponges or squeeze toys which make noises.

2. Use firmer items for the hypersensitive child, avoiding furry and tickly textures.

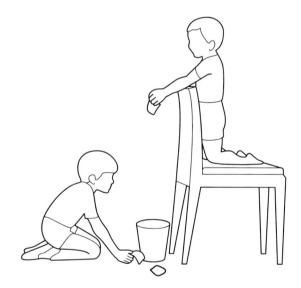

Figure 19.22 • Grasp and release. The back of a sturdy chair may be used to support upright kneeling whilst throwing or dropping bean bags into a bucket.

3. Encourage the child to grasp and release objects by dropping them repeatedly into a container such as a can which makes a sound each time the child lets go (Figure 19.22).

4. If the child shows an excessive clenched grasp, tap, rub or stroke the back of the hand, in the direction from the finger joints to the wrist, to encourage hand-opening.

Refined fine manipulative skills emerge when the child can move the fingers separately from each other, particularly the index finger.

1. Provide toys which encourage poking and pressing with one finger only.

2. Numerous push-button toys, toy pianos and pop-up surprise toys are available commercially.

3. Alternatively make holes in the sides of a box and place pegs or unsharpened pencils in the top for the child to poke into the box.

4. Allow the child to pinch and pull playdough or pastry with the thumb and index finger.

5. Turning knobs and keys for wind-up toys will also encourage the rotary movements of the fingers

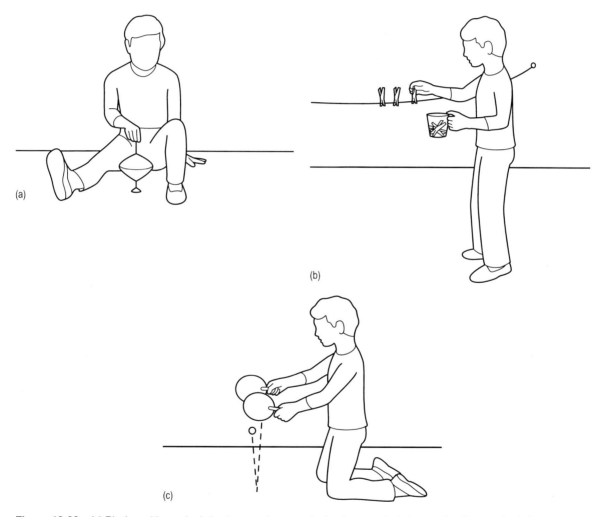

(a)

(b)

(c)

Figure 19.23 • (a) Playing with manipulative toys such as a spinning top may help to practise fine manipulation movements. (b) Encouraging a child to hold with one hand still whilst moving the other in functional activities may lead to more difficult bimanual tasks in which the hands need to do different movements. (c) Playing with two hands holding bats to lift, bounce and catch a ball. If the child is able to hold the bats with the index finger pointing along the back of the bat, the movement may be a good preparation for writing and eating with a knife and fork.

necessary for moving items within the hand (Figure 19.23a).

6. To encourage pincer grasp, use tiny objects which do not easily roll away and provide finger foods at snack times.

7. For the child who has developed thumb to fingertip control but continues to have poor skill, pinching clothes pegs to place notes or pictures on the rim of a can will develop strength and timing (Figure 19.23b).

More advanced manipulative skills such as pencil control, sewing, buttoning and fastening zippers may remain difficult for the child with CP (Figure 19.23c). The decision to move towards compensatory equipment such as adapted handles on cutlery, adapted clothing and also keyboards to support written work should be considered when the effort and energy required to perform the task are excessive and the accuracy remains poor and undermines the confidence and self-esteem of the child. Switch-accessing computer technology or modified keyboards, for example slowing key response times or use of key guards, is recommended even if the child has the basic motor ability, as the effort of learning academic concepts alongside performing motor tasks often undermines the child's learning progress. Practice and development of motor skills may be undertaken more effectively if separate from cognitive and academic work.

Play and having fun with movement are imperative in developing all aspects of motor competence. Encouraging the child to imitate your actions, with consistent rewards for effort, is a first step in supporting understanding of the impact the child can have on his or her environment with the execution of simple movements. Repetition and practice are important, particularly when trying new movement tasks, but care should be taken to avoid the child becoming exhausted with attempts that lead to failure and demotivation. As the child progresses to learning more complex fine motor skills, some aspects of the environment or postural demands may need to be simplified to enable the child to concentrate on the new task. Thus even if the child has mastered independent sitting, it may still be appropriate to place the child in supportive postural systems when working on new cognitive, social or fine motor skills so that the child can give

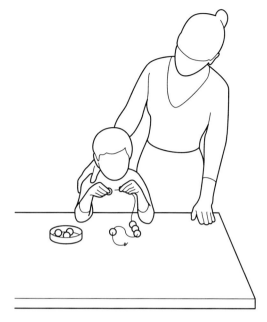

Figure 19.24 • The child may find it easier to prop on the elbows on a table when practising fine manipulative tasks or playing with toys needing two hands.

undivided attention to the appropriate challenge rather than having to worry about losing balance or more basic motor demands (Figure 19.24). This is similar to the learner driver who needs to concentrate on the mechanics of driving and is unable to hold a conversation simultaneously. Once the child masters a skill and is able to repeat that skill consistently with success, new challenges can be added. For example, once the child can grasp a toy when seated securely, encourage the child to reach just outside his or her centre of gravity (postural base) to grab a toy or food. In cases where the child seems uninterested in toys or objects and does not engage in play consider:

1. The qualities of the toy or object, size, weight, colour and ease of manipulation

2. The demands of the environment, including social and sensory demands

3. Postural demands

4. The level of cognitive maturity (complexity of knowledge) needed to use or manipulate the toy

Further consultation with medical professionals may be needed if the child seems frustrated, uninterested or detached after a variety of attempts to encourage play.

Complementary or alternative strategies

Striking the right balance between effort, practice and success is important when harnessing the children's interest to master their environment. Traditional therapies have usually emphasized engagement in activities along a developmental model within the family unit, adapting these where necessary to assist posture and grip control. When appropriate, other therapeutic interventions such as rhythmic exercise programmes (Conductive Education) and targeted training for specific movement patterns (MOVE programme) have been incorporated to help the child move more easily. Other specialized treatments may help relax overly active muscles through medication, may provide more rigid assistance to hand and arm position (casting and splinting) or may provoke more active use of a weaker arm. In some cases surgical intervention to the upper limb may also be warranted. Determining which of these additional or alternative approaches will best support skills whilst minimizing pain and discomfort should be discussed with your child's medical practitioners and therapists. There are no hard and fast rules suggesting which child with CP with what type of motor involvement would benefit from what type of input. Research has suggested some clinical indicators.

Muscle relaxants

Children with excessively high tone in their arms and hands which persistently prevents them from reaching forward and opening their hands may benefit from a systemic muscle relaxant such as baclofen. This may be administered orally or by intrathecal infusion to the spine to relax many postural muscles and major muscles of the arms and legs. Localized injections of botulinum toxin A (BTX-A) to specific muscles have been shown to be of benefit in certain instances of upper-limb spasticity, especially when tolerance to wearing hand splints is recommended to lessen the risk of deforming hand positions (Lowe et al. 2007).

BTX-A is more frequently administered to upper-limb muscles when there is an abnormality in tone resulting in poorly controlled movements and where there is no evidence of loss of range of movement due to sustained hypertonicity. After BTX-A injections to the upper limb a need for intensive therapy to strengthen muscles has been suggested. Regular monitoring and stretching are needed postinjection as some of the functional benefits may wear off as BTX-A loses its potency. Helpful, but not permanent, results have been achieved across age ranges, intellectual ability and types of movement disorders except if severe hypertonicity with contractures is present. It is not really known how many courses of injections are maximally beneficial or potentially detrimental if localized resistance builds up.

Splinting and casting

Some children may need external support to hold their wrist and hand in a good position to support functional grips. The disadvantage of applying a splint or cast is that it reduces the surface area for receiving important sensory information about an object for grip control. Needless to say, there may be an indication for splinting if there is a risk of deformity or pain when a child remains in a fixed posture, such as a flexed and clenched grasp, which may also make it difficult to maintain hand hygiene. Different splint materials may be used varying from rigid thermoplastic materials to more flexible neoprene and Lycra or a mix such as a neoprene hand splint with an aluminium support for wrist extension. The advantages of achieving what appears to be a more 'cosmetic' or appropriate hand position need to be offset against any loss of voluntary use of the hand to prop or support objects or discomfort with increased heat and sweating.

Serial casting – casts to maintain a constant stretch across a joint or joints such as the elbow and wrist, and changed each week to increase the tension – may be used, especially after a course of BTX-A. A dynamic bivalved brace which provides a constant torqued force across a joint but allows movement within a set range, defined by the locks and tension of the hinges, may be considered in cases where there is still a good range of movement in the muscles of the arm and wrist but where hypertonicity may lead to a permanent contracture as the child is unable to move actively to the full extent of the joint range. These braces are quite heavy and therefore the child needs to have fairly good musculature across the trunk and upper arm to tolerate their use.

Surgery

There are occasions, particularly as the child reaches adolescence, when surgery to the upper limb may be indicated. This may take the form of a wrist arthrodesis (fixation) to stabilize the wrist in a more functional extended position or tendon transfer to shift flexor muscles to the back of the hand, again to support more active wrist extension and finger opening. It is often worth a trial with a cast to 'mock' the surgery and see if the improved position has any functional or cosmetic benefit. Tendon lengthening may also be recommended, especially when a permanently bent elbow or clenched fist is affecting skin hygiene. Surgical intervention on the upper limb is rarely indicated for the younger child, especially while there is continuing bone growth.

Constraint-induced movement therapy

Children with hemiplegia may frequently develop alternative strategies, such as using the teeth, to perform tasks and accommodate for the reduced control of one upper extremity. Development and use of the weaker, affected arm and hand are restricted by lack of experience and practice. A protocol for increasing the use of an involved arm whilst restricting the use of the unimpaired limb, is referred to as constraint-induced movement therapy (CIMT) (Taub and Wolf 1997, Eliasson et al. 2005, Gordon et al. 2005, Charles et al. 2006). This allows the child to take advantage of knowledge of the task and task solution to experience attempts to use the involved limb and to force practice. In other words, any attempt to use the affected limb spontaneously will contribute to enhanced perceptual-motor experience and support motor learning.

A number of modifications have been used to restrain the uninvolved limb and encourage use of the involved limb with children. Probably the most child-friendly investigated to date used a thermoplastic paddle splint restricting wrist and finger movements contained within a puppet to allow for some bilateral propping and supporting role of the restrained limb for a period of 2 hours every day for 4 weeks whilst simultaneously engaging the child in one- and two-handed tasks.

This therapeutic approach is intensive and requires significant commitment of the family. Subsequently behaviour difficulties may increase or emerge for the child who is frustrated and having problems focusing attention and persisting with more difficult tasks. Detailed discussion with the family regarding how and when to trial this approach is needed so that any benefits may outweigh any negative impact on family life.

Emerging therapies

The use of robotics and Virtual Reality are showing some promise in the ability to improve upper-extremity control, however empirical evidence is limited, especially with children and, as with CIMT, recommended use should remain within clinical trials until the evidence is clearer (You et al. 2005, Prange et al. 2006, Hoare et al. 2007, Chen et al. 2007).

Summary

The overwhelming contribution of manual dexterity skills to independence in today's modern society is as important as independent mobility. The Dynamical Systems approach to understanding motor development considers that movement is part of a perceptual package enabling the developing child to categorize and recategorize memories of successful motor skills. Therefore, it is suggested that knowledge and skill result from the successive integration of separate modalities that are elaborately intertwined (Thelen and Smith 1994). These are limited not by what children know, but primarily by having adequate opportunities to sample and categorize the world. It is of paramount importance to provide sufficient, enjoyable experiences for children with CP to explore the world through their hands.

References

Amer M, Eliasson AC, Rösblad B et al. MACS manual ability classification system for children with cerebral palsy. Karolinska Institute and CanChild McMaster University, Hamilton 2005.

Bayley N. Bayley scales of infant development, 2nd edn. Therapy Skill Builders, San Antonio, TX, 1993.

Bigelow AE. Locomotion and search behavior in blind infants. Infant Behavior Dev 1992; 15:179–189.

Callaghan TC. Early understanding and production of graphic symbols. Child Dev 1999; 70:1314–1324.

Case-Smith J. Posture and Fine Motor Assessment of Infants (PFMAI). American OT Association, Bethesda, MD, 1992.

Charles JR, Wolf SL, Schneider JA, Gordon AM. Efficacy of a child-friendly form of constraint-induced movement therapy in hemiplegic cerebral palsy: a randomized control trial. Dev Med Child Neurol 2006; 48:635–642.

Chen Y-P, Kang L-J, Chuang T-Y et al. Use of virtual reality to improve upper-extremity control in children with cerebral palsy: a single-subject design. Physical Therapy 2007; 87:1441–1457.

DeMatteo C, Law M, Russell D et al. QUEST Quality of Upper Extremity Skills Test. Chedokee-McMaster Hospital, Ontario, 1992.

Eliasson AC, Forssberg H, Ikuta K et al. Development of human precision grip. V: Anticipatory and triggered grip actions during sudden loading. Exp Brain Res 1995; 106:425–433.

Eliasson AC, Krumlinde-Sundholm L, Shaw K, Wang C. Effects of constraint-induced movement therapy in young children with hemiplegic cerebral palsy: an adapted model. Dev Med Child Neurol 2005; 47:266–275.

Erhardt RP. Developmental hand dysfunction: theory, assessment and treatment. Therapy Skill Builders, Arizona, 1994.

Fitts PM, Posner MI. Human performance. Brooks/Cole, Belmont, CA, 1967.

Folio MR, Fewell RR. Peabody developmental motor scales, 2nd edn. Pro-Ed, Texas, 2000.

Forssberg H. The neurophysiology of manual skill development. In: Connolly KJ (ed.) The psychobiology of the hand. MacKeith Press, London, 1998, pp. 99–122.

Frankenberg WK, Dodds JB, Archer P. Denver II technical manual. Denver Developmental Materials, Denver, 1992.

Goodale MA, Jakobson LS, Servos P. The visual pathways mediating perception and prehension. In: Wing AM,

Haggard P, Flanagan JR (eds) Hand and brain: the neurophysiology and psychology of hand movements. Academic Press, London, 1996.

Gordon AM, Charles J, Wolf SL. Methods of constraint-induced movement therapy for children with hemiplegic cerebral palsy: development of a child-friendly intervention for improving upper-extremity function. Arch Phys Med Rehabil 2005; 86:837–844.

HELP enrichment project for handicapped infants. Hawaii Early Learning Profile. VORT, Palo Alto, CA, 1985.

Krumlinde-Sundholm L, Holmefur M, Eliasson AC. Assisting Hand Assessment Manual: Research Version 4.3 Stockholm. Karolinska Institute, Neuropediatric Research Unit, Astrid Lindgren Children's Hospital, 2006.

Levitt S. Treatment of cerebral palsy and motor delay, 4th edn. Blackwell, Oxford, 2004.

Lowe K, Novak I, Cusick A. Repeat injection of botulinum toxin A is safe and effective for upper limb movement and function in children with cerebral palsy. Dev Med Child Neurol 2007; 49:823–829.

Paillard J. The contribution of peripheral and central vision to visually guided reaching. In: Ingle DJ, Goodale MA, Mansfield RJW (eds) Analysis of visual behavior. MIT Press, Cambridge, MA, 1982, pp. 367–385.

Piper MC, Darrah J. Motor assessment of the developing infant. WB Saunders, London, 1994.

Prange GB, Jannink MJ, Groothuis-Oudshoorn CG, Hermens HJ, Ijzerman MJ. Systematic review of the effect of robot-aided therapy on recovery of the hemiparetic arm after stroke. J Rehab Research Dev 2006; 43:171–184.

Randall M, Johnson C, Reddihough D. The Melbourne assessment of unilateral upper limb function. Arena Printing, Melbourne, 1999.

Shumway-Cook A, Woollacott M. Motor control theory and practical applications. Williams and Wilkins, London, 1995.

Taub E, Wolf SL. Constraint induced movement techniques to facilitate upper extremity use in stroke patients. Top Stroke Rehab 1997; 3:38–61.

Thelen E, Smith LB. A dynamic systems approach to the development of cognition and action. MIT Press, London, 1994.

You SH, Jang SH, Kim Y-H et al. Cortical reorganization induced by virtual reality therapy in a child with hemiparetic cerebral palsy. Dev Med Child Neurol 2005; 47:628–635.

Chapter Twenty

Gross motor development in children with cerebral palsy: what do we know, and how may that knowledge help?

Peter Rosenbaum

Among parents' first thoughts when they are told that their child has cerebral palsy (CP) are questions like 'How bad is it?' and 'Will our child be able to walk?' Doctors and therapists have usually been reluctant to answer either question directly. The reasons for their reluctance have included uncertainty about how to describe severity, and, especially for younger service providers, a lack of experience on which to base an answer about the functional outlook. In addition, we have not always been completely honest. What I mean by that is that, when we can be very certain that a child's motor development is likely to proceed well, we feel comfortable in passing along good news, whereas when we are fairly certain that the outlook for independent mobility is very guarded, we can easily resort to phrases like 'It's too early to tell', 'Children progress at different rates in their development', 'Let's see how therapy works over the next few months', and so on.

It is my guess that we do not fool anyone with these evasions. Furthermore I suspect that by failing to give an honest appraisal of the probability of limited independent mobility, when that is what we expect, we may at times raise parents' hopes inappropriately and in doing so put parents and therapists on trial as the people in whose hands the outcome lies.

The purpose of this chapter is to describe work that has been done over the past decade to provide some facts and evidence about the motor development of children with CP that can be used to answer parents' questions more effectively. While this work is constantly being developed and refined, we believe that, *when parents are ready to ask questions about their child's outlook*, we are now in a position to be able to answer with some confidence.

The Gross Motor Function Classification System (GMFCS) (Palisano et al. 1997 and 2008)

When parents used to ask me how 'bad' their child's CP was, I was always uncomfortable, and never certain what to say. Traditionally, we have described the severity of CP with words like 'mild', 'moderate' and 'severe'. These words might be helpful *if* they were clearly and explicitly defined, and *if* they had a common meaning among parents and service providers – which unfortunately has never been the case. To tell parents that their child's disability is 'mild' might be good news for some and upsetting to others. After all, to this particular family the problems are significant, and to imply (by using the word 'mild') that 'things could be worse' may insult parents, who might hear us saying, 'You are lucky, it isn't as bad as some of the children we see'. At the other extreme, 'severe' CP has little meaning unless the term is accompanied by a description of what that word means in a functional sense – something that has usually not happened.

Based on work that had begun to explore patterns of development of gross motor (whole-body) movement in children with CP (Scrutton and Rosenbaum 1997), a group of researchers at *CanChild* Centre for Childhood Disability Research at McMaster University in Canada created a classification system that we believed would be more useful and meaningful to service providers and parents than the value-laden terms outlined above. Our goal was to describe what children in different levels of the GMFCS could do at different ages, using what was, in effect, a pattern recognition format. The idea was to focus on *function* – what the child was able to do – rather than on what the child could not do, or on the details of which parts of the body were involved. We were interested in creating what we hoped would be meaningful categories of function without using words like 'mild', 'moderate' and 'severe'. We have also been able to show that the body distribution of a child's CP, though important information for many reasons, is not as helpful in describing what a child can do as is the GMFCS (Gorter et al. 2004).

The concept behind the development of the GMFCS is of course not original. In many areas of medicine staging systems have been used for a long time to categorize, for example, different types of cancers, such as Hodgkin's disease. The different stages are based on where the cancer is found in the body, how much spread there is, what the cancer looks like under a microscope, and so on. Different stages are associated with different treatment programmes and certainly

with different expected outcomes. We believed that it should be possible to create such a system, and this has now been done (Palisano et al. 1997). The whole GMFCS is presented in Box 20.1. It can also be downloaded free of charge from the *CanChild* website (www.canchild.ca). The expanded and revised version (Palisano et al. 2008) is presented in Box 20.2.

The creation and field testing of the GMFCS was an international effort, involving CP experts from many countries. We know that, in general, professionals agree quite well with one another when classifying a child into one of the five levels of the GMFCS. More importantly, work from several centres has shown that parents are easily able to identify their child's GMFCS level in a way that is consistent with therapists and doctors (Morris et al. 2004, 2006, Gorter personal communication).

The value of the GMFCS is that it provides a common and widely accepted language by which to describe the motor function of children with CP. As a result it has been taken up and applied around the world (Morris and Bartlett 2004). At the same time it must be recognized that people's ability to agree on classification levels is less good when the children they are classifying are under 2 years of age (Palisano et al. 1997). This may be because in very young children there is simply less motor development on which to make a solid judgement. It may also be the case that the GMFCS descriptions of the motor activities of children under 2 are not yet clear and distinct enough. Work is currently under way by Gorter and colleagues to improve this aspect of the GMFCS.

Ontario Motor Growth (OMG) curves

Following the development of the GMFCS it became possible to undertake a study to look at patterns of gross motor development of children with CP. The purpose of the study was to build on what had been learned in the work reported by Scrutton and Rosenbaum (1997). In the OMG study there were 657 children with CP, ranging in age from 1 to 13 years. They were deliberately

Box 20.1

Gross Motor Function Classification System for cerebral palsy (CP) (reproduced from Palisano et al. 1997)

Introduction and user instructions

The Gross Motor Function Classification System for CP is based on self-initiated movement with particular emphasis on sitting (truncal control) and walking. When defining a five-level classification system, our primary criterion was that the distinctions in motor function between levels must be clinically meaningful. Distinctions between levels of motor function are based on functional limitations, the need for assistive technology, including mobility devices (such as walkers, crutches and canes) and wheeled mobility, and, to much lesser extent, quality of movement. Level I includes children with neuromotor impairments whose functional limitations are less than what is typically associated with CP, and children who have traditionally been diagnosed as having 'minimal brain dysfunction' or 'CP of minimal severity'. The distinctions between levels I and II therefore are not as pronounced as the distinctions between the other levels, particularly for infants less than 2 years of age.

The focus is on determining which level best represents the child's present abilities and limitations in motor function. Emphasis is on the child's usual performance in home, school and community settings. It is therefore important to classify on ordinary performance (not best capacity), and not to include judgments about prognosis. Remember the purpose is to classify a child's present gross motor function, not to judge quality of movement or potential for improvement.

The descriptions of the five levels are broad and are not intended to describe all aspects of the function of individual children. For example, an infant with hemiplegia who is unable to crawl on hands and knees, but otherwise fits the description of level I, would be classified in level I. The scale is ordinal, with no intent that the distances between levels be considered equal or that children with CP are equally distributed among the five levels. A summary of the distinctions between each pair of levels is provided to assist in determining the level that most closely resembles a child's current gross motor function.

The title for each level represents the highest level of mobility that a child is expected to achieve between 6 and 12 years of age. We recognize that classification of motor function is dependent on age, especially during infancy and early childhood. For each level, therefore, separate descriptions are provided for children in several age bands. The functional abilities and limitations for each age interval are intended to serve as guidelines, are not comprehensive and are not norms. Children below age 2 should be considered at their corrected age if they were premature.

An effort has been made to emphasize children's function rather than their limitations. Thus, as a general principle, the gross motor function of children who are able to perform the functions described in any particular level will probably be classified at or above that level; in contrast the gross motor functions of children who cannot perform the functions of a particular level will likely be classified below that level.

Reference: Dev Med Child Neurol 1997; 39:214–223

Gross Motor Function Classification System for CP (GMFCS)	
Before Second Birthday	
Level I	Infants move in and out of sitting and floor-sit with both hands free to manipulate objects. Infants crawl on hands and knees, pull to stand and take steps holding on to furniture. Infants walk between 18 months and 2 years of age without the need for any assistive mobility device
Level II	Infants maintain floor-sitting but may need to use their hands for support to maintain balance. Infants creep on their stomach or crawl on hands and knees. Infants may pull to stand and take steps holding on to furniture
Level III	Infants maintain floor-sitting when the low back is supported. Infants roll and creep forward on their stomachs

Level IV	Infants have head control but trunk support is required for floor-sitting. Infants can roll to supine and may roll to prone
Level V	Physical impairments limit voluntary control of movement. Infants are unable to maintain antigravity head and trunk postures in prone and sitting. Infants require adult assistance to roll

Between Second and Fourth Birthdays

Level I	Children floor-sit with both hands free to manipulate objects. Movements in and out of floor-sitting and standing are performed without adult assistance. Children walk as the preferred method of mobility without the need for any assistive mobility device
Level II	Children floor-sit but may have difficulty with balance when both hands are free to manipulate objects. Movements in and out of sitting are performed without adult assistance. Children pull to stand on a stable surface. Children crawl on hands and knees with a reciprocal pattern, cruise holding on to furniture and walk using an assistive mobility device as preferred methods of mobility
Level III	Children maintain floor-sitting, often by 'W-sitting' (sitting between flexed and internally rotated hips and knees) and may require adult assistance to assume sitting. Children creep on their stomach or crawl on hands and knees (often without reciprocal leg movements) as their primary methods of self-mobility. Children may pull to stand on a stable surface and cruise short distances. Children may walk short distances indoors using an assistive mobility device and adult assistance for steering and turning
Level IV	Children floor-sit when placed, but are unable to maintain alignment and balance without using their hands for support. Children frequently require adaptive equipment for sitting and standing. Self-mobility for short distances (within a room) is achieved through rolling, creeping on stomach or crawling on hands and knees without reciprocal leg movement
Level V	Physical impairments restrict voluntary control of movement and the ability to maintain antigravity head and trunk postures. All areas of motor function are limited. Functional limitations in sitting and standing are not fully compensated for through the use of adaptive equipment and assistive technology. At level V, children have no means of independent mobility and are transported. Some children achieve self-mobility using a power wheelchair with extensive adaptations

Between Fourth and Sixth Birthdays

Level I	Children get into and out of, and sit in, a chair without the need for hand support. Children move from the floor and from chair-sitting to standing without the need for objects for support. Children walk indoors and outdoors, and climb stairs. Emerging ability to run and jump
Level II	Children sit in a chair with both hands free to manipulate objects. Children move from the floor to standing and from chair-sitting to standing but often require a stable surface to push or pull up on with their arms. Children walk without the need for any assistive mobility device indoors and for short distances on level surfaces outdoors. Children climb stairs holding on to a railing but are unable to run or jump
Level III	Children sit on a regular chair but may require pelvic or trunk support to maximize hand function. Children move in and out of chair-sitting using a stable surface to push on or pull up with their arms. Children walk with an assistive mobility device on level surfaces and climb stairs with assistance from an adult. Children are frequently transported when travelling for long distances or outdoors on uneven terrain

Level IV	Children sit on a chair but need adaptive seating for trunk control and to maximize hand function. Children move in and out of chair-sitting with assistance from an adult or a stable surface to push or pull up on with their arms. Children may at best walk short distances with a walker and adult supervision but have difficulty turning and maintaining balance on uneven surfaces. Children are transported in the community. Children may achieve self-mobility using a power wheelchair
Level V	Physical impairments restrict voluntary control of movement and the ability to maintain antigravity head and trunk postures. All areas of motor function are limited. Functional limitations in sitting and standing are not fully compensated for through the use of adaptive equipment and assistive technology. At level V, children have no means of independent mobility and are transported. Some children achieve self-mobility using a power wheelchair with extensive adaptations
	Between Sixth and 12th Birthdays
Level I	Children walk indoors and outdoors, and climb stairs without limitations. Children perform gross motor skills including running and jumping but speed, balance and coordination are reduced
Level II	Children walk indoors and outdoors, and climb stairs holding on to a railing but experience limitations walking on uneven surfaces and inclines, and walking in crowds or confined spaces. Children have at best only minimal ability to perform gross motor skills such as running and jumping
Level III	Children walk indoors or outdoors on a level surface with an assistive mobility device. Children may climb stairs holding on to a railing. Depending on upper-limb function, children propel a wheelchair manually or are transported when travelling for long distances or outdoors on uneven terrain
Level IV	Children may maintain levels of function achieved before age 6 or rely more on wheeled mobility at home, school and in the community. Children may achieve self-mobility using a power wheelchair
Level V	Physical impairments restrict voluntary control of movement and the ability to maintain antigravity head and trunk postures. All areas of motor function are limited. Functional limitations in sitting and standing are not fully compensated for through the use of adaptive equipment and assistive technology. At level V, children have no means of independent mobility and are transported. Some children achieve self-mobility using a power wheelchair with extensive adaptations

Distinctions between levels I and II

Compared with children in level I, children in level II have limitations in the ease of performing movement transitions; walking outdoors and in the community; the need for assistive mobility devices when beginning to walk; quality of movement; and the ability to perform gross motor skills such as running and jumping.

Distinctions between levels II and III

Differences are seen in the degree of achievement of functional mobility. Children in level III need assistive mobility devices and frequently orthoses to walk, whereas children in level II do not require assistive mobility devices after age 4.

Distinctions between levels III and IV

Differences in sitting ability and mobility exist, even allowing for extensive use of assistive technology. Children in level III sit independently, have independent floor mobility and walk with assistive mobility devices. Children in level IV function in sitting (usually supported) but independent mobility is very limited. Children in level IV are more likely to be transported or use power mobility.

Distinctions between levels IV and V

Children in level V lack independence, even in basic antigravity postural control. Self-mobility is only achieved if the child can learn how to operate an electrically powered wheelchair.

selected to represent all five GMFCS levels in approximately equal numbers. The motor function of these children and youths was assessed systematically several times over a period of 4 years. Using a valid change-detecting measure of motor function developed specifically for children and youth with CP, we were then able to create what we called 'motor growth curves' (Rosenbaum et al. 2002).

Like the growth curves that allow people to look at changes in height and weight of children over time, the motor growth curves were meant to describe different patterns of motor development taking account of children's ages and their GMFCS levels. An additional feature of the curves is that they describe what motor function can be expected, on average, for children in each GMFCS level. The curves are reproduced in Figure 20.1. The curves are also available on the *CanChild* website (www.canchild.ca).

It is obvious that there is variation in motor progress within each level, as well as between levels. We know that age and GMFCS level are the most powerful factors that determine how well a child develops motor function, but it is less certain what else influences motor development. Many people have asked about the types of therapy the children in the OMG study were receiving. The best we can say is that they were receiving a wide variety of developmental therapies, that some had aids and orthoses, and that 91 of the 657 had some form of orthopaedic surgery during the time the study was being done. What we cannot say, because this study was not designed to answer the question, is what effect any specific therapy had on motor development. Work is under way to explore what role surgery had on measured motor function; and it has been possible to report on the clear measurable impact of aids and orthoses on motor function (Russell and Gorter, 2005). In general, however, a study to evaluate the effect of any specific treatment should be designed and carried out in a very different way from the way the OMG study was done.

What use are the OMG curves?

We believe that the OMG curves represent the expected patterns of motor development and function of children with CP, based on currently available treatments. As such, they offer parents at least part of an answer to the question: 'Will our child walk?' More generally, the curves provide information about the outlook for mobility in children with CP *based on GMFCS level*. The GMFCS level can be determined quite reliably after the age of 2, simply by looking at what that child does in independent mobility. Therefore, we are in a position to predict what level of mobility independence a child might be expected to develop. In this way we have been able to describe more than simply walking, which children in level I and II do without aids, and children in level III can often do with a walker or other mobility aids. Children in level IV are likely to be primarily wheelchair users for functional mobility in school and community, and depending on other factors (such as hand control, vision and level of cognition), many children in level IV may be able to use either a manual or power chair.

It might be worrying for parents to see that at the age of around 6 or 7 years the OMG curves seem to level off. Does this mean that children should stop receiving therapy because no more

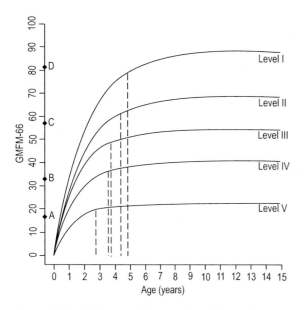

Figure 20.1 • Motor growth curves for children with cerebral palsy. (Adapted from Rosenbaum et al. JAMA 2002; 288:1357–1363. Copyrighted 2002, American Medical Association.)

changes in gross motor function were observed in the OMG study?

No! In fact it is important to emphasize several points. The curves report only *gross motor function* as measured by the Gross Motor Function Measure (GMFM) (Russell et al. 2002), and the GMFM only looks at what one might call basic mobility skills up to activities such as climbing stairs. The study to create the curves did not measure factors such as quality of movement and motor control, or skill development, or the amount of effort that a child uses to get around. These are all areas of motor function and motor development that may be the focus of therapies and other interventions, once the child has achieved a basic level of motor capacity. Furthermore, as children grow up they usually develop their own interests. Therapy should take account of children's mobility needs to meet those goals and help them to achieve the things that are important to them. In fact, a study from the Netherlands showed how parent- and child-directed goal-setting for physical therapy was associated with better outcomes – and with less overall therapy – than treatment directed at therapists' goals (Ketelaar et al. 2001).

Another important concept for both parents and therapists to note is how much a child's function can vary from one environment to another. As therapists and doctors we usually focus on what is sometimes called 'capacity', what people can do at their best; for example, what we hope to see in an assessment at the clinic or in a therapy session, where the environment is set up to elicit the best a person can do. However, 'performance', what people do under ordinary circumstances, can be quite different. Performance can be strongly influenced by motivation, environmental barriers or supports, and personal factors such as how bold or cautious a child might be (Tieman et al. 2004). For example, consider a child trying to use a stairway. If the child needs a railing and there is none on the stairway to be used, the child's performance may be quite different from what is done at home or at Granny's house when railings are available. If the child is an outgoing and adventurous person something might be tried that has not been done before and the child may attempt to climb; whereas if the child

has fallen previously the child may appear unable to do an activity accomplished in a therapy session. In other words, we need to consider more than what a child's capacity might be, and reflect on environmental factors, including, of course, technical mobility aids that might enhance performance.

Do the OMG curves give parents and therapists specific intervention recommendations? The brief answer is 'no'. However, it is obvious that if we know that a child is functioning in level I, our interventions might be less active because the outlook for independent motor function is good, and may be aimed primarily at enhancing the quality of motor function and the development of more advanced motor skills such as running, jumping and climbing stairs. On the other hand, if it is clear, for example, that a child is functioning in level IV, early attention to the skills associated with seating and wheelchair use should be considered along with other aspects of therapy.

Does this mean that some children should not have, or worse, do not deserve, therapy? Again, no. What it does mean is that it should be easier than it used to be to advise parents about the motor function outlook for their child with CP, and then to tailor therapies to functional targets that are consistent with the motor abilities usually associated with children in that GMFCS level. In other words, armed with clearer ideas about 'how bad it is' (GMFCS levels) and 'whether this child is likely to walk' (OMG curves), today's therapists and doctors can address parents' questions with current evidence that has been specifically collected to provide answers to these questions.

Finally, let me repeat that it is important that service providers only review this information about GMFCS levels and motor function outlook *when parents ask*. Some parents are clear that they do not want to know the answers to these questions, or at least, not until they are ready. However, it is our impression that the majority of parents find this type of information helpful when making intervention decisions for their child. Now that the information is available, we hope that both parents and service providers are in a better position than we have previously been to communicate effectively with each other about motor development of children with CP.

Box 20.2

Gross Motor Function Classification System for cerebral palsy (CP) – expanded and revised (reproduced from Palisano et al. 2008)

Introduction and user instructions

The Gross Motor Function Classification System (GMFCS) for cerebral palsy is based on self-initiated movement, with emphasis on sitting, transfers, and mobility. When defining a five-level classification system, our primary criterion has been that the distinctions between levels must be meaningful in daily life. Distinctions are based on functional limitations, the need for hand-held mobility devices (such as walkers, crutches, or canes) or wheeled mobility, and to a much lesser extent, quality of movement. The distinctions between levels I and II are not as pronounced as the distinctions between the other levels, particularly for infants less than 2 years of age.

The expanded GMFCS (2008) includes an age band for youth 12 to 18 years of age and emphasizes the concepts inherent in the World Health Organization's International Classification of Functioning, Disability and Health (ICF). We encourage users to be aware of the impact that **environmental** and **personal** factors may have on what children and youth are observed or reported to do. The focus of the GMFCS is on determining which level best represents the **child's or youth's present abilities and limitations in gross motor function**. Emphasis is on usual **performance** in home, school, and community settings (i.e., what they do), rather than what they are known to be able to do at their best (capability). It is therefore important to classify current performance in gross motor function and not to include judgments about the quality of movement or prognosis for improvement.

The title for each level is the method of mobility that is most characteristic of performance after 6 years of age. The descriptions of functional abilities and limitations for each age band are broad and are not intended to describe all aspects of the function of individual children/youth. For example, an infant with hemiplegia who is unable to crawl on his or her hands and knees, but otherwise fits the description of level I (i.e., can pull to stand and walk), would be classified in level I. The scale is ordinal, with no intent that the distances between levels be considered equal or that children and youth with cerebral palsy are equally distributed across the five levels. A summary of the distinctions between each pair of levels is provided to assist in determining the level that most closely resembles a child's/youth's current gross motor function.

We recognize that the manifestations of gross motor function are dependent on age, especially during infancy and early childhood. For each level, separate descriptions are provided in several age bands. Children below age 2 should be considered at their corrected age if they were premature. The descriptions for the 6 to 12 year and 12 to 18 year age bands reflect the potential impact of environment factors (e.g., distances in school and community) and personal factors (e.g., energy demands and social preferences) on methods of mobility.

An effort has been made to emphasize abilities rather than limitations. Thus, as a general principle, the gross motor function of children and youth who are able to perform the functions described in any particular level will probably be classified at or above that level of function; in contrast, the gross motor function of children and youth who cannot perform the functions of a particular level should be classified below that level of function.

Operational definitions

Body support walker – A mobility device that supports the pelvis and trunk. The child/youth is physically positioned in the walker by another person.

Hand-held mobility device – Canes, crutches, and anterior and posterior walkers that do not support the trunk during walking.

Physical assistance – Another person manually assists the child/youth to move.

Powered mobility – The child/youth actively controls the joystick or electrical switch that enables independent mobility. The mobility base may be a wheelchair, scooter or other type of powered mobility device.

Self-propels manual wheelchair – The child/youth actively uses arms and hands or feet to propel the wheels and move.

Transported – A person manually pushes a mobility device (e.g., wheelchair, stroller, or pram) to move the child/youth from one place to another.

Walks – Unless otherwise specified indicates no physical assistance from another person or any use of a hand-held mobility device. An orthosis (i.e., brace or splint) may be worn.

Wheeled mobility – Refers to any type of device with wheels that enables movement (e.g., stroller, manual wheelchair, or powered wheelchair).

General headings for each level

LEVEL I – Walks without limitations

LEVEL II – Walks with limitations

LEVEL III – Walks using a hand-held mobility device

LEVEL IV – Self-mobility with limitations; may use powered mobility

LEVEL V – Transported in a manual wheelchair

Distinctions between levels

Distinctions between levels I and II – Compared with children and youth in level I, children and youth in level II have limitations walking long distances and balancing; may need a hand-held mobility device when first learning to walk; may use wheeled mobility when traveling long distances outdoors and in the community; require the use of a railing to walk up and down stairs; and are not as capable of running and jumping.

Distinctions between levels II and III – Children and youth in level II are capable of walking without a hand-held mobility device after age 4 (although they may choose to use one at times). Children and youth in level III need a hand-held mobility device to walk indoors and use wheeled mobility outdoors and in the community.

Distinctions between levels III and IV – Children and youth in level III sit on their own or require at most limited external support to sit, are more independent in standing transfers, and walk with a hand-held mobility device. Children and youth in level IV function in sitting (usually supported) but self-mobility is limited. Children and youth in level IV are more likely to be transported in a manual wheelchair or use powered mobility.

Distinctions between levels IV and V – Children and youth in level V have severe limitations in head and trunk control and require extensive assisted technology and physical assistance. Self-mobility is achieved only if the child/youth can learn how to operate a powered wheelchair.

Gross Motor Function Classification System – Expanded and Revised (GMFCS – E & R)	
Before Second Birthday	
Level I	Infants move in and out of sitting and floor sit with both hands free to manipulate objects. Infants crawl on hands and knees, pull to stand and take steps holding on to furniture. Infants walk between 18 months and 2 years of age without the need for any assistive mobility device.
Level II	Infants maintain floor sitting but may need to use their hands for support to maintain balance. Infants creep on their stomach or crawl on hands and knees. Infants may pull to stand and take steps holding on to furniture.
Level III	Infants maintain floor sitting when the low back is supported. Infants roll and creep forward on their stomachs.
Level IV	Infants have head control but trunk support is required for floor sitting. Infants can roll to supine and may roll to prone.
Level V	Physical impairments limit voluntary control of movement. Infants are unable to maintain antigravity head and trunk postures in prone and sitting. Infants require adult assistance to roll.

Between Second and Fourth Birthdays	
Level I	Children floor sit with both hands free to manipulate objects. Movements in and out of floor sitting and standing are performed without adult assistance. Children walk as the preferred method of mobility without the need for any assistive mobility device.
Level II	Children floor sit but may have difficulty with balance when both hands are free to manipulate objects. Movements in and out of sitting are performed without adult assistance. Children pull to stand on a stable surface. Children crawl on hands and knees with a reciprocal pattern, cruise holding onto furniture and walk using an assistive mobility device as preferred methods of mobility.
Level III	Children maintain floor sitting often by "W-sitting" (sitting between flexed and internally rotated hips and knees) and may require adult assistance to assume sitting. Children creep on their stomach or crawl on hands and knees (often without reciprocal leg movements) as their primary methods of self-mobility. Children may pull to stand on a stable surface and cruise short distances. Children may walk short distances indoors using a hand-held mobility device (walker) and adult assistance for steering and turning.
Level IV	Children floor sit when placed, but are unable to maintain alignment and balance without use of their hands for support. Children frequently require adaptive equipment for sitting and standing. Self-mobility for short distances (within a room) is achieved through rolling, creeping on stomach, or crawling on hands and knees without reciprocal leg movement.
Level V	Physical impairments restrict voluntary control of movement and the ability to maintain antigravity head and trunk postures. All areas of motor function are limited. Functional limitations in sitting and standing are not fully compensated for through the use of adaptive equipment and assistive technology. At level V, children have no means of independent movement and are transported. Some children achieve self-mobility using a powered wheelchair with extensive adaptations.
Between Fourth and Sixth Birthdays	
Level I	Children get into and out of, and sit in, a chair without the need for hand support. Children move from the floor and from chair sitting to standing without the need for objects for support. Children walk indoors and outdoors, and climb stairs. Emerging ability to run and jump.
Level II	Children sit in a chair with both hands free to manipulate objects. Children move from the floor to standing and from chair sitting to standing but often require a stable surface to push or pull up on with their arms. Children walk without the need for a hand-held mobility device indoors and for short distances on level surfaces outdoors. Children climb stairs holding onto a railing but are unable to run or jump.
Level III	Children sit on a regular chair but may require pelvic or trunk support to maximize hand function. Children move in and out of chair sitting using a stable surface to push on or pull up with their arms. Children walk with a hand-held mobility device on level surfaces and climb stairs with assistance from an adult. Children frequently are transported when traveling for long distances or outdoors on uneven terrain.
Level IV	Children sit on a chair but need adaptive seating for trunk control and to maximize hand function. Children move in and out of chair sitting with assistance from an adult or a stable surface to push or pull up on with their arms. Children may at best walk short distances with a walker and adult supervision but have difficulty turning and maintaining balance on uneven surfaces. Children are transported in the community. Children may achieve self-mobility using a powered wheelchair.

Level V	Physical impairments restrict voluntary control of movement and the ability to maintain antigravity head and trunk postures. All areas of motor function are limited. Functional limitations in sitting and standing are not fully compensated for through the use of adaptive equipment and assistive technology. At level V, children have no means of independent movement and are transported. Some children achieve self-mobility using a powered wheelchair with extensive adaptations.
Between Sixth and 12th Birthdays	
Level I	Children walk at home, school, outdoors, and in the community. Children are able to walk up and down curbs without physical assistance and stairs without the use of a railing. Children perform gross motor skills such as running and jumping but speed, balance, and coordination are limited. Children may participate in physical activities and sports depending on personal choices and environmental factors.
Level II	Children walk in most settings. Children may experience difficulty walking long distances and balancing on uneven terrain, inclines, in crowded areas, confined spaces or when carrying objects. Children walk up and down stairs holding onto a railing or with physical assistance if there is no railing. Outdoors and in the community, children may walk with physical assistance, a hand-held mobility device, or use wheeled mobility when traveling long distances. Children have at best only minimal ability to perform gross motor skills such as running and jumping. Limitations in performance of gross motor skills may necessitate adaptations to enable participation in physical activities and sports.
Level III	Children walk using a hand-held mobility device in most indoor settings. When seated, children may require a seat belt for pelvic alignment and balance. Sit-to-stand and floor-to-stand transfers require physical assistance of a person or support surface. When traveling long distances, children use some form of wheeled mobility. Children may walk up and down stairs holding onto a railing with supervision or physical assistance. Limitations in walking may necessitate adaptations to enable participation in physical activities and sports including self-propelling a manual wheelchair or powered mobility.
Level IV	Children use methods of mobility that require physical assistance or powered mobility in most settings. Children require adaptive seating for trunk and pelvic control and physical assistance for most transfers. At home, children use floor mobility (roll, creep, or crawl), walk short distances with physical assistance, or use powered mobility. When positioned, children may use a body support walker at home or school. At school, outdoors, and in the community, children are transported in a manual wheelchair or use powered mobility. Limitations in mobility necessitate adaptations to enable participation in physical activities and sports, including physical assistance and/or powered mobility.
Level V	Children are transported in a manual wheelchair in all settings. Children are limited in their ability to maintain antigravity head and trunk postures and control arm and leg movements. Assistive technology is used to improve head alignment, seating, standing, and/or mobility but limitations are not fully compensated by equipment. Transfers require complete physical assistance of an adult. At home, children may move short distances on the floor or may be carried by an adult. Children may achieve self-mobility using powered mobility with extensive adaptations for seating and control access. Limitations in mobility necessitate adaptations to enable participation in physical activities and sports including physical assistance and using powered mobility.
Between 12th and 18th Birthdays	
Level I	Youth walk at home, school, outdoors, and in the community. Youth are able to walk up and down curbs without physical assistance and stairs without the use of a railing. Youth perform gross motor skills such as running and jumping but speed, balance, and coordination are limited. Youth may participate in physical activities and sports depending on personal choices and environmental factors.

Level II	Youth walk in most settings. Environmental factors (such as uneven terrain, inclines, long distances, time demands, weather, and peer acceptability) and personal preference influence mobility choices. At school or work, youth may walk using a hand-held mobility device for safety. Outdoors and in the community, youth may use wheeled mobility when traveling long distances. Youth walk up and down stairs holding a railing or with physical assistance if there is no railing. Limitations in performance of gross motor skills may necessitate adaptations to enable participation in physical activities and sports.
Level III	Youth are capable of walking using a hand-held mobility device. Compared to individuals in other levels, youth in level III demonstrate more variability in methods of mobility depending on physical ability and environmental and personal factors. When seated, youth may require a seat belt for pelvic alignment and balance. Sit-to-stand and floor-to-stand transfers require physical assistance from a person or support surface. At school, youth may self-propel a manual wheelchair or use powered mobility. Outdoors and in the community, youth are transported in a wheelchair or use powered mobility. Youth may walk up and down stairs holding onto a railing with supervision or physical assistance. Limitations in walking may necessitate adaptations to enable participation in physical activities and sports including self-propelling a manual wheelchair or powered mobility.
Level IV	Youth use wheeled mobility in most settings. Youth require adaptive seating for pelvic and trunk control. Physical assistance from 1 or 2 persons is required for transfers. Youth may support weight with their legs to assist with standing transfers. Indoors, youth may walk short distances with physical assistance, use wheeled mobility, or, when positioned, use a body support walker. Youth are physically capable of operating a powered wheelchair. When a powered wheelchair is not feasible or available, youth are transported in a manual wheelchair. Limitations in mobility necessitate adaptations to enable participation in physical activities and sports, including physical assistance and/or powered mobility.
Level V	Youth are transported in a manual wheelchair in all settings. Youth are limited in their ability to maintain antigravity head and trunk postures and control arm and leg movements. Assistive technology is used to improve head alignment, seating, standing, and mobility but limitations are not fully compensated by equipment. Physical assistance from 1 or 2 persons or a mechanical lift is required for transfers. Youth may achieve self-mobility using powered mobility with extensive adaptations for seating and control access. Limitations in mobility necessitate adaptations to enable participation in physical activities and sports including physical assistance and using powered mobility.

References

Gorter JW, Rosenbaum PL, Hanna SE et al. Limb distribution, type of motor disorder and functional classification of CP: How do they relate? Dev Med Child Neurol 2004; 6:461–467.

Ketelaar M, Vermeer A, Hart H et al. Effects of a functional therapy program on motor abilities of children with CP. Phys Ther 2001; 81:1534–1545.

Morris C, Bartlett DJ. Gross Motor Function Classification System: impact and utility. Dev Med Child Neurol 2004; 46:60–65.

Morris C, Galuppi BE, Rosenbaum PL. Reliability of family report for the Gross Motor Function Classification System. Dev Med Child Neurol 2004; 46:455–460.

Morris C, Kurinczuk JJ, Fitzpatrick R et al. Who best to make the assessment? Professionals and families' classifications of

gross motor function are highly consistent. Arch Dis Child 2006; 91:675–679.

Palisano R, Rosenbaum P, Bartlett D et al. Content validity of the expanded and revised gross motor function classification system. Dev Med Child Neurol (in press).

Palisano R, Rosenbaum P, Walter S et al. Development and validation of a gross motor function classification system for children with CP. Dev Med Child Neurol 1997; 39:214–223.

Rosenbaum PL, Walter SD, Hanna SE et al. Prognosis for gross motor function in CP: creation of motor development curves. JAMA 2002; 288:1357–1363.

Russell DJ, Gorter JW. Assessing functional differences in gross motor skills in children with CP who use an ambulatory aid or orthoses: can the GMFM-88 help? Dev Med Child Neurol 2006; 48:158.

Russell DJ, Rosenbaum PL, Avery LM et al. Gross Motor Function Measure (GMFM-66 and GMFM-88) user's manual. Clinics in Developmental Medicine no. 159. MacKeith Press, London, 2002.

Scrutton D, Rosenbaum PL. The locomotor development of children with CP. In: Connolly K, Forssberg H (eds) Neurophysiology and neuropsychology of motor development. MacKeith Press, London, 1997, pp. 101–123.

Tieman BL, Palisano RJ, Gracely EJ et al. Gross motor capability and performance of mobility in children with CP: A comparison across home, school, and outdoors/community settings. Phys Ther 2004; 84:419–429.

Chapter Twenty One

21

Chairs, pushchairs and car seats

Revised by Eva Bower

One of the most helpful things a therapist can do for your child with cerebral palsy (CP) is to advise on and provide, if able, suitable seating. A good chair may improve communication and feeding and assist with mobility in a non-ambulant child.

Most importantly, sitting upright in a suitable chair may enable your child to establish eye contact and socialize.

Adaptive seating for your child with CP aims to try to correct and control postural abnormalities in sitting and thereby improve voluntary upper-limb function and enhance communication, feeding, social skills and learning in the widest sense.

Different types of chairs and pushchairs or strollers provide different amounts of support and stability and the chair required by a particular child will depend upon the abilities and problems of that child.

The designs of chairs and pushchairs or strollers are continually being modified and updated by manufacturers using new technology, materials and ideas from engineers, orthotists and therapists. Therefore in this chapter I shall confine myself to describing a few basic chairs, simple seating you could make yourself and basic pushchairs/strollers and car seats.

Chairs and pushchairs/strollers involve a considerable financial outlay for parents and are certainly not items that should just be chosen from a catalogue. They should be purchased following an evaluation of your child's abilities and problems by a physiotherapist or occupational therapist, discussion between you, your child if appropriate, and the therapist, and if at all possible practically trying out the chair to find out if it is appropriate for your child, you and your environment.

There have been many clinical observations, much research and publication on the subject of adaptive seating but I would like to suggest that primarily a seating system should ensure that your child has:

1. A stable postural base – the position of the pelvis is an important factor

2. Postural trunk control and alignment

3. Postural head control

The chair should be appropriately adapted for ability, ensuring sufficient control of your child's posture yet at the same time it should encourage your child to develop as much independent sitting ability as possible.

All seating systems should be adaptable for growth, easy to handle, easily kept clean, fit into the child's environment, and most importantly, comfortable for your child.

General considerations

Sitting becomes a truly functional position for play when a typical child is about 8–9 months old. By this time the typical child has good trunk control, balance in sitting and hip mobility. The typical child no longer has to rely on the hands for support, can reach out in any direction to get toys and is able to develop and practise manipulative hand skills when sitting.

One should not wait until a child with CP has developed all these abilities before allowing the child to sit and play and, of course, some children with CP may never attain independent sitting. By choosing the right basic chair, adapted for the individual child's needs, the child can be enabled to maintain a stable, symmetrical sitting posture so that the child can use the hands for play, feeding, communication and learning.

No child should spend prolonged periods of the day in a chair.

The child with severe involvement (levels IV and V on the Gross Motor Function Classification System or GMFCS: Palisano et al. 1997) will require a lot of postural support to sit securely in a chair. This can be compared with one of us sitting in a seat in a cinema where there is no room to stretch our legs for 3 hours. Although we are able continually to adjust our position, when we do eventually get up we often feel rather stiff. It is therefore obvious that a child who is unable to move or adjust position will not only become very stiff but in time will be in danger of becoming chair-shaped or, to put it another way, develop deformity. Consequently it is important that children who are limited in their ability to move should spend their day in a variety of positions including on the floor and be encouraged to move about freely. If possible they should also spend time in an upright position using one of the many standing systems available.

The position in which a chair is placed in a room and the occasions a child needs to sit on the chair will depend upon the stage of the child's development, family and environment. At meal times the best position for a child who can sit in a highchair would be at the table with the family, a practical position for the mother while she feeds her child and later when helping the child to eat independently. This is also a good place for the child to play alone while the mother is nearby.

If the child has siblings who prefer playing on the floor or at a low table the child may become unhappy or frustrated if unable to play beside them. To avoid this happening, if the highchair is not of a type that converts into a low chair, it is better to find another position for the child, perhaps on the floor, so that the child can play at the same level as the siblings for at least some of the time. A child who has some sitting balance, although able to sit on the floor or on a stool when self-supporting with the hands, may not have sufficient balance to play with siblings but only to watch. The child might be able to play if sat in the corner of the room on the floor or on a stool, especially if a low table is placed in front of the child on to which the child can lean. A non-slip mat for the feet might help further.

Some children, even when they have good sitting balance, often find dressing and undressing easier if sitting on a bench rather than a regular chair or their bed, as the width of the seat provides a good supporting surface.

It is worth remembering that when you are playing with your young child, your lap or the corner of the sofa is softer and more comfortable than a chair.

Assessment

All seating needs to be continually evaluated and your observations of your child's achievements or difficulties when sitting in a chair are invaluable. For example, you may have noticed that when using the hands your child slips down in the chair and it becomes impossible for your child to see what he or she is doing, or perhaps that when trying to reach for toys, your child bends forward from the trunk rather than from the hip joints and you may wonder if there is some way of stabilizing the pelvis. On the other hand you may feel that your child's sitting balance when sitting on the floor has improved so much that the minimal support previously suggested is no longer necessary. Rather than just waiting for your child's next reassessment, make a note or, if you have a video camera, take a short sequence of any points you may wish to consider so that you and your therapist can discuss the points and make any changes that are necessary.

It is also a good idea to check the chair itself to see if there is any uneven wear on the seat or armrests as this will indicate that the postural support recommended may need to be reassessed.

The ideal sitting position for a typical child sitting on a regular chair is as shown in Figure 21.1:

1. The head slightly forwards
2. The spine straight
3. The pelvis touching the back of the chair
4. The legs slightly apart with the knees vertically above the feet
5. The feet placed on the floor

Difficulties which can prevent sitting being a useful functional position and for which adaptations are usually required are:

1. Pushing backwards and sliding out of the chair
2. Falling forwards out of the chair

The first may require the seat of the chair to be tilted backwards plus lap or groin straps.

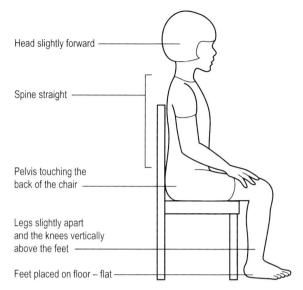

Figure 21.1 • An ideal sitting position for a typical child on a regular chair.

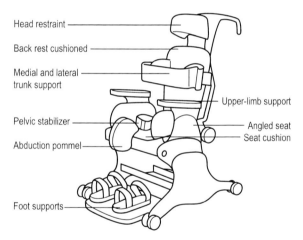

Figure 21.2 • Adapted chair with all the more usual types of support available. Most children are unlikely to need them all.

The second may require a tray which fits around the chair and supports the child's trunk in an upright position plus a piece of non-slip mat to anchor the pelvis.

If straps are used it is important to ensure that they are padded and that the child does not get red or sore skin (Figure 21.2).

Box 21.1

Children's needs for supportive seating as predicted by classification on the Gross Motor Function Classification System (GMFCS)

Before 2nd birthday

Children at level I do not usually need different seating from their peers without abnormality
Children at level II may need a chair with some extra support at the back/pelvis at 7–10 months
Children at level III will need a chair with some extra support, probably at the back/pelvis, and a tray fitted around their front at about 7–10 months
Children at level IV will need a chair with trunk and pelvis support at 7–10 months plus a tray
Children at level V will need a chair with head, trunk and pelvis support at 7–10 months plus a tray

Between 2nd and 4th birthdays

Children at level II should no longer need a chair with extra support
Children at level III may still need a chair with some extra support
Children at level IV will still need a chair with extra support as above
Children at level V will still need a chair with extra support as above

Between 4th and 6th birthdays

Children at level III should no longer need a chair with extra support

An assessment chart which may be helpful to therapists evaluating the most suitable type of chair and adaptations for a child is the Box Sitting Assessment Chart, which is part of the Chailey Heritage Clinical Services Levels of Abilities and is obtainable from Beggars Wood Road, North Chailey, East Sussex BN8 4JN, UK.

As has been suggested above, children with CP should be given the opportunity to sit at the same age as their typical peers using adaptive seating. Bearing this suggestion in mind, Box 21.1 lists children's needs for supportive seating as predicted by classification on the GMFCS.

Measuring for a regular chair

See Figure 21.3.

Chairs

Baby seats

Until a baby reaches the age of being able to bring the trunk forward and self-support on the hands when sitting, regular baby seats are often found quite adequate (Figure 21.4).

The young child who has just developed sitting balance

For a young child who has just developed sitting balance a regular child's box seat when placed in a cardboard box or plastic storage box is an excellent way of giving confidence (Figure 21.5). The fact that the child has the sides of the box to hold on to if balance is lost makes the child feel safer and encourages the child to lean forwards automatically when reaching for toys.

Inflatable chairs

Inflatable chairs in various shapes such as a triangle or a round seat may be useful for very small children but a word of warning as they are generally rather light: for safety they should always be placed where there is additional stable support.

Never leave your child unsupervised in an inflatable chair.

The triangular inflatable chair shown in Figure 21.6a is most useful for the young child who

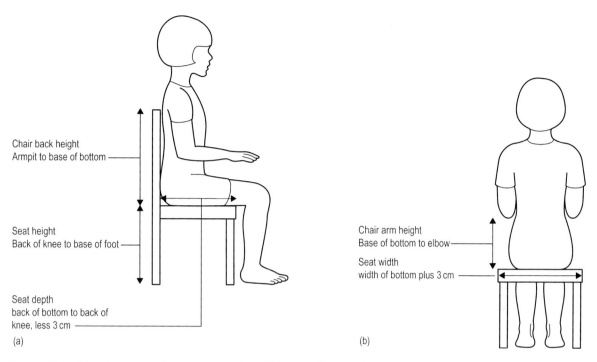

Chair back height
Armpit to base of bottom

Seat height
Back of knee to base of foot

Seat depth
back of bottom to back of
knee, less 3 cm

(a)

Chair arm height
Base of bottom to elbow

Seat width
width of bottom plus 3 cm

(b)

Figure 21.3 • How to measure for a regular chair. (a) Side view. (b) Rear view.

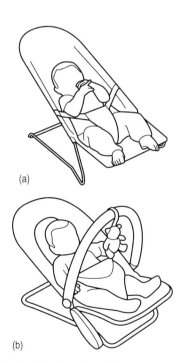

(a)

(b)

Figure 21.4 • (a, b) Examples of baby seats.

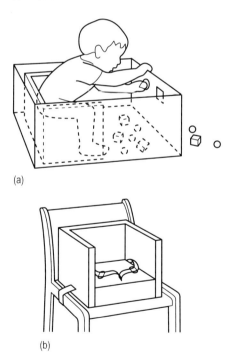

(a)

(b)

Figure 21.5 • (a) Seat in a cardboard box. (b) Box seat strapped on to a dining-room/kitchen chair for use at table.

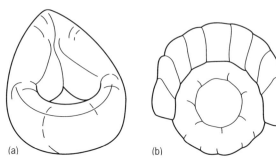

Figure 21.6 • (a) Triangular inflatable chair; (b) Round inflatable chair for young children with one-sided stiffness or those who are just gaining sitting balance.

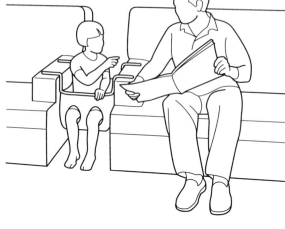

Figure 21.7 • Safa bath seat for young children with one sided stiffness or those who are just gaining sitting balance.

pushes backwards when sitting as the lack of stimulation on the buttocks, due to the hollow seat may minimize the extension and the triangular-shaped back helps to keep the head up and shoulders forward.

The round inflatable chair shown in Figure 21.6b should only be used for a small child and can be placed in a chair or pram, but not a pushchair. It may be useful as a chair in which to feed your child.

Safa bath seat for young children with one sided or those who are just gaining sitting balance

This seat was originally designed by a father as a bath seat for his child but it is also useful as a regular seat for young children who are just beginning to get sitting balance and particularly so for the young child with stiffness involving one side of the body (hemiplegia).

The seat gives the child a feeling of security as the feet are on the ground. It also has the advantage that, if children feel that they are losing their balance they can hold on to the metal bar at the front of the seat and therefore no additional support is necessary. If wished, a table can be placed in front of the seat for play.

This type of seat is *not recommended* for any child with strong extensor or flexor stiffness or intermittent spasms.

The most satisfactory way of suspending the seat is between two chairs, as shown in Figure 21.7.

A seat for the young child (levels 4 or 5 GMFCS) with low truncal tone and poor head control

The seat shown in Figure 21.8 has been designed to provide postural support and a stable sitting base for a child in the age range of 6 months to 4 years who has low truncal tone and poor head control. The modular seat can be purchased with an extensive range of positional pads which can be easily adapted for a child's changing needs. The range of adjustments to the angle of the chair means that the child can be placed in a more upright position at the appropriate time in the child's postural development. The chair is supported in a light-weight,

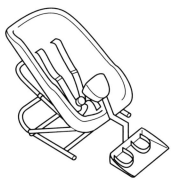

Figure 21.8 • Modular seat for the young child with low truncal tone and poor head control.

strong, steel frame with a stable base and can easily be moved from place to place, enabling your child to interact with you in different environments. Although this seating is a good, supportive system for young children with poor head control and low truncal tone who flop forward when placed in sitting, as soon as the child starts to extend the head and back actively the child should be seated in a more upright chair with good pelvic stabilization.

A seat for the more severely involved young child (levels IV or V GMFCS) with stiffness and asymmetry

The floor sitter shown in Figure 21.9, as a result of its contour shape, is often the only type of seating that a young child with severe involvement finds comfortable because of stiffness and asymmetry. The seat is covered with soft, washable material over firm-density foam that retains its shape and includes an integral abductor pommel to keep the thighs apart, pelvic positioning belt to keep the hips back and down and a shoulder and chest harness. A separate wedge holds the unit in an upright or inclined position. This chair can be useful for feeding a child in.

The contour shape of this seating module is designed to fit the fleshy contours of the buttocks and is therefore comfortable for a child with this level of involvement. This shape will not provide sufficient stabilization to counteract asymmetry that may present at the pelvis and care must be taken to check that any asymmetry is corrected by a hip positioning belt and some pads.

As the centre of gravity is behind the sitting base, there is a tendency for the pelvis to tilt backwards and the child to slip down and forwards in the chair. This must be carefully monitored.

Corner seats

Corner seats are useful for children with changing tone and involuntary movements or moderate stiffness who can sit in long sitting (with their legs out straight) but lack sufficient balance to use their hands in this position (levels III or IV GMFCS).

Corner seats usually come with:

- Upholstered, adjustable back and lateral wing supports
- Padding that extends over the top of the seat for neck and head support
- Wedge-shaped abductor pommel with positional changes
- Seats that can be raised by locking in an extra sitting base
- Trays that are adjustable in both height and angle

Any of these additional supports can be easily moved and adjusted as the child develops more sitting balance.

Figure 21.10 illustrates a corner seat with padded head, back and side supports. The oblong, reversible pommel is adjustable in depth. A tray could be fitted that is adjustable in both height and angle.

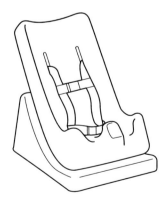

Figure 21.9 • Floor sitter for the young child with stiffness and asymmetry.

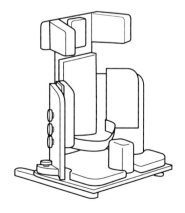

Figure 21.10 • Corner seat.

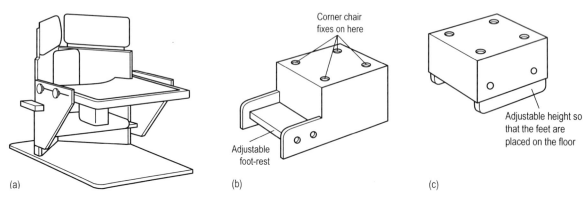

(a)　　　　　　　　　　　　　　　　(b)　　　　　　　　　　　　　　　　(c)

Figure 21.11 • (a) Corner seat with raised sitting base, enabling the child to sit with legs flexed and feet flat on the floor. (b and c) Alternative ways of raising the seat height off the ground.

Children with extensor stiffness and tight hamstring muscles who sit back on their sacrum with a flexed spine should not use a corner seat unless the sitting base is raised so that the child can sit with legs flexed and feet flat on the floor, as shown in Figure 21.11.

Folding seats for children with milder stiffness who can sit supported but lack balance (level III or IV GMFCS)

The main advantage of this seat is that it is light and portable and can be easily transported. The design of the seat encourages the legs to roll outwards and when the seat is raised off the ground the child's feet can be flat on the floor. It slopes backwards to reduce the necessity of strapping. To prevent the seat being pushed backwards there are two extensions at the back well behind the corner.

Roller chairs

If a child's thighs push inwards sitting astride a roller may remedy the situation.

The roller chair was originally designed by Nancie Finnie for children with extensor stiffness who were unable to achieve pelvic and trunk alignment or to sit with their hips flexed, legs abducted and outwardly rotated and feet flat on the floor. These problems made it difficult for such children to bring their arms forwards plus the fact that often, as they brought their hands together towards midline, adduction and extension of the legs increased. Groin straps and

round abduction pommels often used in such a scenario were considered inadequate. Although it holds the child's knees apart, a pommel does not solve the basic problem of extension, adduction and internal rotation at the hips. Thus the idea of the roller chair, with help from a parent in the design, was born. The design was later amended, adding a back to the chair and making its height, and that of the roller itself adjustable, plus a simple brake for the castors so that the child could push it around (Figure 21.12).

Using the same principles a number of manufacturers have further improved the design and added many other useful features (Figures 21.13 and 21.14).

For the child with mild to moderate seating needs (level II or III GMFCS) its function as a seat can be combined with a means of encouraging dynamic balance by adjusting the amount of freedom of the roller to roll.

For the more severely involved child (levels IV or V GMFCS) adjustable foot and armrests, straps and headrest wings can be added, as shown in Figure 21.14b.

The bean bag chair

Many homes possess bean bag chairs. They make a comfortable chair for a mother to sit in when playing with her baby or young child, although it can be difficult to get into and out of one. Young babies may feel secure on the wide surface and enjoy the movement of the polystyrene bead filling but care must be taken that the baby does not roll or slip off.

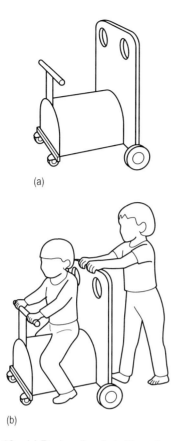

(a)

(b)

Figure 21.12 • (a) Basic roller chair. The roller seat is very stable and can also be used as a walker with a light-weight passenger on board to make it more fun (b).

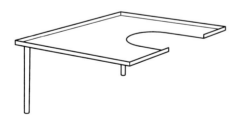

Figure 21.13 • Cut-out table attachment using door bolts to attach the table to the back of the chair.

Few therapists consider the bean bag a suitable seat for an older child as any abnormalities of the muscular skeletal system will be accommodated, not corrected, and the position is usually one of half-lying in which the child looks at the ceiling and not at the surrounding environment.

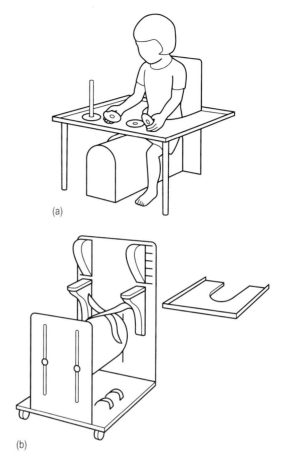

(a)

(b)

Figure 21.14 • (a) Child sitting on the roller chair with a cut-out table in front. Note that the height of the roller is level with the knees. There should be a space of about 55 mm (2 inches) between the child and the table at the front and at the sides. Adjustable foot and armrests, straps and headrest wings can be added (b).

Complete seating systems for children at levels IV or V on the GMFCS

A number of manufacturers have designed complete seating systems which encourage the child to achieve more postural control in the sitting position with external modifications that can be changed or removed as the child grows and abilities change. These chairs are versatile and are supplied with a number of adaptations. Figure 21.2 illustrates a typical example.

Additionally seating systems have been designed in which the child sits in a forward-leaning

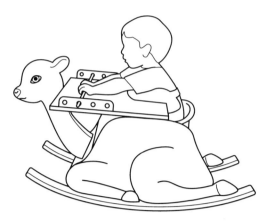

Figure 21.15 • Seating system developed for the young child with postural impairment who is at risk of or has spinal deformity.

position with an extended trunk and the shoulders and arms forwards, thus placing the child in a more functional position. Such seating often comes with chest and lateral supports, abduction seat and adjustable footplates.

The seating system shown in Figure 21.15 has been developed for the young child with postural impairment who is at risk of or has spinal deformity. The child sits in a straddled, forward-leaning position. The seat provides a stable base for the pelvis and thighs, while a thoracic support maintains the alignment of the trunk over the pelvis. The child feels secure and is helped to hold up the head and use the hands.

Seating for the child who can sit unsupported (levels II and III on the GMFCS)

When your child reaches the stage of no longer needing any support, seating is required that provides a good stable base such as the box stool that can be adjusted to different heights and enables the child to get up from the sitting position to standing.

A variable-height ladderback chair can also be helpful. In addition this type of seating, fitted with removable skis, provides a stable walker. It is useful for the child with changing muscle tone, spasms and low truncal tone or moderate stiffness. The ladderback enables the child to reach

forward and grasp the rungs and by 'walking' the hands up them to get into an upright position, as shown in Figure 21.16.

The Tripp-Trapp chair for the child with adequate sitting balance (levels II and III on the GMFCS) is popular with parents as it 'grows' with the child. It has a broad base with steel spacer bars for adequate strength and safety (Figure 21.17). The two platforms can be altered in height and depth, the footrest easily positioned.

For a young child with minimal problems a special back rest, deep front rail, activity rail and pommel can be attached.

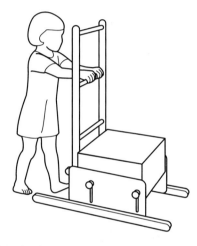

Figure 21.16 • A variable height ladder back chair fitted with skis.

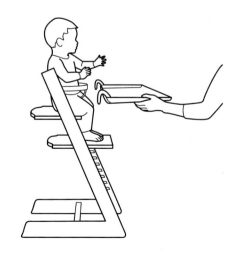

Figure 21.17 • Tripp-Trapp chair.

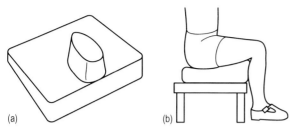

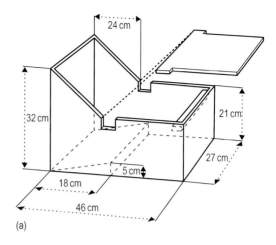

Figure 21.18 • (a) Pommel seat; (b) ramped cushion.

(a)

Chair inserts

There are a wide variety of padded inserts for children's chairs and pushchairs on the market that are made to provide comfort and support. Some have eyelet holes for a safety harness. They are made in a variety of materials and fillings, including 50% cotton and 50% polyester with 100% polyester fillings, or padded foam with PVC covering. Check that the materials conform to fire regulations and that they are easily cleaned or washable.

A pommel seat to use as an insert for a chair or pushchair may be useful for a child who presses the thighs together. The seat is made of foam with a large semi-rigid pommel to provide some pelvic stability and leg abduction, as shown in Figure 21.18a.

Ramped cushions can be useful to give a stable sitting position for the child who tends to lean backwards as a result of tight muscles behind the knees (hamstring muscles). As shown in Figure 21.18b, the ramped cushion may enable the child to come forward in sitting by bending at the hips without rounding the back as the thighs are supported.

Chairs you can make yourself

Box seat

This seat, made of wood, is simple to make and is designed so that a young child can sit with the legs straight out in front (Figure 21.19). The straight back of the box, in combination with the sloping angle of the blunt-ended wedge and

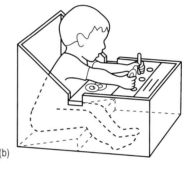

(b)

Figure 21.19 • (a, b) Box seat.

the narrowness of the sides of the box, gives the child with poor sitting balance a stable base and a feeling of security so that additional support is often unnecessary.

The correct angle of the seat is of utmost importance as the child's lower back should rest against the support. If the angle of the seat is too steep the base of the spine will be rounded, the pelvis tilted backwards and the child will be unable to flex at the hips or bring the arms forward to play. If the child's arms have a tendency to press down when sitting make sure that the tray is at chest height or tilted. Different trays can be slotted in to add variety to the child's play.

Mothers who have to apply 'jaw control' when feeding their child often find this seat useful as the child is well supported, leaving the mother's hands comparatively free. Being small, the box seat has

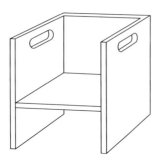

Figure 21.20 • Simple wood chair.

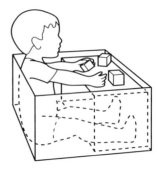

Figure 21.21 • Child sitting in a cardboard box with another inside used as a table.

the advantage that it can be placed on a table at meal times at a helpful height for the mother.

The box seat is not recommended for a child with poor head and trunk control or those who are very flexed. A child with asymmetrical posture may need additional support.

Simple wood chair

This is a stable chair simple in design and easy to make (Figure 21.20). It can be a helpful chair for a child with moderate increased stiffness. Making these chairs with the seating placements at varying heights means that the two seats can be interchangeable over quite a long period of time, using one as a chair and the other as a table. The child's feet should be flat on the floor.

Cardboard and plastic storage boxes

A young child with inadequate sitting balance will often feel more secure when sitting in a confined space. I have made use of large cardboard boxes or plastic storage boxes of varying sizes for both functional activity and play.

A strong cardboard or plastic box can make an excellent play area as toys can be attached across the top or the sides or laid on the floor of the box. A smaller box can be placed inside to form a table (Figure 21.21).

If using a cardboard box make sure that the metal staples used to hold it together are flattened and taped over or, if not required, removed.

Sitting need not be a passive or static function and when a child has reached the stage of moving about in the sitting position and starting to pull up to standing a box can be a good practice area for such activities. When playing in a box, using a far larger box than shown in Figure 21.21, a child may become quite adventurous and begin to practise the movements needed to get up to stand, often using the edge of the box. If this stage is mastered the child may progress to trying to walk sideways around the inside of the box. The box may function as a mobile playpen and being light can be taken into different rooms so that while the mother does various jobs the child can play and move around safely while still being observed. The make-up of the box can be varied to give the child different sensations. For example, the bottom and sides of the box can be lined with pieces of firm carpet or, in contrast, pieces of soft fluffy material such as that which lines bedroom slippers. The contents of the box can be varied too, filling it with tissue paper, newspaper, wrapping up some of the child's toys or putting in odds and ends from around the house such as wooden spoons, empty cartons and squeezy bottles.

Always make sure that none of the articles given for play are hazardous.

The cardboard or plastic box is not recommended for a child who has no sitting balance.

The cylinder chair

The cylinder used for this chair is made of thick reinforced cardboard. The cylinders themselves are produced commercially. With the section cut

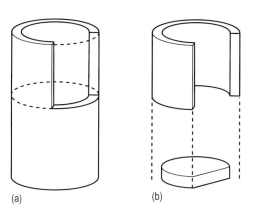
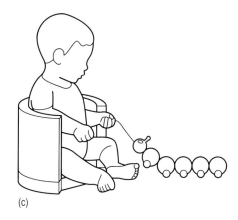
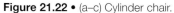

Figure 21.22 • (a–c) Cylinder chair.

out it can form a useful seat. The seat disc of rein-forced cardboard gives the stability necessary to the cylinder. It can be covered in foam and wash-able material with a foam cushion added to the seat (Figure 21.22).

> *All materials used must be approved by fire regu-lations and any staples holding the cardboard box together flattened and taped over.*

This seat may be useful at meal times for chil-dren who have fairly good sitting balance but are still apprehensive when using both hands. The shape of the back of the cylinder keeps the shoul-ders forwards and this makes it easier for the child to bring the arms forwards, especially those chil-dren who tend to fall backwards when they lift a spoon to take food into their mouths. The shape giving good support may also provide a sense of security to the child. For the young child the seat can be placed on the floor.

The cylinder chair is *not recommended* unless a child has fairly good sitting balance. Its main func-tion is to enable the child to bring both arms for-wards for improved hand function.

Tables

Chair and table heights need to relate to one another. The table should be at elbow height so that the upper trunk comes forward which in turn encourages forward movement at the hips, shoul-ders and arms. It also makes it possible for the child to weight-bear on the forearms, providing the child with a position of stability if needed. There is a wide range of different designs of tables on the mar-ket including ones that can be adjusted for height and angle from the horizontal to the vertical which makes it easier for the child to see what the hands are doing. This is important as vision plays a major role in controlling the movements of children.

Optional extras which encourage the devel-opment of basic hand skills such as vertical and horizontal hand grabs and a variety of play frame attachments are also available.

Although it is important to have a washable table top surface this often means that the surface will be slippery and therefore I would advise the use of non-slip mats. These can be purchased in sheets or strips.

Summary

In concluding this section on various types of seat-ing I want to emphasize that the aim should be to have the child sitting without any additional sup-port and in a variety of chairs as soon as the child has developed adequate sitting balance, providing that the hips and spine are regularly monitored for developmental abnormalities and appropriate action taken if needed.

Complete independence will only have been achieved when the child has sufficient balance to use both hands for functional activities, fetch a chair and pull it up to a table independently and get on and off it alone.

Pushchairs or strollers

The principles and critical factors discussed in relation to chairs also apply largely to pushchairs or strollers. In this section I shall use the word 'pushchairs' to mean either. Naturally there are some differences between chairs and pushchairs. In a pushchair you are looking at a child who is sitting but not usually actively involved in using the hands for skilled movements. With a chair the aim is to try to provide a structure that enables a child to function. In those circumstances the chair is a facilitator for daily activities such as eating, playing and learning as well as reinforcing the aims of good positioning, especially symmetry, control and stability. Good upright positioning with symmetry, control and stability are also important features of a pushchair for the child. Nothing can be more conducive to a child's intellectual inertia than lying back in a half-reclining position gazing up at the sky. It is important that on the occasions that your child is out with you experiences should be active rather than passive, and offer opportunities for the child to interact with all that is going on around. To do this your child needs to be in a secure, stable and upright sitting position.

The constantly new developments in design and manufacture already alluded to earlier in this chapter about chairs also apply to pushchairs.

Before buying a pushchair it is always advisable to get professional advice from your therapist rather than just buying one that is recommended by a shop or from a catalogue. If the shop will allow you to have a pushchair on approval, take advantage of this service, as this will give you not only an idea if it meets the needs of your child but also an opportunity to see how practical it is for you to fold, carry, stack in a car boot or take on public transport and whether it is easy to store. Certainly never buy a pushchair without trying your child in it and pushing it around and up and down a kerb or step. You will also be able to see if your child sits as well in the pushchair when you are pushing it as when it is stationary.

General points to bear in mind when choosing a pushchair

1. Choose a light-weight but stable pushchair with an attractive design, padded or rubber hand grips, a good braking system and one that is easy to manoeuvre.

2. Check not only the age and weight range recommended but also the height range.

3. Pick a versatile system, preferably one that has a basic chassis that will take different-sized seats as the child grows.

4. Material used on the seat should be non-slip. Many fabric covers can often only be sponged clean so choose removable covers that can be machine-washed if possible. With a buggy, it will be found easier if you choose a model where the rain gear can remain in place, especially in England.

5. If the pushchair is an imported model, it is important to check that spare parts are available and whether the company provides service agreements for repairs.

6. See that the backrest and seat are firm and that the sides are high enough to give the necessary support.

7. Where adjustments to the angle of the backrest and height and angle of the footrest are available check that they are easy and quick to manage.

8. Accessories add to the cost of the pushchair, so check carefully to see if your child's ability to sit improves with additional support by trying them out first.

9. Finally check that the pushchair, stroller or buggy *meets furniture and fire regulations* and the length of the guarantee.

Having chosen the most suitable pushchair you may find that you need to purchase additional supports similar to those used by your child when sitting in a chair. Manufacturers vary as to the accessories they supply as standard features with their pushchairs. These can be expensive items so ask your therapist to advise whether your child would benefit by having extra support.

Some accessories that may be helpful are shown in Figure 21.2. Others include:

1. Groin straps which may help to stabilize the pelvis when taken in front of the pelvis and over the hip joints at an angle of 45° and pulled down and back and tied under the seat

2. Abduction pommel blocks which may help by keeping the legs apart, providing the child with a wider sitting base

3. Lateral and medial trunk supports which may help keep the trunk in midline

4. A waistcoat (safety jacket) body support or chest pad which may provide a better alignment of the upper trunk in the child whose upper trunk flops forward

5. A retention bar may be a useful addition to a pushchair and can be used by a child as soon as the child has learned to grasp. They often give a child a feeling of security and stability, enabling a child to sit with less support

Footrests on some pushchairs are made in one piece whereas others have a separate support for each foot. If your child has an asymmetrical posture the extra weight pushing down on one side may result in one footrest being lower than the other. It is easy not to notice that this has happened so check regularly and tell your therapist if it has occurred.

Different pushchairs

As there is currently such a wide choice and variety of pushchairs available, each claiming to provide postural control to a different degree, it is now possible following your child's assessment for you and your child's therapist to choose a particular pushchair that is virtually tailor-made for your child, with postural components which can be gradually reduced as your child develops increasing postural control.

Young children with only moderate involvement (levels I, II or III on the GMFCS)

For babies and young children who have only moderate involvement I have found that the wide range of design and choice of pushchairs on the

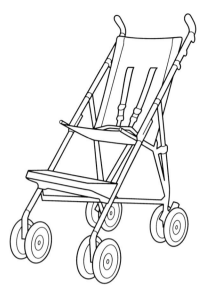

Figure 21.23 • Example of a pushchair suitable for a young child with only moderate involvement (levels I–III on the Gross Motor Function Classification System).

market can be used with little or no modification (Figure 21.23).

Young children with more severe involvement (level IV or V GMFCS)

For young children who have limited pelvic and trunk control an insert into a pushchair, as shown in Figure 21.24a, may provide the support required. It must be used with the pushchair's harness. Alternatively a waistcoat harness, as shown in Figure 21.24b, may be helpful. For babies and young children with limited head control a pushchair as shown in Figure 21.24c may be more helpful.

As mentioned earlier it is important in relation to both chairs and pushchairs that children should be given every opportunity to use whatever abilities they have to control and adjust their positions independently whenever possible, in this way learning to achieve their own balance. Therefore the outside support given and the extra adjustments made to a pushchair should be restricted to the absolute minimum but nevertheless ensuring that the child has a stable base, postural trunk control and alignment. Whereas on the one hand outside support

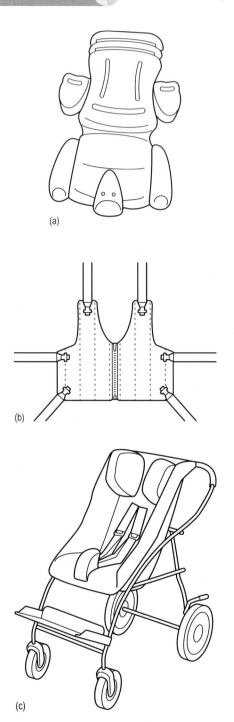

(a)

(b)

(c)

Figure 21.24 • (a) Pushchair insert for young children with limited pelvic and trunk control. (b) Waistcoat harness. (c) Pushchair for young children with limited head control.

should be removed when it is no longer needed, on the other hand hips and spines need to be monitored regularly for any developing abnormalities.

Car seats

In order to ensure your child's safety when travelling in a car, do ask for advice. There is a wide range of car seats available and constant production innovations are ongoing; also regulations are changing frequently. The same safety rules regarding car seats apply to all children: basically the seat must provide adequate restraint and protection with harness straps that fit properly and are easily adjusted. To provide maximum protection it is important when buying a car seat that you get the correct restraint for your child's weight and height as the ages given by the manufacturers are often only approximate guides.

All car seats must be *securely installed into the car* as recommended by the manufacturer's instructions and satisfying legal requirements.

If your child is in a carrycot during the early months it is important that you use a carrycot restraint in the car. This is a legal requirement in most countries.

Rearward-facing car seats are also available. They are stable, should have fully adjustable built-in

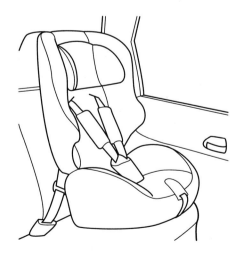

Figure 21.25 • Car seat suitable for children weighing 9–25 kg.

harnesses and often incorporate a head cushion for extra support and safety. They are suitable for children weighing up to 10 kg.

If the passenger seats in your car have an airbag, rearward-facing car seats must not be used unless the airbag can be turned off.

Many parents have found a car seat as shown in Figure 21.25 most satisfactory for children in the weight range of 9–25 kg.

Larger car seats are available with additional controls for children weighing over 25 kg who cannot sit in the car without extra supportive seating.

It is important to try out a car seat before purchasing one, to assess whether it is easy to place your child in it and take your child out of it. This is best carried out with the car seat installed in the car.

If your child needs a car seat when travelling by air it is always a good idea to check with your airline to be sure that the car seat you have is accepted by the Civil Aviation Authority.

Reference

Palisano R, Rosenbaum P, Walter S et al. Development and validation of a gross motor function classification system for children with CP. Dev Med Child Neurol 1997; 39:214–223.

Chapter Twenty Two

22

Aids to mobility

Revised by Eva Bower

For many parents, freedom of independent mobility is one of their main goals for their child. This may be totally free independent mobility or with the assistance of an aid, but it is worth remembering that in adulthood the priorities are likely to be different. As suggested by Bleck (1987), the needs for optimum independent living for adults with cerebral palsy (CP) ranked in order of priority are likely to be:

1. Communication with a yes/no response as the very basic requirement.

2. Independence in activities of daily living facilitated by the availability of one good hand or carers other than the parents.

3. Mobility with a basic requirement of control of just one part of the body (chin, foot, etc.).

4. Walking.

The choice of mobility will be dependent upon a number of factors such as the age of the child, the level of impairment and the situation in which the independent mobility is attempted, for example, at home across the sitting room carpeted floor, outside in the garden on the grass or in the supermarket with a slippery floor and lots of other people around. The important points when choosing an aid that may enable your child to be mobile are that:

1. The mobility aid should challenge your child's ability to improve their independence.

2. The mobility aid should increase your child's potential for independent exploration of the environment with safety.

The usual ages for typical children to crawl are between 9 and 11 months, to stand are between 11 and 13 months, to cruise along furniture are between 12 and 14 months and to walk are between 13 and 15 months. Once a typical child has mastered the skills of crawling and walking independently the child is able to learn more about the world around, both inside and outside the home. The child finds ways into cupboards and drawers, opening and closing doors, inspecting and experimenting with and promptly discarding the contents. No place in the house is left undisturbed. As play becomes more energetic favourite toys are those that can be pushed and pulled, a tricycle without pedals or one of the sturdy toys on wheels that the child can sit astride and propel around the house or garden. However it will be quite a long time before the typical child has the coordination needed to manage a tricycle with pedals – around 3–3½ years.

As a result of the lack of ability and mobility, many children with CP are denied the freedom of exploring and playing in this way. But children with CP should be given the opportunity to move about using aids at the age-appropriate time, thus enabling them to explore in as similar a way as possible to their peers. Box 22.1 lists children's needs for mobility aids as predicted by classification on the Gross Motor Function Classification System (Palisano et al. 1997).

The figures in this chapter illustrate various ideas that may encourage a child to be mobile both inside and outside the home using toys found in the toy departments of shops. Most can be easily adapted if needed. Mobility equipment especially designed to meet the needs of a child with CP is also illustrated.

Box 22.1

Before 2nd birthday

Children at level I do not usually need any different mobility aids from their peers without abnormality

Children at level II may need a walking mobility aid after 13–15 months

Children at level III will need a walking mobility aid after 13–15 months

Children at level IV will need to try a crawling mobility aid after 11–13 months

Between 2nd and 4th birthdays

Children at level II may continue to need a walking mobility aid

Children at level III will continue to need a walking mobility aid

Children at level IV may continue to need a crawling mobility aid; if able to use one and will need a wheelchair, hopefully self-powered electric

Between 4th and 6th birthdays

Children at level II should no longer need a walking mobility aid

Ways of encouraging a child to achieve balance in standing and walking, both with minimal support and independently, are shown. I have also included two types of rollators to be used as walking aids but you will need to ask your therapist to advise which might be the most suitable for your child. Two tricycles are also shown. Advice should again be sought from your therapist as to which might be the most appropriate for your child and when.

Mobility in prone

See Figures 22.1–22.3.

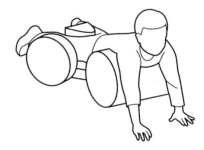

Figure 22.1 • Scooter board with positioning pads to keep the child extended with straight arms and legs.

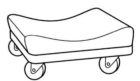

Figure 22.2 • Wooden stool on castors covered with shaped foam which can be used by a child either for lying over and moving about using the arms and/or legs or for sitting on and moving about using the legs.

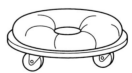

Figure 22.3 • Wooden ring on castors covered with a padded cushion or rubber ring with a dip/hole in the middle which can be used by a child for sitting on and moving around using the legs or for lying over and moving around using the arms and/or the legs.

Mobility in sitting

See Figures 22.4 and 22.5.

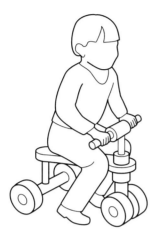

Figure 22.4 • Wooden tricycle on which a child can sit while 'walking' it along with the feet and grasping the handlebars.

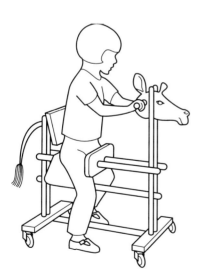

Figure 22.5 • Toy animal on castors which a child can sit astride with support at the spine and pelvis plus adjustable grasp and seat positions. As in Figure 22.4, the child can 'walk' the animal along.

Sturdy trucks which can be used as walkers

See Figures 22.6–22.9.

Walking with support

See Figures 22.10–22.13.

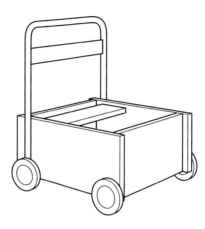

Figure 22.6 • Truck on castors with handle which can be pushed along by a child. The length is about 50 cm, the width about 35 cm and the height about 55 cm.

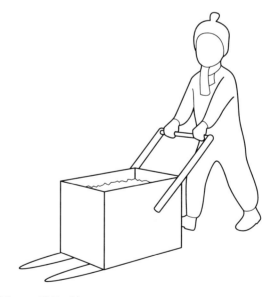

Figure 22.7 • Home-made wooden box with skis on the base plus handle for grasping. The skis will make the box easier to push.

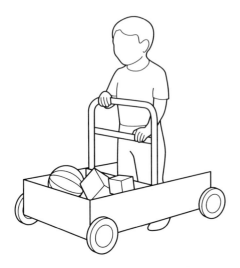

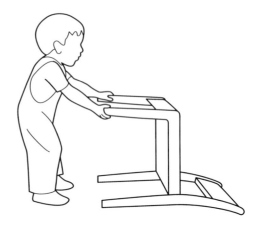

Figure 22.11 • Illustrates how by varying the height and weight of a toy or chair used for pushing along the child's degree of hip flexion (bending) can also be altered.

Figure 22.8 • Truck with variable-height horizontal bars for holding and pushing.

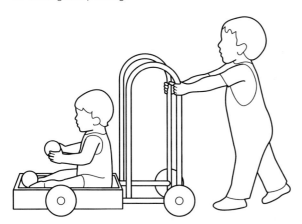

Figure 22.9 • Truck with bars which can be held vertically or horizontally.

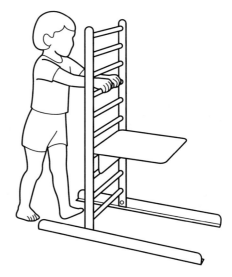

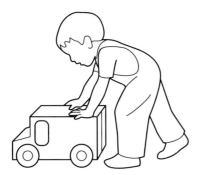

Figure 22.12 • Illustrates how by varying the height and weight of a toy or chair used for pushing along the child's degree of hip flexion (bending) can also be altered.

Figure 22.10 • Illustrates how by varying the height and weight of a toy or chair used for pushing along the child's degree of hip flexion (bending) can also be altered.

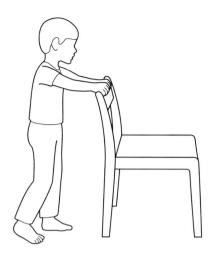

Figure 22.13 • Illustrates how by varying the height and weight of a toy or chair used for pushing along the child's degree of hip flexion (bending) can also be altered.

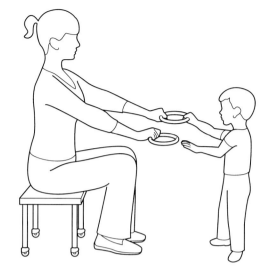

Figure 22.15 • Child grasping a quoit with one hand and about to grasp the second quoit with the other hand. Both quoits are controlled by the mother, who can 'walk' the stool on which she is sitting backwards so that the child takes steps forwards.

Providing support

See Figure 22.14.

Hoops and quoits make useful stable and mobile supports, often bridging the gap from being held when walking to independent walking (Figures 22.15–22.17).

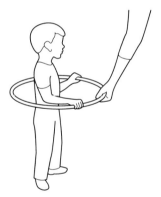

Figure 22.16 • Child using a hoop for support which is controlled by the mother as is needed.

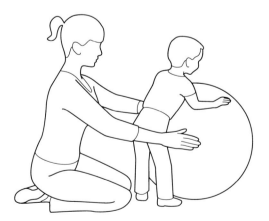

Figure 22.14 • Child walking with a large ball giving some support while the mother controls the movement of the ball.

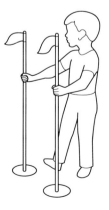

Figure 22.17 • Child, with some standing balance, walking with two poles, each with a large disc on the base for additional stability.

Balance training

See Figure 22.18.

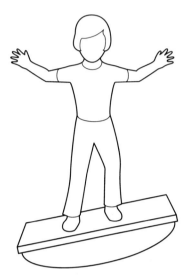

Figure 22.18 • Child with standing balance who is practising transferring weight from one leg to the other on a balance board.

Walking independently

See Figures 22.19 and 22.20.

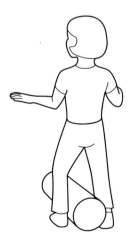

Figure 22.19 • Child practising walking with one leg on each side of a roll, which may encourage a child to transfer the weight from one leg to the other before taking a step.

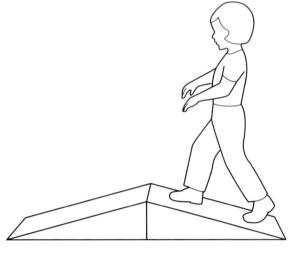

Figure 22.20 • Child practising walking up and down an incline on a foam wedge, the softness of which may also encourage balance reactions in the feet.

Walking trainers

See Figures 22.21–22.24.

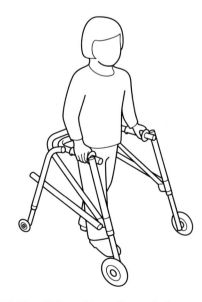

Figure 22.21 • Child walking with a pull-along rear postural control walker, often called a Kaye walker.

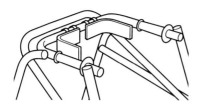

Figure 22.22 • Hip location pads which can be fitted to the walker shown in Figure 22.21 to help control the position of the hips.

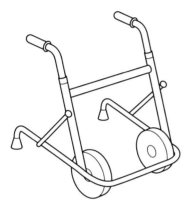

Figure 22.23 • Folding rollator which is pushed forwards.

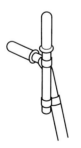

Figure 22.24 • Vertical hand holds which can be fitted to the rollator shown in Figure 22.23 instead of horizontal hand holds.

Walking with elbow crutches

See Figure 22.25.

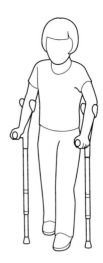

Figure 22.25 • Child walking with elbow crutches.

Tricycles

See Figures 22.26 and 22.27.

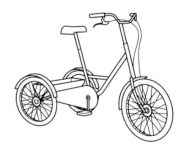

Figure 22.26 • Child's tricycle.

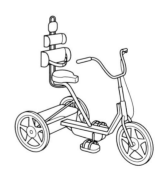

Figure 22.27 • Custom-made child's tricycle with head, upper and lower trunk supports and foot plates. Such a tricycle could be power-assisted.

References

Bleck EE, Orthopaedic management in cerebral palsy. Clinics in developmental medicine no. 99/100, Mackeith Press, Oxford, Blackwell Scientific Publication, with Philadelphia, J. B. Lippincott.

Palisano R, Rosenbaum P, Walter S et al. Development and validation of a gross motor function classification system for children with CP. Dev Med Child Neurol 1997; 39:214–223.

23

Play

Revised by Eva Bower

It is mainly through play that a child learns during the early years. As discussed earlier, a child begins to learn about the world from what is heard, seen, touched and tasted, with parental help and interaction provided only as needed. Once self-aware, the child learns about others in relation to the self. As eye–hand coordination develops, the child begins to explore nearby objects, grasping and putting them into the mouth; the child starts to become aware of their shape and texture, and that some taste pleasant whereas others are unpleasant.

As the physical abilities and hand skills develop, the fingers become the main source of information and the child starts to concentrate on what is being done with the hands, learning first by chance and later by repetition and practice.

The typical child

The typical child learns what can and cannot be done with toys and familiar objects. Familiar objects and toys are now the tools a child uses for further exploration and development. The child finds that these objects have a top, a bottom, an inside and an outside. If an object is hard it cannot be squeezed, but if it is soft it can. The child learns that objects can be put into and out of a container, first emptying them all out at once and, at around 18 months, in an orderly and systematic manner. The child discovers that by putting one thing on top of another, building can be undertaken, making a tower of two small bricks, or that one can hold an object steady with one hand while using the other. The child also discovers how to assess the amount of effort needed to get the desired result, for example, that some toys move more easily and go faster when pushed, others when pulled. Able to make choices, the child now only plays with those toys that are of interest, discarding others.

The child with cerebral palsy

Play also provides a child with CP with a medium through which intellectual, emotional, communication, gross and fine motor skills can develop. As a result of the child's physical difficulties, and depending on the severity and type of CP, including any impairment of vision and/or learning, progress may be slow. Poor perceptual ability, a short attention span and difficulty with recall or short-term memory, if present, will all mean that to gain the most enjoyment and benefit from play, the child with CP will need considerable help, guidance and support.

Although a child with CP may lack many of the typical gross motor movements that are necessary to use the hands in a skilled coordinated manner, if helped to make use of existing skills, however

limited they may be, the child will be able to learn through play. This may be helped by:

1. Seeing that the position that the child is in is a position which provides a secure base, and the necessary stabilization, so that arm and wrist fixation is possible

2. Choosing toys that are at the child's developmental level and ability and are the correct size for the child to handle

3. Paying attention to preferences by allowing the child to choose those toys that are enjoyed and of interest

4. Being aware of the child's tolerance level and ability to concentrate

5. Allowing the child to explore at the child's own speed and initiative, giving help only where necessary

6. Giving simple directions using short sentences

When playing with your child, always remember that the important thing is your child's interest and curiosity in the toys played with while tackling the problems they present, not that the child necessarily completes what has been set out to do.

The importance of concentration

Children are often easily distracted and it is difficult to hold their attention even for a short time. They soon tire of their toys or games and want to move on to something else, and with a child with CP, this stage is often prolonged.

It is helpful if we know and appreciate the maximum amount of concentration a child is capable of giving, for if we ask too much of children, they will lose interest, become frustrated and cease to try. Lack of achievement will soon lead to boredom. The child will return to the toys and games known and understood, and so be deprived of learning and gaining new experiences. The frustration and tolerance of a child with CP are often low, and if the child does not succeed at the second or third attempt, the child often gives up. This especially applies to children of higher intelligence who know what they want to do, but cannot control movements sufficiently to enable them to do it.

Here are two suggestions that may help your child to concentrate. When giving toys, offer only two from which to choose, then put away the one not wanted. See that your child is not surrounded by things that will distract, such as an open toy cupboard, a pet or other activities going on in the room, or playing by the window. Eventually, of course your child will need to get used to things going on around without interruption of play. One has to remember that, although typically a child can pick up a new toy and play with it, often quite a lot of help is needed to understand how it works and this help has to be repeated not once, but several times. Stay with your child, see if your child can manage and that your child understands what you have explained. You may find that your child would play and use the hands more easily in another position or if there was more support giving better balance and stability.

Play that involves sensory motor learning

A child needs to become aware of objects as a whole before being able to appreciate their parts and their relationship one to another. A good way of starting to help to do this is to explore the everyday objects that the child would typically get hold of and play with. For example, you could use unpeeled fruit such as an apple, orange or banana, helping the child to hold the fruit, feel its shape and texture, name the fruit and get to know the way it feels when handled.

The more severely disabled child

As play only really starts when a child succeeds in making something happen, if the child seems to have no interest in toys, we need to think of activities that will get a reaction with little effort. Examples are simple commercial toys such as a jack in the box or pop-up men. The latter only needs the slightest pressure for the men to pop up, and later may be used for colour matching and imaginative games. For a young child, you could try a discovery mat, with its surprising sounds and soft textures, or encourage the child to splash the hands in the bath, resulting in floating toys moving about in the water.

A way I often use is either to put a collection of toys on a child's lap, or have the child sit in a confined space and crowd toys around, even letting the child sit on some of them. This often stimulates the child to look and start to push them away. Seeing something happen as a result of the child's own actions may stimulate the child to try again. Watching and touching and later trying to get hold of a balloon or bubbles blown into the air are other simple ways of getting the interest of the more severely involved child.

If a child frequently just throws toys on the floor, you can try either tying them to a chair, a belt or thick piece of string around the waist of the child, or attaching smaller toys to an old cushion.

Even if a child cannot use the hands or speak, the child is likely to have some way of indicating what is wanted. For example, if you are building a house with bricks, have a book with different pictures of houses and get your child to act as 'foreman' and 'direct proceedings', choosing the type of house the child wants you to build, the type of roof, the number of windows, and where your child wants the door to be. In this way, when the house has been built the child will know that he or she took an active part in its construction.

The more moderately disabled child

It is up to us to see that play activities are presented in such a way that children are able to succeed, to make their own choices and to vary the way they wish to play, experimenting on their own, not directed by us. We should only help when the child gets into difficulties or asks for our help.

The following are some ideas you might like to try.

Water play

Use a large basin of water or, in the summer, if you have a paddling pool let the child play in the pool. See that the objects for playing with are as varied as possible: ones that sink or float, and those that make a noise when banged together. Later a plastic bottle funnel, sieve or colander, all giving a different effect as they are taken into and out of the water, can be used. Playing in this way, the child learns about how liquids behave and how they behave in a container. Making the water cloudy with some bath foam is a good way of getting a child to use both hands automatically while playing with the bubbles and searching for objects that have sunk to the bottom. A squeezy bottle cut in half makes a good home-made chute to send things down into the water.

Sand play

Again you need a variety of objects for the child to play with. Different-size spoons make good spades. A wooden spoon can be used for stirring and a soup ladle to pour sand from one container to another. A Perspex or plastic box is fun for the child to fill as the child can see how much is in it.

Play buckets are ideal for water and sand play – one which sprinkles, one which pours and one which empties through a spout at the side (but you may need to pad the handle if the child has insufficient grasp). A collection of brightly coloured small boats in a variety of types and sizes are fun to use too.

Simple items

Newspaper or tinfoil can be made into a light, safe ball. One can hide a favourite toy in a loose paper parcel and play 'pass the parcel'. Make a mask or a simple spy hole in the paper. You can also make simple finger puppets by either drawing faces on them or using transfer stickers.

Play foam can be used for making patterns on a mirror. Finger paints are good for making hand, finger and foot prints.

Books

Looking at a book together is a special quiet time for parents whose child has CP. To begin with, look at the pictures in the child's scrapbook or photograph album, then progress to one picture to a page, with objects which are familiar to the child such as a cup, spoon, shoe, ball or car. Avoid those that have pictures of animals or things the child may never have seen.

Show your child and name just two pictures at any one time, until the child becomes familiar with them. If there is a picture of a dog or cat, make the noise these animals make and get the child to copy the noise.

Encourage the child to hold the book with you, but as learning to turn the pages is difficult for a child, start with a book with a hard back or practise with an old magazine, as inevitably pages will get torn at first.

Play throughout the day

All children are curious and learn not only by playing with their toys but by exploring familiar objects in the environment, both inside and outside the home.

There are a number of children with CP who, although able to use their hands while sitting, are not sufficiently mobile to explore their environment on their own. This, I think, highlights the importance of encouraging play throughout the day in everyday situations, rather than putting aside a special time for a play session.

Make use of things around you

When in the bedroom let your child look in the mirror, play with the brush, bounce and roll about on the bed. While your child is being dressed, encourage play with a sock or shoes. In the bath, give the child the flannel or sponge to play with, and let the child help you put the towel back on the rail when drying has been finished. When you are both in the kitchen, give a saucepan and wooden spoon, empty cereal box, yoghurt container or empty squeezy bottle for play. Let your child taste hot and cold food while you cook. Many children with CP dislike getting dirty. If you are making pastry, give your child a bowl, moisten the flour and encourage your child to copy you as you knead the flour. Let your child take a finger around a bowl that has held custard or a mixture that is liked. In the garden, if you are potting a plant, encourage your child to help you put the soil in the pot, brush the leaves, and later have the child's own small garden plot to cultivate.

Integration between gross motor abilities and play

As a child becomes more mobile, play extends to learning about moving through space, by climbing in and out, up and down, under and over objects. The child learns to judge the size of a space for squeezing through, which heights are dangerous to jump from and which are safe.

If a ball rolls under a chair, the child works out the best way to get it out. If the child climbs on to a chair to get a toy, the child decides how to get down without dropping it. The child bumps into furniture until realizing that it is solid and a way round it needs to be found.

The young child with cerebral palsy who has the ability to balance and is mobile

A young child who has the ability to balance and is mobile should not only play in a sitting position. If this happens, the chance of gaining many new experiences will be missed. By moving around while playing, the child will make new movements and acquire new experiences and skills. For example, if the child has learned to move from sitting to kneeling upright, play games and place toys in such a way that the child can practise this sequence of movement.

Organization of self

It is very important at this stage for a child to become aware of surrounding space during play. This should include the space behind the child. Encourage the child to move in different ways – backwards, forwards and sideways, crawling, upright kneeling and walking. Games that include throwing a bean bag over the shoulder or passing

a ball over the head and guessing from a sound behind what object you are holding are all ways of encouraging this awareness. Miming to nursery rhymes, conducting or moving to music, and playing on seesaws, slides and swings are ways of playing that will help children to understand the relationship between space and their own constantly changing position.

Games such as 'London bridge is falling down', 'Ring-a-ring o'roses', 'Oranges and lemons' and 'statues' will assist in teaching the concept of up and down and round and round. Obstacle courses are a good way of teaching a child to climb over and under, through, sideways and around objects. Hide and seek, and getting the child to roll over and crawl on verbal command, are good active games.

The transition from play to function

In time, a child uses the basic skills that have been learned and practised when playing with toys to manipulate simple functional objects in the home. For example, the child may like to open and close cupboards, drawers and doors, but will not be able to manage objects that screw and unscrew until later.

The child starts to enjoy self-feeding, if in a somewhat messy manner, and begins to cooperate more when washed, bathed, dressed and undressed. Later, the child often likes to imitate the mother while she cleans, picking up things when they fall over, be with her when she gardens, pass her the shopping when she puts it away in the cupboard. The child begins to follow short verbal commands, e.g. 'Put your mug on the table', 'Bring me your shoes so I can clean them', 'Sit on the chair so that I can put your socks on'.

Choice of toys

The following are ideas for simple toys found mostly in the home. No attempt has been made to state any particular age group, as so much depends on the ability of the individual child to use the hands, as well as on the level of intelligence, and powers of concentration and comprehension. Your therapist will advise you on the most suitable toys and games to use with your child.

A heavy ball is easier for children with involuntary movements and intermittent spasms to play with, as their movements are so disorganized and clumsy that a light ball is apt to roll away. A child with spasticity, on the other hand, can play best with a smaller solid ball, as their grip is apt to be firm and there will be difficulty in lifting and letting go of a heavy ball. A child with a spastic hemiplegia should play with a large beach ball to encourage the use of both hands together. When a child can only grasp a bat or stick, a ball attached by elastic enables play with the ball. For the child who may want to throw and catch a ball but is unable to hold it, a bean bag can be used instead of a ball. Bean bags are easy to make and can be made of bright washable material, in many shapes, weights and sizes. Velcro mitts and contrasting ball are also good for encouraging the use of both hands and make catching easier and more fun.

A medium-sized ball can be used for a young child to push when first starting to walk, and as a movable base for an adult to sit on with a child sitting on the lap, when encouraging balance reactions.

Velcro or a magnetic strip attached to building bricks will make it easier for the child to build. Large light-weight wooden bricks can be used for games as well as building. It is as well to remember that children get as much fun knocking down as they do building up. Many early learning games designed to help the child with activities, such as grouping and matching, involve the use of cards with pictures of, for example, different fruits, or all the articles associated with bathing. The child is required to pick out and place the appropriate card with its picture in the correct place or group. For the child with CP, this may be more difficult because it is difficult to manipulate the thin card. However, by gluing the cards to bricks the child may then be able to play the game.

Poor or clumsy coordination of the child's arms, hands and fingers often makes it difficult to hold toys and at the same time to move them around. If, for example, your child enjoys playing cars, either give a friction car or place a magnetic strip on the car, and on the end of a short stick. Felt stuck on the bottom of a toy will make it easier to move over a polished surface.

A doll's house made from large wooden or cardboard boxes can be used for the child with CP, as the rooms will be big enough to put the hands inside, and by using larger furniture it may be easier to move the objects about. In a similar way, a simple garage can be made at home.

Coloured wooden or plastic cotton reels make excellent counters and can easily be fitted over a board of wooden pegs. Small empty plastic bottles (make sure that they have not previously contained anything toxic) can be used for guessing games and are useful sizes for the child to hold. Fill them with different things to smell and make them of varying weights and sounds. Squeezy bottles can also be used as a home-made set of skittles.

Something that is found in most kitchens – a kitchen plunger with a suction cap – can be used to give a child a lot of amusement while at the same time learning. By fixing it either perpendicularly or horizontally and using different-sized rings, the child can be encouraged to stack them on the stick plunger. We have found varying sizes of curtain rings useful.

A popular toy with many children is an activity centre. For children with CP, a home-made activity centre can be made on a larger scale and designed specifically to meet their needs.

Discovering shapes

Once a child begins to discover that objects have a shape (i.e. round, square, triangular, oblong), collect objects of different shapes with the child, and then find pictures of the shapes to cut out. Get the child to draw round them with a pencil, then later encourage copying and drawing the various objects. In this way the child may not only learn the names of objects, but also what they are used for, why they are made in a certain shape, the different colours in which they are made and what you can do with them.

If the child gets to the stage of recognizing shapes, start by getting the child to master one shape at a time. You can do this by having a series of cardboard boxes that will only take one shape, starting with a round; when this has been mastered, a box that will only take a square. Then a box that takes a round and a square. Then a box that takes a round and a square so that the child has to make a choice.

A good posting box can be made from any square transparent-type container so that the child can enjoy the pleasure of watching the pieces as they fall through. The container can be divided into three or four sections with firm pieces of cardboard, so that apart from posting different shapes the child can be encouraged to fill each section with, for example, dried peas, beans, macaroni pieces or different-sized buttons. See whether the child can name, or even point to, the section you name, then see what happens when you take away the cardboard divisions and the contents become mixed – ask the child to try to pick out pieces of similar objects.

Keeping a scrapbook

Encourage your child to keep a scrapbook of common objects around the house, including the food eaten. Begin with a room in the house, perhaps the kitchen. First show and name the objects, then see if the child can find them in a magazine or paper, and cut them out and paste them in a book. You can enlarge on this idea when you go out for a walk together, colleting leaves, and flowers, and press them in the scrapbook. If you have a camera, take photographs and make a special album of family, friends, pets and familiar places, all of which may encourage recollection and speech.

Making a collection

In addition to the toys brought for children, they often get great pleasure in playing with the odds and ends found around the house, or collected in the garden or on walks. All children are collectors and hoarders, and if they cannot walk or move around the house they are not only denied the pleasure of exploring and finding out things for themselves, but also of acquiring a private collection of their own. If a child is severely disabled, it is up to us to take the child out to explore the surroundings or bring things to the child so that the child can find out all about them and keep those particularly liked. A large magnifying glass is a good way of helping to look at and explore the collection in greater detail – especially interesting if you have visited a pond or river and have a jar of water to put the objects in. An outsized magnifying glass with small 'legs' at each corner can also be of interest if placed over a patch of earth.

Making music

Most children love music. Listening to the radio or stereo is fine, but it is far better to encourage them to make their own music. Severely disabled children who cannot hold a stick to bang a drum or bang it with their hands can make a satisfactory noise if a piece of elastic is tied over the top and bottom of the drum. Squeezy bottles filled with sand, buttons and dried beans can give a variety of sound effects when shaken. Bracelets for the wrists and ankles can be made of leather or felt and small bells sewn securely on to them. This is a good way to encourage music-making and movement at the same time.

When choosing toys, do not always go to a toy shop. The kitchen and general sundries department of a store will often have things that can be fun for your child and easily adapted as toys. Shops that sell products from India and Asia often have a variety of doorchimes, mobiles and handbells. Craft shops with products from continental Europe and Russia often have a good selection of simple games and toys.

Simple games using everyday objects

Many of the everyday objects in the home can, with the application of a little thought and sometimes adaptation, be used in an interesting and amusing way to encourage learning, at no or little cost to you.

For matching

Use food or soft-drink tins or cans, and preferably brightly patterned and coloured ones, making sure that there are no sharp edges. As a moving object often presents a problem for a young child to follow, roll the tin towards the child from different angles in the hope that the child will follow it with the eyes, then later see if the child can push the tin back using both hands. If an added stimulus is needed, put some dried beans and peas into the tin – the sound will help attract attention. Take a number of tins and fill two of each of them with similar objects; by shaking them the child may be able to match similar sounds.

A helpful way to teach the child to learn how to match is by sticking sets of transfers, drawings and cut-out pictures on the lids and bottoms of margarine or yoghurt cartons, then getting the child to match the picture on the lid with the same picture on the base.

Strips of materials such as carpet, emery paper, silk, woollen or fluffy materials stuck on a tin can be used to help a child identify the texture of the material by feeling. See that the strips are broad and do not put more than three different materials on one tin. Sew or bind together 12-cm (5-inch) squares of knitted material, carpet and curtains, then take loose pieces of similar materials to encourage the child to match them.

The shoes and socks of the family can also be used for sorting and pair-matching or helping you sort out the washing. For the older child, folding up dusters or dishcloths and sorting them into appropriate piles can be helpful.

For manipulation

Many food packs of the same product can be bought in different types and sizes, some with screw-on lids and others with lift-off lids. These can all be used to encourage fine movements of hands and fingers.

Bowls and containers, or, if you have one, an old shoebox, are also useful in helping to get fine coordination of the fingers. Tie pieces of wool, ribbon, string or plastic twine together in a length and put it in the container. Then cut a small slit in the lid, pull one end of the wool or whatever through the slit as a 'starter', and encourage the child to pull the length through the slit. As it

comes through, the child should wind it over a stick or something similar – a little competition could be devised to see which of two children completes the winding over the stick first.

Children are fascinated with objects that seem to disappear and reappear. One way to do this is to take a large empty matchbox, either square or oblong, with divisions in it; place different objects in each compartment, then let the child open the box by pushing. Another way is to make a hole in the lid of a small cardboard box and another one at the side of the box near the bottom. The child then puts a marble or something similar into the box and then has to shake it to try to get the marble out of one of the holes.

It is hoped that the foregoing will be sufficient to prove that everyday objects in one's home can provide many sources of ideas to combine simple play with learning. My experience with children, whether they have or have not got a disability, satisfies me that young children get as much enjoyment playing with simple things found in their homes as with expensive toys. This is probably one of the reasons why, when a child borrows a toy from a toy library, the toy is returned but the box is often missing.

Some dos and don'ts when playing

Keep advice and help to a minimum

In our efforts to improve the physical function of children with cerebral palsy we may tend to interfere with and direct their play too much. When a child is playing with bricks, for example, we all tend to make the mistake of advising, to 'Try the small one on top of the large one', or when the child tries to take the lid off a jar, 'Don't pull, turn the lid round and unscrew it'. Then again, as the child attempts to push a large model car through a narrow tunnel, 'You will never manage that, try the little car'. The point stressed here is that the child will learn far more seeing the large brick fall off, or failing to get the lid off the jar by pulling or failing to push the big car through the tunnel.

As a child with CP does not learn as spontaneously and easily as a child typically would, it is important that we balance this help by allowing children to make their own mistakes, asking for help when they feel it is needed. All this calls for patience. Some children can only manage to play for 5 minutes at a time, whereas others may play the same game quite happily for 20 minutes. Try always to understand what new things your child is attempting to do and give the appropriate materials and opportunities, helping only when there is a real difficulty.

Far too often, children with CP, lacking in experience and in imagination, never get past the stage, when playing with their cars, for example, of lining them up and then returning them straight to their box, or pushing their trains around and around in the same direction. A good way of helping a child use imagination is by building a garage for the cars, so that the child can pretend to fill them up with petrol and oil and to wash them, as may have been seen at a garage. No child learns unless interested, and it is therefore up to us to stimulate interest by helping them think of new ideas and situations while playing. Make sure that it is possible for the child to participate actively in the various games, for this is a good way by which there will be benefit and learning.

Imitative play

The typical child

Between 2 and 3 years of age, children begin to be interested in activities going on around them as well as playing with their toys. Anything that Mummy uses or does is fascinating and must be examined and tried. They continually watch and imitate their mother as they play; they want to polish with a duster, to stir with a spoon; to try to wash, dress and undress and take care of their dolls in the same way as their mother looks after them.

Play now becomes more varied, and symbolic play develops – dolls have tea parties, are put to bed, scolded and praised. If there is a new baby, they are only too anxious to have a live 'doll' to play with, if given the chance. When there are older children in the family, they watch and copy them, listen to stories about school and enact the various episodes with their toys.

The child with cerebral palsy

The child with CP often has the same desire to join in the activities of the mother, brothers and sisters, but the disability prevents this happening. If the child is to have a chance of enjoying these new experiences, help must be available.

If you are polishing and dusting, give your child a duster; even the more severely disabled child can polish for you while sitting in a chair. A child who drags the toes of the shoes when walking may be put in charge of cleaning and polishing them. It may even encourage the child to try harder to lift the feet. A child who can walk, but does so in a rather disorganized manner, can help polish the floor if you wrap dusters over the child's shoes. This should help to improve coordination and balance, as well as giving pleasure in helping you.

The kitchen is another place where your child can help and learn at the same time; let your child help to cut out some pastry cases, give something to stir, put the salt in the potatoes for you, let your child make buns. Show and explain what you are doing; for example, when you make a cake or dessert, give some of the ingredients to pour into the bowl or let your child help you to weigh them. The child will be learning all the time while watching and helping you.

Remember that there will be many questions the child would like to ask, but, either because speech is poor or it takes time to put ideas into words, the child loses the opportunity. The head of a school for disabled children told me that often when children are asked at school, for example, how pastry is made, the reply comes back: 'You get it from a frozen packet and roll it out', or when asked where milk comes from, 'From a milk bottle'. This is what they have seen and, if the first answer is accepted without question, may remain the full extent of their knowledge.

Shape recognition

The typical child

At around 4 years of age a child begins to group together similar shapes and objects, and later to identify them when asked, for example, which is the circle, the square? This is done by matching shapes, picking one out from a group of shapes, seeing the shape in three dimensions, imitating, copying and finally reproducing the shape when asked.

The child with cerebral palsy

Difficulty in recognizing and differentiating between various shapes and forms is one of the many factors which may prevent the child with CP from learning to read and to write. It is therefore worthwhile spending time helping the child to feel, to recognize and match different shapes while playing. This can be done by teaching about one shape at a time, mastering and recognizing that one shape before introducing another. The following example illustrates how you might do this with a circle.

Give your child a ball and describe its shape, then take the child's fingers and place them round the ball, letting the child feel it in the hands. Let your child see, because of its shape, how it rolls, then take a square and show why, because the square has corners, it cannot roll. Find objects of the same shape, i.e. different-sized balls, an orange. Later, get your child to make the shape in play dough or flour dough. You can then show the round shape in a quoit or other ring and how this circle is a space through which your child can see, pass things through or place over objects. Then point out the same round shape in cups, lids, saucers, saucepans.

When out for a walk, collect some round stones, point out the round of the wheels of the cars and buses, the round flower beds in the park. In this way your child may learn to associate a particular shape with many objects, thus extending awareness of the things around. Place a round sweet among some square ones and ask your child to find the round one. Later, collect together a mixture of round and square objects and ask your child to place them into two different groups. Your child should then be encouraged to make the same shapes with the fingers in sand, flour, with finger paints and with a pencil or crayons. A supermarket is also an excellent place for a child to learn colour, size, shape and texture, and also when unloading your shopping basket at home.

Some children find it difficult to grasp and lift an object but are nevertheless ready to learn about the concept of shape and form. A magnetic board is useful for such children. It can be placed flat on a table or propped up at any angle from the perpendicular to the horizontal, or even attached to a pegboard on the wall. The makers of magnetic boards also supply figures, letters, shapes and a variety of designs which are easy for the child to handle as little effort is required to move them around the board. You can buy magnetic strips for use on a flat magnetic board that can be attached to any toy.

When a child is learning to place shapes in a simple form board, the child will sometimes find handling them easier if you start by giving shapes that have a knob on the top. These should not be too large or they may distort the outline of the shape for the child. Begin by taking one shape at a time out of the board and letting the child put it back; then take two, and when the child has mastered three shapes take them all out at once and let the child replace them. Later, turn the board around and ask the child to replace the shapes again.

When a child has difficulty in using the hands this will take time and patience, but continue to persevere, as the learning and understanding of shape is a very important step for many skills, including when starting to read and write. Your occupational therapist will analyse the particular difficulties your child presents with and show you exactly how you can help.

Simple puzzles

A child's first puzzles should have clear simple pictures with a well-defined background and foreground, as a picture with too much detail will only be confusing for the child. Before trying to do the puzzle let your child really get to know the picture, then take one piece out and let the child replace it, immediately becoming familiar with each shape. In this way it will be much easier to understand how each piece fits the whole.

The field of perception is a most specialized one and your child's occupational therapist, and later teachers, will give you expert advice on how to follow up training. This will include, for example, learning how to distinguish between tall and short objects, a comparison difficult for the child with CP who spends much time on the floor or sitting in a chair, and therefore builds up a concept of the size and height of things around in a limited way. This point has been demonstrated to us by a child of 11 years who, when stood up for the first time, was amazed to find that the refrigerator, tables and chairs were so much smaller than this child had thought.

Colour awareness

A child learns about colour in a definite sequence, first by learning a primary colour, which will soon be recognized, although when shown another colour in comparison will often find it difficult to identify the second. Once the child has learned to identify the primary colours, matching similar colours should be started, describing them by name and, finally, naming the colour of things around.

Toy libraries

Toy libraries have been set up in many countries throughout the world. Some are run by volunteers, others by parents themselves or by professionals with a special interest in play, such as nursery and school teachers, health visitors, therapists and psychologists. They may be found in a variety of locations: in nursery and primary schools, health centres, hospitals, public libraries, mobile vans and play buses.

Toy libraries provide a selection of good-quality toys for children with physical, speech and language difficulties, visual impairment and learning problems. Many also have a reference library of books, booklets and catalogues which specialize in various aspects of play activities and toys.

The advantages of using a toy library are two-fold. Firstly, it enables a child to have a variety of toys of particular value for developing special skills at different stages in development; and secondly, it enables parents to discuss the various learning situations possible with each toy and gives an opportunity for an exchange of ideas between parents and members of the library and parents with one another.

Parents in England can apply to become a member of the National Association of Toy and Leisure Libraries (NATLL) which will enable them to receive mailings, including the quarterly membership magazine *Play Matters*, discounts on the NATLL's publications, advice, support and information. International links are maintained by the NATLL through the International Toy Library Association, and they can provide the addresses of toy libraries throughout continental Europe and the rest of the world.

It is hoped that, in the foregoing, it has been made clear how learning through play is essential for all children, and that in the process they are being prepared for the basic learning experiences which they gain when they go to nursery school.

Activities which may encourage motor skills through play

The following illustrations may be helpful as a means of utilizing positions and activities towards greater independence in gross and fine motor activities. Depending upon their level of severity, many children with CP will not be able to progress through the spectrum of motor skills described but will get stuck at one of the earlier stages.

Ways to encourage play in sitting

Practising and refining the skill of sitting up may help the child with communication and socialization plus eating, drinking, washing and playing. It may enable the child to see both hands more easily and to use them more effectively (Figures 23.1–23.8).

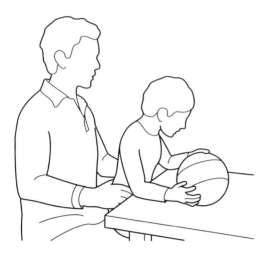

Figure 23.1 • Child sitting securely on the father's lap. The child is able to bend forward and self-support on the elbows and forearms. If given a toy such as a ball, the child is able to move it around with the hands and make something happen without someone else's assistance.

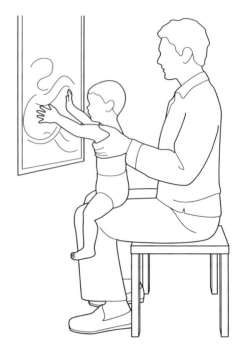

Figure 23.3 • Child sitting astride the father's knee and being supported at the shoulders. The child is playing with both hands using play foam on a mirror.

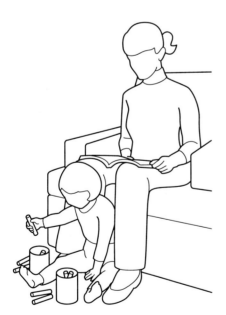

Figure 23.2 • Child sitting between the mother's legs, which are controlling the child's shoulders while the mother's feet provide stability to the child's hips. The child is sorting red and blue rods while the mother is reading.

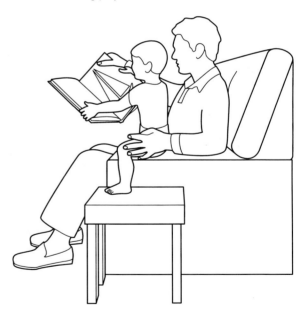

Figure 23.4 • Child sitting across the arm of an armchair with one foot supported on a stool and the other on the base of the armchair. The father is stabilizing the child's pelvis. The child is helping to hold the book, pointing to pictures in it and naming them with some prompts from the father.

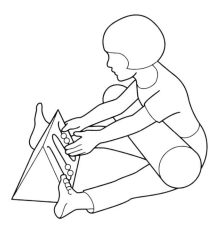

Figure 23.5 • Child sitting on the floor with a small roll placed over the thighs over which the child can bend forward and play with the activity toy.

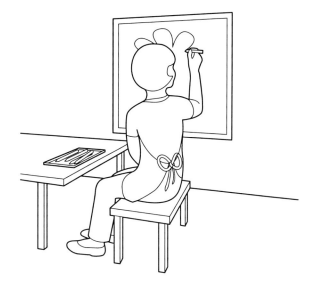

Figure 23.7 • Child sitting on a low stool placed in front of a table and next to the wall. The child is drawing with chalk on to the blackboard placed at a low level on the wall.

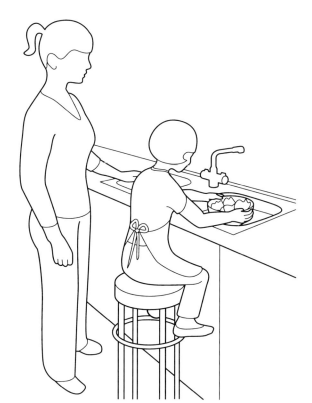

Figure 23.6 • Child sitting on a high stool supporting the elbows on the kitchen surface, the knees against the kitchen cupboards and the feet on the rung of the stool, washing the vegetables in a colander. A parent is nearby.

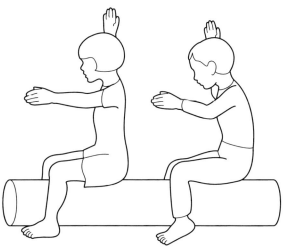

Figure 23.8 • Child sitting over a roll behind a friend copying the movements that the friend makes.

Ways to encourage play on the floor

Figures 23.9–23.11 may be helpful in encouraging a child to move and explore on the floor when creeping/commando crawling/crawling are the methods of locomotion.

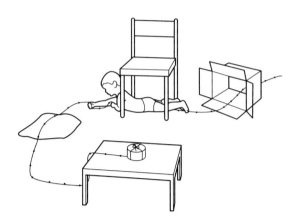

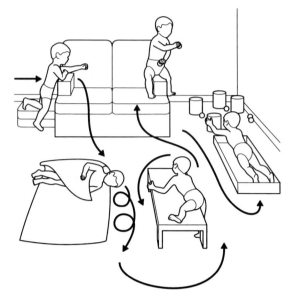

Figure 23.9 • Obstacle course made by using various objects under and over which the child is encouraged to creep/commando crawl. The sequence is determined by a line drawn with coloured chalk. As an incentive a small prize, put into a box so that it is a secret, may be placed at the end of the course.

Figure 23.11 • Obstacle course made by using various objects around which the child is encouraged to scramble and partake in certain activities in competition with siblings or friends.

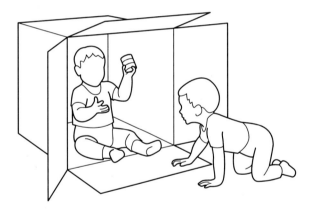

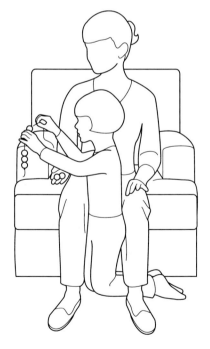

Figure 23.10 • A large cardboard box which can be used as a house for crawling into, out of and around with a sibling or friend.

Ways to encourage play in upright kneeling

Practising and refining the skill of upright kneeling may help the child to balance in standing later (Figures 23.12–23.18).

Figure 23.12 • Child in an upright kneeling position supported and controlled by the mother's legs. The child is busy threading cotton reels.

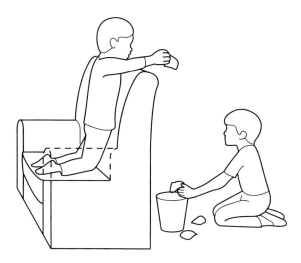

Figure 23.13 • Child using the back of a stable armchair for support in upright kneeling and throwing bean bags into a bucket below.

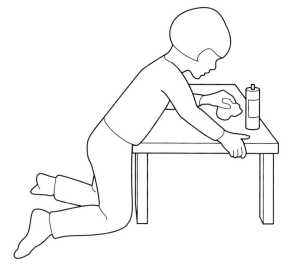

Figure 23.15 • Child upright kneeling using a low table for trunk support, holding on with one hand while wiping the table with the other.

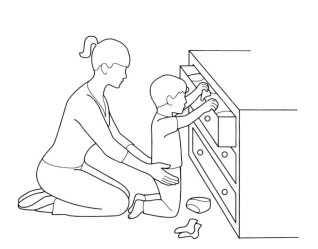

Figure 23.14 • Child getting clothes out of a low chest of drawers in the upright kneeling position. The mother is holding the child around the hips to support as needed so as to prevent the child wobbling at the hips.

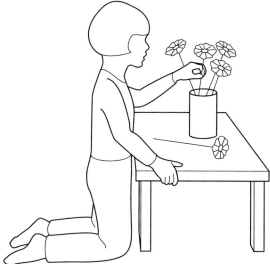

Figure 23.16 • Child holding the low table with one hand only in the kneeling position and arranging flowers with the other hand.

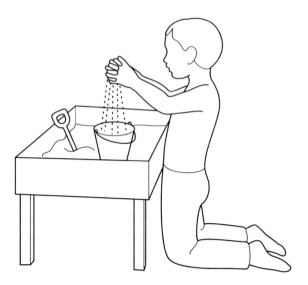

Figure 23.17 • Child playing with sand with two hands in the upright kneeling position.

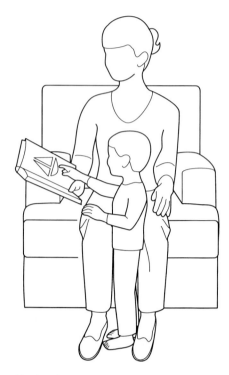

Figure 23.19 • Child standing supported by the mother's legs and holding on to her thigh with one hand while the other is used to point at pictures in a book, maybe even tracing around the pictures with a finger.

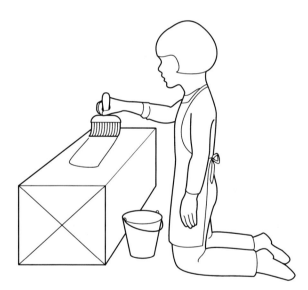

Figure 23.18 • Child painting a large cardboard box in the upright kneeling position without support apart from that gained through the painting hand.

Ways to encourage play in standing

Practising and refining the skill of standing may help the child with weight-bearing and transferring from one position or place to another position or place (Figures 23.19–23.24).

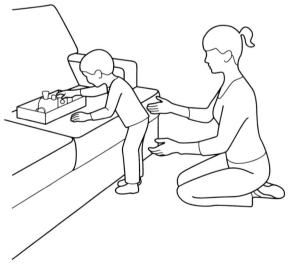

Figure 23.20 • Child standing at a sofa leaning on it with one arm and the chest and playing with some toys in a box with the other arm and hand. The mother is behind the child in case of a fall.

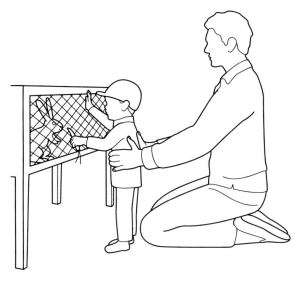

Figure 23.21 • Child standing with support from the father at the trunk and leaning against a rabbit hutch with one hand while giving the rabbit a carrot with the other hand.

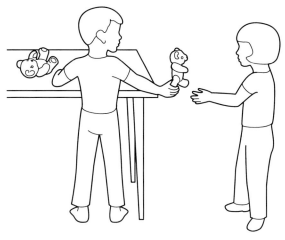

Figure 23.23 • Child playing at a table with one hand supporting on the table while turning to give a toy to a friend slightly behind and to the right of the child.

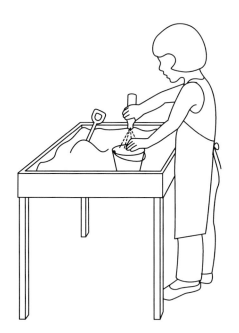

Figure 23.22 • Child standing at a sand pit supporting with one hand and playing with the other.

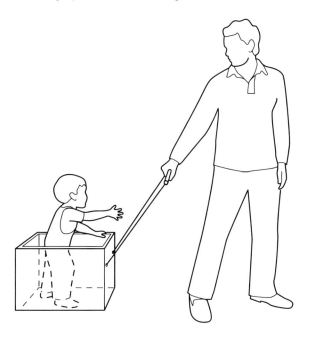

Figure 23.24 • Child standing in a box holding on with one hand while being pulled along.

Ways to encourage a child to get from sitting to standing

Getting from sitting to standing and vice versa is a useful skill if getting on and off a chair or toilet. It is generally easier for a child to get to standing from sitting on a stool or chair than from sitting on the floor. This is especially true if the child is offered a pair of hands or a bar which can be grasped by the child and from which the child can pull up to standing (Figures 23.25–23.29).

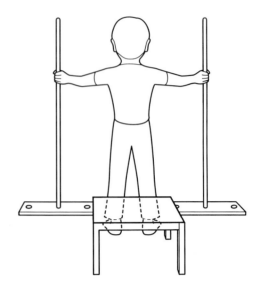

Figure 23.27 • Child grasping two well-secured sticks placed slightly in front of the child and the child grasping the sticks and pulling up from sitting to standing. This movement can also be practised using a ladderback chair.

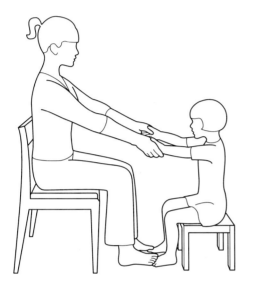

Figure 23.25 • Child sitting on a stool, hands outstretched to the mother, ready to pull up to standing holding on to the mother's hands.

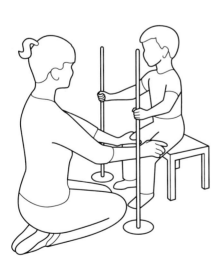

Figure 23.26 • Child grasping two well-secured sticks placed slightly in front of the child and the child grasping the sticks and pulling up from sitting to standing. This movement can also be practised using a ladderback chair.

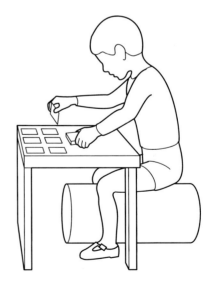

Figure 23.28 • Child sitting over a roll at a low table playing with cards and pulling to stand at the table by pushing up using one hand while still playing with the other.

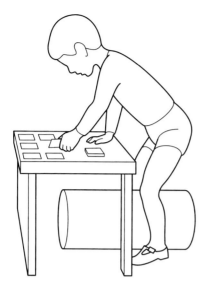

Figure 23.29 • Child sitting over a roll at a low table playing with cards and pulling to stand at the table by pushing up using one hand while still playing with the other.

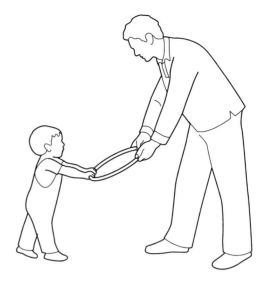

Figure 23.31 • Child walking forwards holding on to a hoop with two hands. The hoop is supported by another person walking backwards.

Ways to encourage a child to walk (Figures 23.30–23.37)

As stated at the beginning of this section on encouraging motor skills through play, many children with CP will not be able to progress through all the

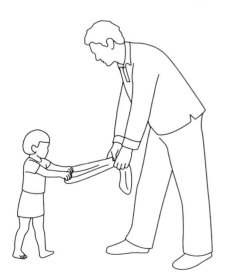

Figure 23.30 • Child walking forwards holding on to a towel with two hands. The towel is held by another person in front of the child who walks backwards.

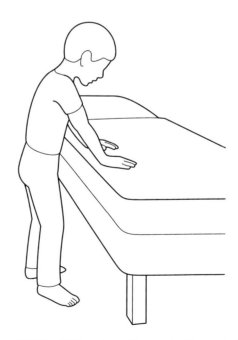

Figure 23.32 • Child walking sideways holding on to the edge of a bed.

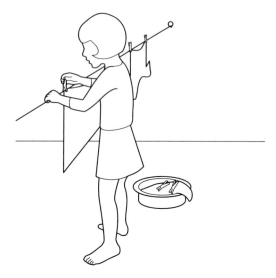

Figure 23.33 • Child walking sideways holding on to a washing line.

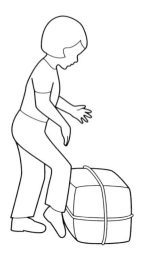

Figure 23.36 • Child walking forwards kicking a large parcel at each step.

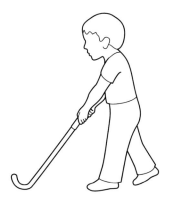

Figure 23.34 • Child walking forwards with a hockey stick.

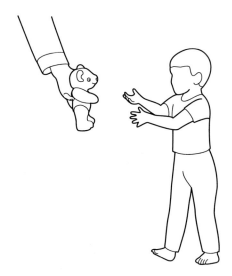

Figure 23.37 • Child walking forwards encouraged by a parent holding a soft toy in front, which the child can always grab if needed for balance or support.

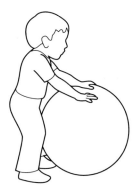

Figure 23.35 • Child walking forwards with two hands on a large ball.

stages described above. The Gross Motor Function Classification System (Palisano et al. 1997) described in Chapter 20 may give you an idea of how far your child with CP is likely to progress in gross motor activities. The amount of encouragement needed by individual children with CP to reach their likely motor ability level will be largely determined by their particular cognitive, behavioural and visual characteristics. Nevertheless some of the positions described may be helpful in counteracting the development of deformity.

Reference

Palisano R, Rosenbaum P, Walter S et al. Development and validation of a gross motor function classification system for children with CP. Dev Med Child Neurol 1997; 39:214–223.

Chapter
Twenty Four

Leisure and fitness

Revised by Eva Bower

Most children enjoy taking part in a physical hobby or activity, even if they are not particularly good at it. We are now beginning to realize how important it is for all children and adults to exercise regularly to promote better health and fitness. This fact applies to all children, whether they have cerebral palsy (CP) or not. In fact it is probably even more important for children with physical movement problems as in CP to exercise as actively as possible as they are likely to have a more sedentary lifestyle or, to put it another way, to move about less and more slowly and to spend more time sitting than their peers. Such physical inactivity may lead to a lowering of energy levels, increasing fatigue and increasing movement difficulties so that the less children with CP move, the harder it becomes for them to move.

Physical activity may promote physical health and fitness in a child with CP by:

1. Controlling weight and discouraging obesity

2. Encouraging the development of muscles and the growth of bones

3. Improving cardiovascular endurance and physical stamina

4. Improving respiratory function and the control of breathing

5. Protecting against osteoporosis and fractures in the bones

Physical activity or exercise may also promote emotional health and fitness in a child with CP by:

1. Being enjoyable and fun

2. Being part of a team or group activity which may encourage sharing and turn-taking

3. Encouraging a sense of achievement, which is important for good self-esteem

Care must always be taken that your child does not overstrain or overtrain and that the joints are protected from potential damage.

Damaged joints lead to pain in later life.

Before your child with CP undertakes a new physical activity it is necessary to check with your paediatrician or general practitioner that it is a good idea and that the professional thinks it is a suitable physical activity for your child. This is especially important if your child has epilepsy or a sensory problem in addition.

It is also important to ensure your child is supervised by an instructor who is, firstly, qualified in the particular activity to be undertaken by your child and, secondly, knowledgeable about the condition and problems of your child. This person may be a therapist or a teacher.

The more common physical activities organized for children with movement problems under 5 years of age are music and movement, swimming and horse riding. In addition to improving general health, music and movement may encourage children to improve their spatial relationships, such as up and down and left and right, their visual and auditory discrimination, eye–hand coordination and fine motor skills. Swimming and horse riding may also encourage children to improve their body symmetry, trunk control and overall mobility and balance.

Music and movement

From the very early days in a child's life most mothers and fathers sing to and with their child, adding in gestures, actions and movements appropriate to the words of the songs. At first the parent performs these gestures, actions and movements with the child, helping the child to point an arm upwards, stretch a leg downwards or collapse into a bodily heap and then rise again stretching upwards. As the child develops independent movement the child will take over and increasingly respond actively and spontaneously with the appropriate gestures, actions and movements. Many songs and nursery rhymes lend themselves well to such exercise and give enjoyment to both parent and child. As the child gets older the activity will be continued at nursery or playgroup together with other children.

Examples are:

1. Mother sings 'How big are you?' to her child and then responds for her child with 'So big', raising both her child's arms gently upwards towards the ceiling. Gradually as able her child takes over the words and actions. This song can be sung with the child sitting supported on the mother's lap.

2. Mother sings 'Row, row, row the boat, gently down the stream. Merrily, merrily, merrily, merrily, life is but a dream.' During this song the mother and her child sit on the floor facing each other and the mother holds the child's hands and together they rock their trunks gently forwards and backwards. Initially the movement and posture are controlled by the mother but gradually her child takes over.

3. 'Head and shoulders, knees and toes, knees and toes. Head and shoulders, knees and toes, knees and toes. And eyes and ears and mouth and nose. Head and shoulders, knees and toes, knees and toes.'

   While the nursery nurses and children sing this song the children are encouraged to point to the body parts named with both hands.

   This song can be sung in sitting or standing, either supported or not as necessary.

4. 'As tall as a house, as wide as a bridge, as small as a mouse, as thin as a pin.'

   While the nursery nurses and children sing this song the children are encouraged to:
   (a) make themselves as tall as possible;
   (b) make themselves as wide as possible;
   (c) make themselves as small as possible; and
   (d) make themselves as thin as possible.

   This song can be sung in supported or free sitting or standing.

5. 'Can you walk on tiptoe as softly as a cat? Can you stamp along the road, stamp, stamp, stamp, like that? Can you take some great big strides just like a giant can? Or walk along so slowly like a poor old, bent old man?'

   While the nursery nurses and children sing this song the children are encouraged to:
   (a) walk on tiptoe;
   (b) stamp their feet on the ground noisily;
   (c) walk with very long steps; and
   (d) walk along very slowly and carefully.

   This song can be sung in supported or non-supported standing or walking.

Box 24.1 lists some other songs which can be used in English or translated into another language.

Music and movement action songs should be repeated several times each day. Young children love the repetition of such activity. It is however important to remain aware of your child's

Box 24.1

Action songs

Incy wincy spider, climbing up the spout
Down came the rain and washed the spider out
Out came the sunshine and dried up all the rain
Incy wincy spider climbed the spout again

Two little dicky birds sitting on the wall
One named Peter, one named Paul
Fly away Peter, fly away Paul
Come back Peter, come back Paul

One, two, three, four, five
Once I caught a fish alive
Six, seven, eight, nine, ten
Then I let it go again
Why did you let it go?
Because it bit my finger so
Which finger did it bite?
This little finger on the right

I hear thunder, I hear thunder
Hark! Don't you? Hark! Don't you?
Pitter patter raindrops, pitter patter raindrops
I'm wet through, so are you

I'm a dingle-dangle scarecrow
With a flippy-floppy hat
I can shake my hands like this
And stamp my feet like that

Tommy Thumb, Tommy Thumb
Where are you?
Here I am, here I am
How do you do?

Jack-in-the-box
Still as a mouse
Deep down inside
Your little dark house
Jack-in-the-box
Resting so still
Will you come out?
Yes, I will!

Other action songs

The grand old Duke of York
Here we go round the mulberry bush
Ring a ring of roses
Humpty Dumpty sat on a wall
Hickory, dickory, dock

chronological age and to advance the songs and movements appropriately. The natural progression is towards pop songs with older children and movements may progress to dance, if required in wheelchairs. Another natural progression is to aerobic exercises from earlier music and movement sessions.

Swimming

Most children love playing with water and find it great fun. If your child is apprehensive and not quite sure, encourage gentle splashing in the bath with both hands and feet, cupping water in the hands and then letting it trickle out through the fingers, progressing to putting water on the face and lying down supine in the bath and getting the hair wet. If the weather is sufficiently warm, supervised play in a paddling pool in the garden is another good preliminary activity before swimming.

When to start swimming

If there are no contraindications the best time to start swimming with children is between 9 and 12 months old as at this stage there is generally little fear of water.

Where to start swimming

If possible it is probably best to start by joining a small group organized by a qualified swimming instructor, who should always be present, for mothers and/or fathers and their children. Such a lesson would take place in the local teaching or therapy pool where the water is kept at about 30°C (86°F).

Swimming pools are often noisy places so if your child is sensitive to noise try to choose a quieter, less busy corner of the pool.

Flotation or buoyancy aids

There are conflicting views on the use of flotation and buoyancy aids. Most mainstream swimming instructors recommend their use. Figure 24.1

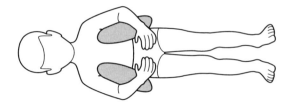

Figure 24.1 • Using this swimming float enables the child to lie on the back with the legs horizontal in the pool.

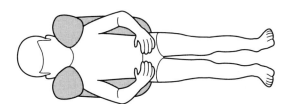

Figure 24.2 • Child using a buoyancy aid.

illustrates one type of swimming float which enables the child to lie on the back with the legs horizontal in the pool. If the float is repositioned the child can lie on the tummy horizontal in the pool, but *always watch the child carefully in this position and be sure that the face remains out of the water*.

Figure 24.2 shows a child floating in the pool on an aid and enjoying a newfound independence, but again *never leave a child unwatched on such an aid*.

The Halliwick method for teaching the disabled to swim, evolved by James McMillan and championed by Margaret Reid, suggests that the use of flotation or buoyancy aids is undesirable. They say that the aids hamper the child's ability to move freely in water and to learn to control the body independently. They suggest instead a number of different ways of holding the child in the water.

Getting into the swimming pool

If there is a ramp down into the pool and your child is small it is probably best to walk down the ramp carrying your child into the water.

If your child is heavy and there is a hoist available use it to lower your child gently and slowly into the water, telling your child all the time what you are doing.

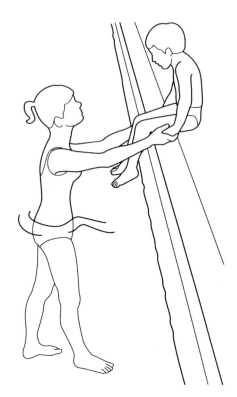

Figure 24.3 • Getting into the swimming pool: step 1.

If neither of these facilities is available or appropriate, sit your child at the edge of the pool and let yourself into the water first, gently and without splashing while holding on to your child sitting at the edge, as shown in Figure 24.3.

Figure 24.4 shows you standing in the water putting your child's hands on to your shoulders and placing your hands around your child's trunk.

Figure 24.5 shows that you have made sure that your child's feet are dangling freely and are not hooked into the side of the pool. Stepping back, you bring your child forwards and downwards towards you and into the water.

Holding your child in the swimming pool

Never grip your child but hold firmly with both hands just below your child's waist whether your child is lying as shown in Figure 24.6 or is sitting facing you, or with their back to you in an upright position as shown in Figure 24.7.

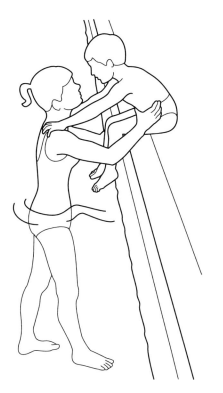

Figure 24.4 • Getting into the swimming pool: step 2.

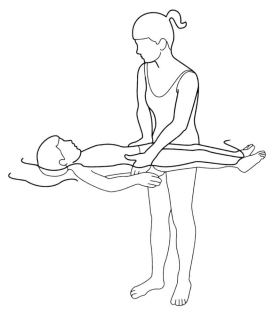

Figure 24.6 • Holding a child who is lying.

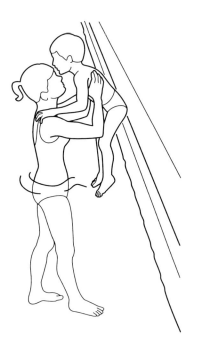

Figure 24.5 • Getting into the swimming pool: step 3.

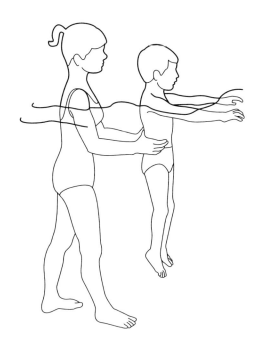

Figure 24.7 • Holding a child in an upright position.

While in the water activities usually take the form of games, the ultimate goal of which is to produce a competent swimmer.

Getting out of the swimming pool

If neither a ramp up and out of the pool nor a hoist is available or appropriate, bring your child to the edge of the pool and holding your child around the pelvis with both of you facing the edge of the pool, put your child's hands up on to the edge of the pool (Figure 24.8).

Figure 24.9 shows you lifting your child upwards and forwards on to the edge from the hips and your child ready to wriggle forwards, pushing on the arms.

Figure 24.10 shows that having taken a step backwards, you lift the child's legs clear of the water and your child continues to wriggle forwards.

Figure 24.11 shows you helping your child to roll on to his or her back by crossing the legs. The child may then creep or crawl away from the pool if able. Figure 24.12 shows you helping your child to sit up if this is required.

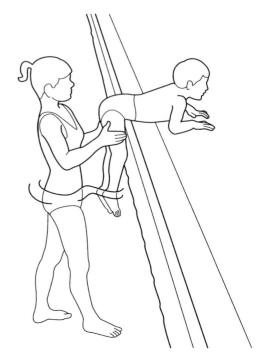

Figure 24.9 • Getting out of the swimming pool: step 2.

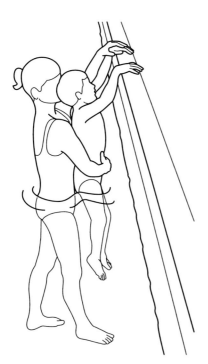

Figure 24.8 • Getting out of the swimming pool: step 1.

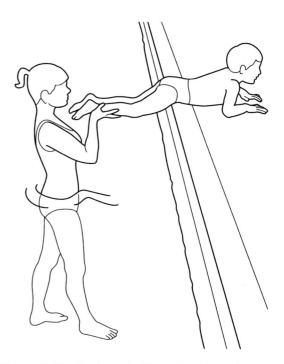

Figure 24.10 • Getting out of the swimming pool: step 3.

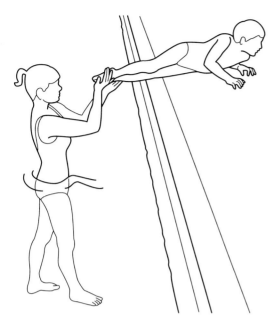

Figure 24.11 • Getting out of the swimming pool: step 4.

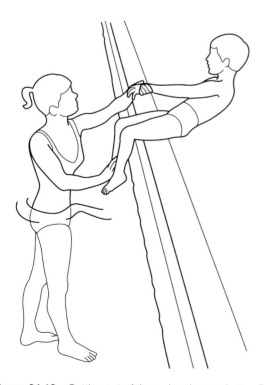

Figure 24.12 • Getting out of the swimming pool: step 5.

This set of manoeuvres is not suitable for a child with a lack of head control or an inability to commando crawl.

Swimming is a sport that can be started young and continued throughout life. It can be socially beneficial in that it can become a family pastime or a competitive sport against non-disabled peers.

Horse riding

Riding a horse can be a very pleasant, recreational activity for a child with CP, providing good exercise and the opportunity to develop a rapport with an animal and enabling the child to learn to care for an animal by joining in the general stable management which includes grooming, feeding and watering the horse plus cleaning or mucking out the stable and cleaning the tack or equipment. These activities may help to promote self-confidence and esteem in a child so long as the child is not frightened of horses, in which case horse riding is probably not an appropriate activity until the problem is resolved.

If a child is to ride a horse it is imperative that a correctly fitting hard riding hat manufactured according to the necessary British Safety Authority standard is worn.

In addition many instructors, riding schools and parents like their child to wear a well-fitting, waistcoat-like back protector. Apart from shoes or boots with a slight heel, no other special clothing is essential. Older boys find boxer shorts uncomfortable.

The horse or pony selected for a child to ride should be of a quiet disposition and an appropriate size. Suitable arrangements must be in place to enable the child to mount and dismount the horse safely.

Riding for the child with CP falls into three basic categories – hippotherapy, therapeutic riding and recreational riding.

Hippotherapy

The purpose of hippotherapy is not to teach riding but to use a horse and its movements to meet specific therapy objectives and goals. The session is usually supervised by a certified riding instructor. Each child works individually with a physiotherapist or occupational therapist and many positions on the horse are used, for example:

1. Lying over the horse to try to develop head and trunk control and relax the extremities

2. Sitting backwards on the horse with the hands on the rump to try to develop weight-bearing

3. Lying supine over the rump to try to mobilize the spine and shoulder girdle

Therapeutic riding

In therapeutic riding the child is usually a member of a small group. A therapeutic group is usually taken by a specially trained, certified riding instructor. A physiotherapist or occupational therapist may also be part of the team advising on suitable warm-up and cool-down exercises as well as any specific group activities that would enable all the children in the group to participate.

Riding is taught but there is an emphasis on symmetry, head and trunk control and sitting balance as well as sensorimotor skills and educational objectives. Children may be kept on a leading rein and aided by one or more assistants if needed.

Recreational riding

Recreational riding is usually reserved for the child who will be able to ride independently. The child needs to be safe but also to have fun. It can be taught on a one-to-one basis or in a group but instruction needs to be given by a qualified person. As everyone who has ridden a horse will know, riding a horse with expertise exercises the muscles of the legs, the pelvis, the trunk and the arms. On the one hand it can be an exhilarating and satisfying experience for a child – on the other it can be very tiring.

Summary

Music and movement may encourage the development of muscles and the growth of bones and, if weight-bearing through the legs is included, may protect against osteoporosis.

Swimming may improve cardiovascular function and breathing control.

Riding may encourage the development of muscles and the growth of bones.

All three activities use up energy and therefore may control weight and discourage obesity.

They all encourage much-needed active movement.

Fitness is needed for life and to this end exercise should be started early. Music and movement is one way to start exercising at a young age with a progression on to leisure and recreational activities such as swimming, horse riding, dancing and aerobic exercise.

Exercise needs to be continued throughout life.

Chapter Twenty Five

Deformity: growth and the problems of getting taller

David Scrutton

CHAPTER CONTENTS

A child with cerebral palsy (CP) is no more likely to be born misshapen than any other child but, because CP is likely to restrict the amount and the range of movement regularly used, some structures may gradually develop disproportionately. These changes, which occur as children grow, can be so mild as to be unnoticeable and of no consequence, or be mildly restricting, or become a major aspect of their life and the management of their CP. Health workers call these changes *deformities*.

Deformities

Why does the body grow like this? Our bones grow but our muscles, tendons, ligaments (around joints), veins, arteries, nerves and skin just gradually elongate to keep up, adapting to the forces applied to them by the bones' growth and by our movements and habitual postures. Muscles do not get longer unless they are stretched. Stretched too much, they get too long and stretched too little they become too short; and both happen in CP. The term *deformity* is usually only used to describe structures which are too short, *because they restrict movement and so can limit a child's postural and movement opportunities.*

The word *contracture* is frequently used to describe short muscles and tendons but it is really incorrect for young children with CP and it may be of interest to explain why. *Contracture* implies that something has shortened: it *was* a certain length and *is now* shorter; but this is not what happens in CP until perhaps later in life. A newborn baby's body tissues are the lengths determined by intrauterine postures and movements and as the infant develops and bones grow they adjust their lengths to the new (extrauterine) situation. Children lacking typical movement and postural development adapt to their (different) experiences and so some of their tissues may fail to keep up and are 'short'. They have not contracted – they have probably grown longer – but they have failed to lengthen enough to allow a full range of movement. That difference between contracting and not growing quite enough is important as it relates to the way in which we treat the child.

Where do deformities occur?

At a joint

1. *Temporary or postural*, when the range of movement is *not* limited but the muscle action allows postures or movements of only limited range

2. *Fixed deformity*, when the range of movement is *always* limited because soft tissues (muscle, tendon, ligaments) are not long enough to allow a full range of movement

3. When the joint surfaces have changed shape or are no longer fitting together properly (dislocated)

In a bone

1. The bone has become wrongly shaped. Sometimes (e.g. in the thigh bone) it is not immediately obvious that the problem is within the bone rather than limited joint range

2. The bone is the wrong length (seldom by very much, but it can be a problem)

Secondary deformity

Some postural deformities are compensating for a deformity somewhere else. The child adopts an unusual posture, as this makes a movement or posture easier. It is important to recognize that the real (primary) problem is elsewhere. For instance, if the knee will not straighten fully the child may stand or walk with a bent hip, but there may be nothing wrong with the hip.

Movements, postures and muscle action

Movements, positions and muscle actions have names and it is worth becoming familiar with them because physiotherapists and orthopaedic surgeons use them in clinic.

Movements and positions

In general *flexion* means bending and *extension* means straightening. Bending forwards from the waist is flexing the spine and standing erect is extending it. Bending the spine to the side is called left or right *side flexion*.

Different words describe movements at the ankle and wrist: standing on tiptoe is extension but is more usually called *plantarflexion* and the opposite movement (when crouching) *dorsiflexion*. If the foot is fixed or always used in tiptoe it is called *equinus* and the opposite posture is *calcaneus*. Equinus and calcaneus imply a deformity (rather than a normal use) of a position or movement. At the wrist, these two movements are called *palmarflexion* and *dorsiflexion* and there is no different name for any deformity. The wrist also has some sideways movement: to the little-finger side it is called *ulnar deviation* and to the thumb side *radial deviation* (because the two forearm bones are the radius and the ulna).

The hips and shoulders can move in almost any direction and movement of a leg or arm away from the body is called *abduction* whereas movement taking the limb towards or across the body is *adduction*. In CP these terms are most often used about the hip, as hip deformity is a major problem for many children with CP. Some joints can also twist: movement of the hip can turn the knee inwards (*internal rotation*) or outwards (*external rotation*) and the same at the shoulder. The similar forearm movements have been given different names: when you hold your hand so you look at the palm the forearm is *supinated* and when you turn your palm away the forearm is *pronated*. Twisting the body to face right or left (called trunk rotation) is *right rotation* and *left rotation*.

Feet have more movements than being plantar-flexed and dorsiflexed at the ankle. They can *invert* (so the soles face each other) or turn out – *evert*. When the position of the foot cannot be corrected, an inverted foot is said to be *varus* and an everted foot is *valgus*.

Muscle action

A group of muscles which moves a part of the body in a direction is given the name of that direction. As a result, the muscles which straighten the knee are called knee extensors and those which move the thigh into abduction are called hip abductors.

There is no need to know these terms, but hospital visits can be more understandable and often less worrying if they are familiar.

Physical examination (looking for deformity)

Never use force to try to get greater range of movement. Keep light pressure to hold the position and either the muscles will gradually relax on their own, or there is no further movement possible in that situation.

Examining a child with CP for deformity requires skill and experience. It is not always easy or possible to overcome muscle spasm or control the body position properly so as to get a true range of movement. Assessment is the role of a physiotherapist, occupational therapist or orthopaedic surgeon. However it is useful for carers to understand what deformity is, how it is assessed and some of the likely problems. This part of the chapter will very briefly describe how you can see for yourself any of the physical limitations making movements difficult.

There will be greater detail about the legs than the arms and spine because, although the elbow and wrist are easily assessed, the ranges of movement of the shoulder blade and shoulder and of the hand are complex and require skilled examination. Apart from the very limited safety checks given below, examination of the spine requires someone experienced in managing the spine of children with CP and is quite outside the purpose of this chapter.

Arms

Can the fingers be straightened with the wrist in any position or only if the wrist is not stretched back (dorsiflexed), indicating tight finger flexor muscles? Can the thumb be moved fully, the tip touching the base of the little finger and out to the side, making a right angle with the index finger? Can the wrist be palmar- and dorsiflexed almost to a right angle?

With the elbow bent to a right angle (to make certain the movement is in the forearm and not the shoulder), can the hand turn palm to face and also turn 180° to face away? Elbow movements are straightforward but the shoulder is rather more difficult as the wide range of movement occurs in both the shoulder joint and the whole shoulder girdle.

Spine

For a carer there is one important spinal check. With support if necessary, sit the child on a chair or stool and bend the spine straight forwards with the head between the knees or as far as it will easily go. The spine should make a straight curve forward without deviating to left or right and the ribcage should be symmetrical right and left (Figure 25.1). Minor deviations are not unusual and need not be a cause of worry, but you should *always* demonstrate any twist, turn or asymmetry to your physiotherapist who can *either set your mind at rest or refer the child for further examination.*

Pelvis

The position of the pelvis is important and can be affected by the legs and the spine as it can transfer a problem from the legs to the trunk and vice versa (Figure 25.2). Asymmetric leg posture can

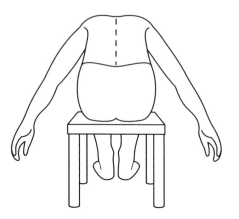

Figure 25.1 • Examination of the spine. The child is bent forward with the head between the knees. The spine should curve forwards in a straight line and not deviate to one side. The ribcage should be symmetrical right and left.

twist the pelvis and spine. Look at the position of the pelvis in lying, sitting and, if possible, standing. Is it symmetrical? If not, discuss this with your physiotherapist.

Legs

Examining the legs will be described in greater detail as they are common sites for deformity and affect total body posture in lying, sitting, standing and walking. Consequent spinal posture affects the postural stability needed for arm use and head control. CP varies in severity, the parts of the body affected and the type of movement disorder. The examination of the legs depends to some extent on whether the child is walking, has the possibility of walking or almost certainly will never walk. What is described below is a checklist

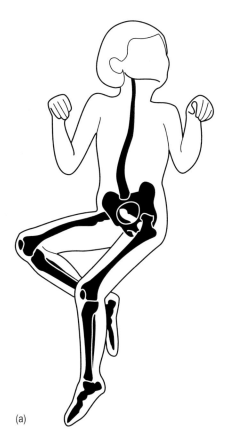

(a)

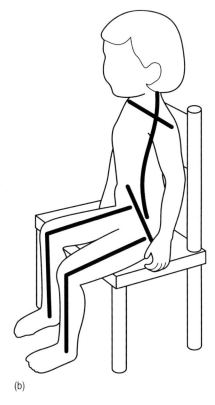

(b)

Figure 25.2 • (a, b) Although the body might appear straight when clothed, trunk side flexion or asymmetry of the hip posture can cause the pelvis to be oblique and by transmitting the asymmetry to the hips or spine respectively create a secondary postural deformity.

to give carers an insight into what physiotherapists and orthopaedic surgeons are looking for and thinking about when they examine a child.

Foot/ankle

When sitting, does the child have both feet flat on the floor? If not, is this because the heel is raised, the foot is turned in facing the other foot or rolled over into a flat-footed position? Can you correct the foot position with your hands? Strong muscle spasm can prevent you from correcting the position, but there may be a fixed deformity. If you can correct the position, but it springs back when you let go, it is muscle spasm which might be controlled with an orthosis.

Ankle joint

Getting the heel down on the floor is an ankle movement rather than in the foot. This position may be easier in sitting than in standing, because one of the calf muscles being stretched (the gastrocnemius muscle) also goes across the knee and so is relaxed when the knee is flexed for sitting. Lie the child face up, bend the hip and knee (Figure 25.3a) and correct the foot position as much as possible. Can the foot go past a right angle? If not, the whole calf muscle may be short. If it can, slowly straighten the leg (Figure 25.3b). Could you keep the corrected position? If not, standing with the heel down may not be possible because the gastrocnemius muscle is too tight.

Shin bone (tibia)

If a child walks with some difficulty, particularly if the knees point inwards all the time, the shin bone can gradually twist so than the foot turns in or out more than is normal. Lie the child face-down, bend one knee vertically and, with the foot held gently in a normal standing position, see which direction the foot points (Figure 25.4). If the bone is twisted, it is not something your child can correct when standing or walking.

Knee joint

Can it straighten? There are two tests which need to be done: the first relates to the knee when

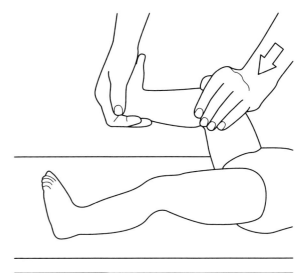

(a)

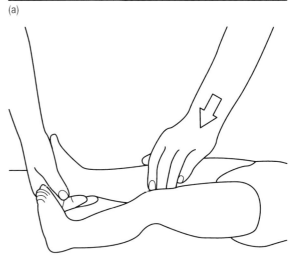

(b)

Figure 25.3 • Examination of the ankle. The range of dorsiflexion is often limited. (a) Check with the knee flexed to a right angle and then (b) gradually extending the knee to see whether the gastrocnemius muscle is tight.

standing: the maximum knee extension. Lie the child face up. Can you fully straighten the knee? Next check the tightness of the knee flexor muscles. The most important of these (hamstrings) also cross behind the hip joint and so are stretched when the hip is flexed (Figure 25.5). Flex one hip to a right angle and slowly extend the knee

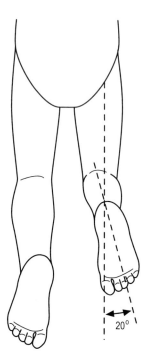

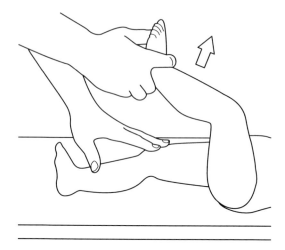

Figure 25.5 • Examination of the knee flexor muscles (hamstrings), tested one leg at a time while ensuring that the opposite leg is held on the floor to prevent rotation of the pelvis. Keeping the hip bent to 90°, gradually extend the knee. It needs to extend to more than 90° to allow sitting and perhaps a further 30° for walking.

Figure 25.4 • Examination for twist in the shin bone (tibia). Bend the knee to a right angle and, holding the foot in a normal position, look at the angle its midline makes with the thigh. The normal range is between a few degrees turned in to about 20° turned out.

(making sure that someone holds the other leg down). The range of movement is very different across the general population, but needs to be more than a right angle for those in wheelchairs and preferably more than 30° greater for those walking.

Can the knee joint bend fully? Lie the child face up and push the knees up to the tummy. The calf muscle should touch the back of the thigh. When the hip is extended tightness of one of the knee extensor muscles (rectus femoris, which also flexes the hip) can limit the flexion range. To test this, lie the child face-down and slowly bend the knee while gently pushing down on the buttocks to keep the hip straight (Figure 25.6). If there is no shortening of the muscle a full range of knee flexion can be reached without the buttock trying to rise (i.e. the hip flexing). Lack of a full range is usually only a problem for children who are walking. For sitting 90° flexion with the hips at 90° is needed.

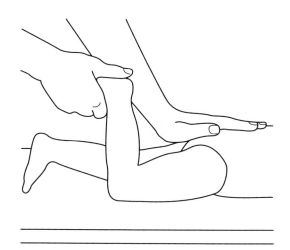

Figure 25.6 • Examination of knee flexion with the hip extended (rectus femoris muscle), tested one leg at a time ensuring that the buttocks do not rise (and so allowing greater knee flexion).

Hip joint

Joint ranges

The hip is a very mobile joint: it can flex, extend, abduct, adduct and rotate.

Rotation

Rotation of the thigh at the hip (seen as turning the knee inwards or outwards) depends on two things: the range of movement in the hip joint and the *position* of that range. The total range is usually about 90° but how much of that is externally or internally rotated varies markedly in the population. For example, some children have a genetic tendency to have much greater internal than external rotation and frequently use only a between-heel sitting position. This posture is sometimes discouraged for children with CP as it is thought to increase the internal rotation twist in the femur, but it seems unlikely to be the cause, as sitting in that position is very uncomfortable *unless you can already do it*. It is also a position with many advantages for children with CP:

1. It provides a secure base

2. It allows both hands to be used

3. It encourages good spinal and head posture

Put at its simplest, the *range* of movement comes from the hip joint, but *where* that range is comes from the amount of twist in the thigh bone (femur).

Thigh bone

In CP the twist in the thigh bone usually gives greater internal rotation so that the knee faces inwards when standing. Since this is primarily a problem for walking it is tested with the hips extended (the child lying face-down, as in Figure 25.7a and b). Bend both knees up to a right angle and, using the shins as pointers, rotate the thighs so as to separate the feet, making sure that the pelvis does not twist. This gives the ranges of internal rotation. External rotation is checked one leg at a time as otherwise they get in each other's way. Bend up one knee only and, again using the shin as a pointer, turn the leg the other way. Note any marked difference between the amount of internal and external rotation, as children usually walk most comfortably with their hip about halfway between the two extremes of the range (Figure 25.7c). Children who can *only just* take up a normal standing position will not use it when walking, but revert to their mid-position of rotation.

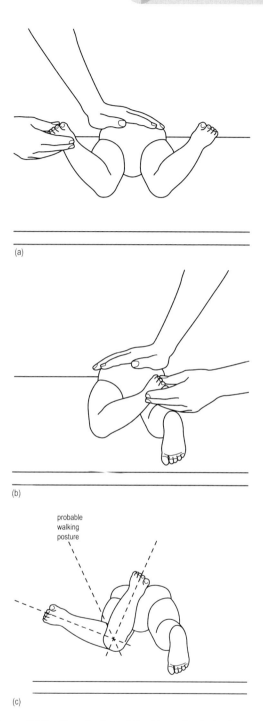

(a)

(b)

probable
walking
posture

(c)

Figure 25.7 • Examination of the hip and twist in the thigh bone (femur). (a) Internal rotation right and left legs together: ensure that the pelvis does not rotate. (b) External rotation one leg at a time: keep one hand on the buttocks to prevent the pelvis twisting (c).

Rotation in flexion for sitting (rotation with the hip extended has just been described)

Lie the child face-up and, keeping the one leg as flat as possible on the floor, bend the other leg so the hip and knee are at a right angle (Figure 25.8a). Now rotate the hip by using the shin as the hand of a clock to show the angle of external rotation. Testing internal rotation is easier done on both legs at the same time (Figure 25.8b). The ranges are very variable in the general population and testing in this position is mainly done to see that the child can take up a proper sitting position easily. A few severely affected children cannot rotate their hips in flexion sufficiently to allow correct sitting without twisting their pelvis (Figure 25.8c).

Extension

The full range of extension allows the thigh to go slightly beyond being straight and is examined one leg at a time in supine (Figure 25.9) by pushing the opposite leg up towards the tummy. The thigh should be able to touch the tummy without the straight (tested) leg coming off the floor. The angle that the tested leg makes with the floor is the hip's *fixed flexion*. Most children with hypertonic CP have a small amount of fixed flexion which may not matter unless it affects their walking. Significant limitation can affect hip joint stability.

Flexion

As just described, the thigh should be able to bend up to touch the tummy. Two things may prevent this: tight hip extensor muscles or a hip already dislocated. However it is important that the hip can flex to a right angle without encountering spastic or fixed resistance, as this is the range needed for good sitting posture. Ensure that the movement is happening at the hip and not in

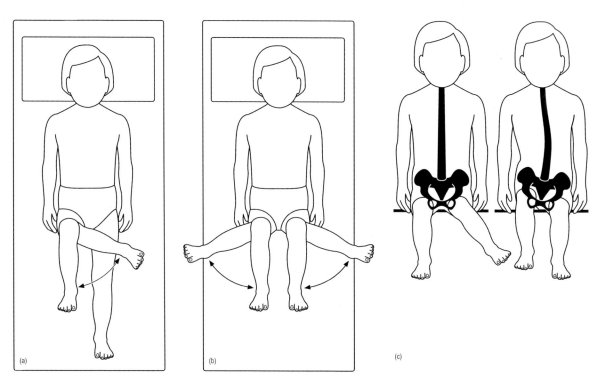

Figure 25.8 • Examination of the hip. Rotation in flexion (for sitting). (a) External rotation one leg at a time: ensure the pelvis does not rotate with the thigh. (b) Internal rotation right and left legs together: twist both legs so that the feet go to either side of the body. (c) Some children's rotation range does not allow for a normal sitting position without twisting the pelvis.

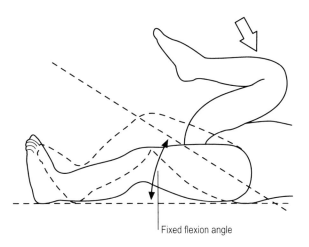

Fixed flexion angle

Figure 25.9 • Examination of the hip. The extended leg should be able to remain on the floor when the other leg is bent up to the child's tummy. Any fixed flexion is shown by the angle the thigh makes with the floor.

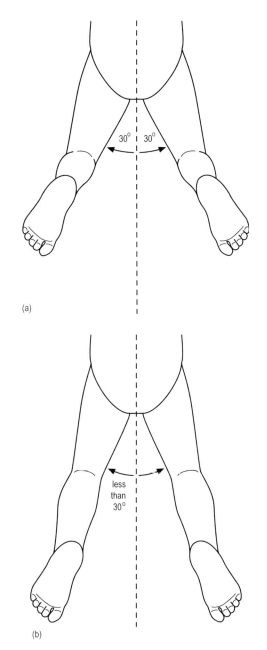

(a)

(b)

Figure 25.10 • Examination of the hip. Abduction range with the hip extended. (a) The knees are flexed to 90° to relax some of the hamstring muscles. The knees are separated, taking care that the pelvis remains flat on the floor. There should be at least 30° each side. Next (b) slowly straighten the knees and check the range when they are straight. The hamstrings may have reduced the range of abduction considerably and this (extended hips and knees) position is of course the one used for standing or walking.

the lumbar spine (by holding the other leg down to fix the pelvis).

Abduction

Abduction is tested with the hips extended and flexed to 90°.

Extended

Lie the child face-down, flex the knees so that the shins are vertical (Figure 25.10a), hold the knees and slowly pull them apart. Watch that the buttocks do not lift (hip flexion). The range is rather variable but should be more than 30° each side. You are also checking to see if there is a marked difference in range right and left. Then, with the legs still apart, slowly straighten the knees and see whether muscle tightness reduces the range of abduction (Figure 25.10b). The range (with straight knees and hips) is needed for standing and walking.

Flexed

With the child lying face-up, bend the hips and knees to 90° and slowly pull the knees apart (Figure 25.11), watching the pelvis to see that it is not rotating to one side. With the pelvis level, the thighs should be able to make at least

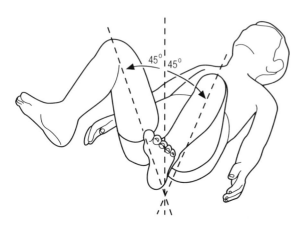

Figure 25.11 • Examination of the hip. Abduction range with the hip flexed to 90° (for sitting). Separate the knees, making sure that the pelvis does not rotate to one side. The thighs should be able to make a right angle between them, 45° each side.

a right angle between them, each being over 45° abducted. Note any marked difference between the two sides, particularly if one hip can abduct much more than 45° and the other much less, which may indicate a problem known as *windswept hips* (see below) and needs to be examined more fully.

Windswept hips

The legs of some children with severe CP fall always to the same side when lying and sitting (Figure 25.2). They develop abduction with external rotation of one hip and adduction with internal rotation of the other. It is a problem not only for overall posture but puts the adducted and internally rotated hip at great risk of dislocation. Any tendency to this posture should be brought to the attention of your physiotherapist as in the long run the spine and hips can be at risk.

Leg length difference

Any child who has one side of the body more affected than the other (e.g. hemiplegia, asymmetric diplegia) may have one leg slightly shorter than the other. This is usually in both the thigh (femur) and the shin (tibia). It can appear while the child is still an infant, but be assured that it

very seldom increases greatly as the child grows. A difference of 1.25 cm at 18 months usually increases to no more than 2 cm by adulthood and by then is a much smaller proportion of the total leg length. Measuring leg length can be difficult, but its effect can be clearly seen in standing and by looking to see if the pelvis is tipped to one side and the spine curving to compensate (Figure 25.12). Putting a book under the foot of the short leg can measure the difference and correct the posture. Some children just bend the leg and keep the pelvis in the same position, but many benefit from having a raise fitted to their shoe to compensate for some of the difference in length.

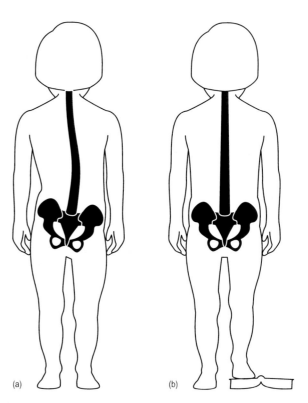

(a)   (b)

Figure 25.12 • Checking for leg length difference. (a) Note that the pelvis is lower on one side and there is a compensatory spinal curve. (b) Using a book to stand on, correct the pelvic and spinal posture: note the amount of leg length difference.

Preventing deformity: what do we know?

All the evidence points to the fact that the body, particularly the growing body, adapts to become the shape of its habitual posture.

Muscles and tendons

A child who habitually adopts the same posture can develop muscle lengths to match. It does not always happen as it also depends on the type of hypertonus (overactivity) in the muscle. There is nearly always some deformity with *spastic* hypertonus, possibly because spastic muscles are seldom, if ever, fully stretched, whereas *dystonic* hypertonus does allow full stretch to occur spontaneously as part of the child's natural movement repertoire.

Understanding that deformity can be caused by the habitual posture, although rather obvious, only began to be accepted in the mid-1970s (Scrutton and Gilbertson 1975, Fulford and Brown 1976); before that it had been assumed to be due to different muscle strengths acting across a joint, as had been seen in polio (Sharrard 1979). In the 1980s research, well summarized by O'Dwyer et al. (1989), showed how the change of length in muscles and tendons occurs: *any muscle/tendon units which are consistently kept in a shortened position will become too short, and muscle/tendons which are stretched all the time will become too long.* Both of these situations can cause problems in CP, but we will concentrate on the short muscles only as they limit movement range. So it is clear that muscles need to be stretched to their full length to prevent deformity. There is also evidence of two other things:

1. Spastic muscles become different in their structure (Frank et al. 1984, Williams et al. 1988, Cornall 1992, Booth et al. 2001).

2. When stretching a muscle/tendon continuously over more than a few days the tendon lengthens more than the muscle, leaving the child with *short* muscles and *long* tendons (O'Dwyer et al. 1989). This is not necessarily a good thing as a short muscle is less extensible and so has a shortened range of action.

However the main message seems to be very clear and simple: stretch tight structures – but how often and for how long? Is it enough to stretch a muscle/tendon and keep it stretched or should it be stretched and relaxed repeatedly? At the moment we are still not sure as the evidence from clinical experience and from research trials is not fully consistent. Tardieu et al. (1988) demonstrated that to maintain the calf muscle length of children with spastic diplegia the muscles needed to be stretched for about 6 hours a day. This does not necessarily mean 6 hours continuously: the muscle may be stretched intermittently, e.g. as it normally would be while walking around. Indeed, some people consider that without activity (relaxing and contracting the muscles) continuous stretch has little effect, but the clinical situation appears to contradict that view. Those wanting greater detail might read the articles listed in the Further Reading section.

What is written above concerns only the muscles and tendons: deformities of the hip, limb bones and the spine are also posturally caused, but by different mechanisms. Short bone length probably has a separate causation altogether.

Hip

Hip subluxation or dislocation is very common in CP. By the age of 5 years over a third of children with bilateral CP will have a hip problem requiring an orthopaedic opinion and follow-up (Scrutton et al. 2001). If one hip dislocates it will create an asymmetry of posture which is very likely to distort the pelvic position (and eventually the pelvic bones), causing a postural asymmetry of the spine which may become a scoliosis. Hip stability needs to be considered quite separately from all the other deformities because when dislocation occurs it cannot be considered an isolated event similar, say, to severe fixed knee flexion. It cannot be treated so easily and with any certainty of success. If both hips dislocate, the pelvis and spine may remain symmetrical, but there may not be sufficient hip flexion for sitting and, with the pelvis in the wrong position, comfortable and functional sitting can become impossible. Many dislocated hips cause pain, perhaps not in young children but all too often as they grow older (Cooperman et al. 1987). Caring for a child with dislocated hips can be difficult as the thighs cannot be easily separated for nappy changing and washing, and moving the legs can be painful.

An adult hip is a very secure joint and the socket has to be fractured to dislocate it. Children are different: young bones are made of cartilage (gristle) which only gradually develops into bone. Cartilage can be distorted and develop into a wrongly shaped bone, so the hip socket may not be as deep as it needs to be and the upper part of the thigh bone can be distorted. Unfortunately many children with CP adopt hip postures of adduction, slight flexion and internal rotation (Figure 25.13) which make the joint shallow and unstable, because to get the *head* of the femur right into the pelvic socket the thigh needs to be *abducted* (Figure 25.13c).

It appears that the onset of dislocation, called *subluxation* as the old word for dislocation was 'luxation', can occur very early in life and be well established by 3–4 years old (Kalen and Bleck 1985), although actual dislocation, which may happen as early as the first year of life, often occurs many years later as children approach or are in their teens.

Any child with CP affecting both sides of the body is at risk of hip dislocation. The risk is very much smaller if the child is walking and even less for early walkers. How early? Each child must be considered as an individual; but in our study of all the children with bilateral CP born over 4 years in south-east England, none of the 69 children who had walked alone by 30 months had a hip problem at 5 years; 8 (15%) of the 52 children who walked between 30 months and 5 years had a problem, as did 109 (54%) of the 202 children still unable to walk at 5 years.

The ranges of movement of the hip are important, but of far greater importance is to establish the stability of the hip joint itself – whether it is subluxed or dislocated. Examination of the hip joint's stability requires not only skill and experience but, if the child has CP affecting both sides of the body, *must* include an X-ray at some time early in the child's life, certainly by around 30 months (Scrutton and Baird 1997, Scrutton et al. 2001, Paterson 2003).

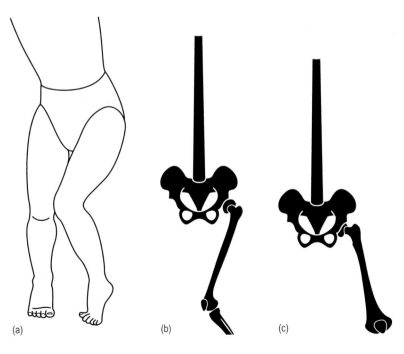

(a) (b) (c)

Figure 25.13 • (a) Typical posture seen in many children with cerebral palsy. The adduction and internal rotation of the hips put the hips at risk of not developing securely. (b) Representation of how this prevents the femoral head fully entering the acetabulum (socket). (c) Representation of the effect of hip abduction on the position of the femoral head in the socket.

Spine

The spine is a miracle of muscles working in harmony to balance 24 bones one upon another and still allow this tall column to flex, extend, side flex and rotate while supporting the head, ribcage, shoulder girdle and arm activity. The surprise is not that it sometimes distorts, but that it so seldom does. Many children with CP have minor spinal deformity which may not affect their lives or their function, and others who spend their lives in wheelchairs have minor spinal deformities which may give them pain or discomfort as they grow older; but there is a group of profoundly disabled children with CP for whom sitting properly is impossible and difficult for any support system to control, and they are at risk of a severely disabling spinal deformity called scoliosis.

Scoliosis is not just the slight sideways curvature seen quite often, for instance, in children with hemiplegia. Not only is there sideways curving but each of the vertebrae is rotated on the one above and below it. Untreated, deformity can develop rapidly and, by distorting the cavity containing the lungs and heart, become a major and life-shortening deformity. Treatment in this instance means an orthopaedic consultant *with experience of CP spines*, for these spines need rather different management from ordinary childhood scoliosis. The reason why some of these spines deform readily while others appear to be more resistant is not fully understood.

Short bones

It is not unusual for children with severe movement problems other than CP (e.g. spina bifida) to have slightly short limb bones. In CP this lack of growth really only becomes a problem when only one side is affected (hemiplegia) or one side is much more affected than the other (e.g. asymmetric diplegia). Most of these children walk or are potential walkers and unequal leg lengths can upset the dynamics and look of their gait. However the difference in length is seldom very great. The cause of this undergrowth is still not completely understood. It does not appear to be from less efficient circulation or disuse (Holt 1961).

Prevention, management and treatment

We now move on to what can be done about deformity: prevention and correction. This is divided into two sections: soft tissue and the hip/spine. There will be some overlap as soft-tissue deformity is one cause of hip or spinal problems, but it is easier to separate them.

Soft tissue (mainly muscle and tendon)

Botulinum toxin A (BTX-A)

The use of BTX-A for temporarily paralysing hypertonic muscles has been well established within the treatment of CP for the last 15 years or so. It has been used to make a movement or posture easier while stretching a short muscle to lengthen it (Cosgrove et al. 1994), although there is some evidence that it may not contribute as much as might be supposed in that situation (Glanzman et al. 2004). It can be combined with a number of the methods described below and sometimes for preoperative assessment. The use of botulinum toxin in CP is more fully described in Chapter 27.

Manual stretching

Manual stretching, moving your child's body to ensure that each muscle and joint is taken through its full range, is usually enjoyable for an infant and the carer. Many of the movements are obvious and are done as was described above in the section on physical examination, but ask your physiotherapist to teach you how to move your child's body through its full ranges of movement safely. *Remember never to use force.* Hypertonic muscles will give way to sustained stretch, not violent stretch.

How often and when? Certainly daily, but *when* depends on the age of the child. Young children can be moved at every nappy change and bathing and it can become a natural part of play, whereas some older children may refuse even to allow the possibility. Every family will find its own balance but, if started very young, stretching can become part of life and not a chore. It is usually enjoyed and has three benefits:

1. The muscles, tendons and joints are stretched fully.

2. For children who cannot move much on their own, it relaxes their muscles, feels good and may ease or prevent muscle cramps.

3. Carers are alerted to any change in range of movement or discomfort on certain movements and can tell their physiotherapist.

Serial casting

Stretching a tight muscle/tendon can be done with a series of casts (of plaster of Paris or a variety of mouldable and setting proprietary materials). It requires experience to get the right amount of stretch, the correct position and low skin pressure. The initial cast is left on from a few days to a couple of weeks and then a further cast is applied in an improved position after examination to check that there is no localized pressure and that there has been a gain in range of movement. These may be applied several times in succession and usually, when a good correction has been achieved, an orthosis is made to maintain the corrected position (Phillips and Audet 1990).

Positioning

Positioning children so that certain muscles are stretched for long periods has been used almost since the treatment of CP began. The methods and situations have changed, but it is a long-established approach. Continuous stretch can be applied in many ways and situations depending on the child's age, severity and problems. Positioning is used, not solely to prevent deformity, but also to create different social and functional situations.

1. Prone lying supports. Children unable to sit can play and develop better posture on a prone support. It takes them away from their stereotyped supine posture and can help develop better spinal and head posture (Figure 25.14).

2. Side-lying supports. Some children can lie on their side easily but many need support, sometimes over a curved pad which allows gravity to correct their side-flexed spine. Hip

posture can also be partly corrected (Figure 25.15).

3. Chairs. Most non-walking children with CP sit insecurely, leading to inefficient trunk and head posture, poor arm/hand use and deformity. A correct and secure base is needed for good spinal and head posture. How much support and fixation is needed will vary and requires skilled assessment and the facilities to get things made. Children grow and so equipment needs regular alteration. Hip spine orthoses (Bower 1990) may appear cumbersome but children can then carry most of their postural correction around with them and modified furniture may not be needed.

   Some security of the child's base comes from the feet being on footrests or the floor. So the seat height must be correct and, if necessary, the feet must be attached to the footrests. Examination of the lower limbs is needed as feet do not always fall neatly on to the footrests without wrongly positioning the pelvis.

   Tables or trays can provide some, but seldom sufficient, support on their own and it is better for the child to be sitting securely and correctly first and use a tray or a table as an additional support only (Figure 25.16).

4. Standing frames. Children unable to stand on their own benefit socially from being upright for playing at a table; unsupported, many children stand with plantarflexed ankles, semiflexed knees and adducted, internally rotated and semiflexed hips. Support is needed to control posture and provide a secure base and for some children proprietary standing frames are ideal. In common with any support system they can be restrictive, but they prevent the typically inefficient posture, give a good stretch to the knee and hip flexors, some stretch to hip adductors, allow weight-bearing and give a change of position away from sitting (Figure 25.17).

5. Orthoses (splints). Orthoses are usually named to indicate the part of the body they control: e.g. ankle and foot orthosis = AFO; knee orthosis = KO. They can be used to stretch soft tissue or, at the same time, to position the joint so that other parts of the body can move more efficiently. Using the body more correctly means that other muscles are stretched and strengthened, helping to prevent deformity. The most common sites are to control the ankle/foot (day or night), knee (to prevent flexion at night), hips (to abduct day or night), spine (for non-walking children, day or night) and wrist (to prevent flexion, day or night).

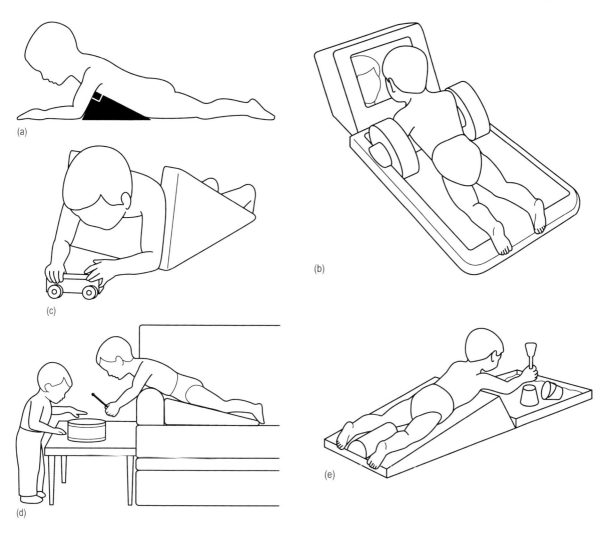

(a)

(b)

(c)

(d)

(e)

Figure 25.14 • (a–e) Children on different prone wedge supports allowing better spinal posture, head control, arm support and hand use.

Where there is still a sufficient range of movement, an AFO can hold the foot in a corrected position for walking, for sitting or at night. Its precise shape and what it is made of will depend on several things and an AFO used for walking is unlikely to be suitable for night use. Fixed deformity may need surgical lengthening of the Achilles tendon, behind the ankle, but even after surgery an orthosis may be used to hold the corrected position. Ankle position is fundamental to gait and an AFO, controlling plantarflexion and so allowing a better heel strike, is frequently used. Ankle plantarflexion not only prevents efficient walking but can make sitting more difficult as feet provide part of our base when sitting, particularly when reaching for something.

When an orthosis is used to improve function, the position of the joint is dictated by the requirements of movements (e.g. of the knee and hip for an AFO), but even when the aim is to stretch tightening structures it is better never to stretch maximally as it is uncomfortable and not well tolerated. It is also unnecessary as the effect on the muscle/tendon can be achieved with comfortably tolerated stretch (Tardieu et al. 1988). See Chapter 26 for more information on this subject.

6. Night positioning with shaped mattresses, moulds or pads can hold the child in a position

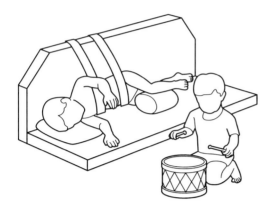

Figure 25.15 • Child on side-lying support.

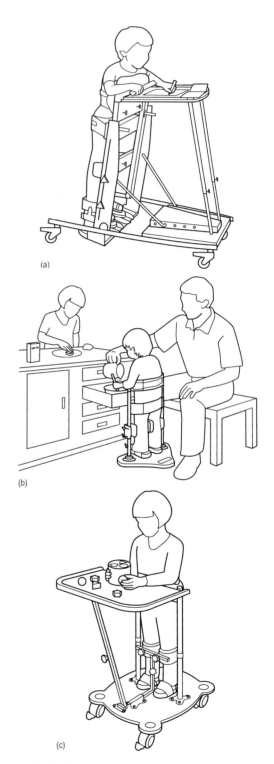

(a)

(b)

(c)

Figure 25.17 • (a–c) Children on three different standing frames.

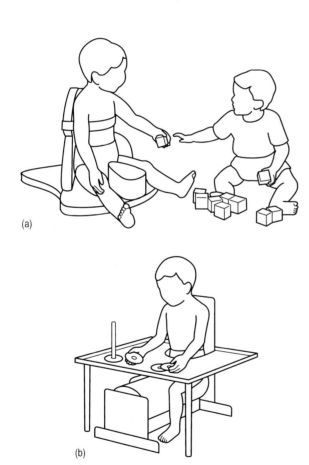

(a)

(b)

Figure 25.16 • Children on different chairs. (a) Corner seat. (b) Roller seat.

which slightly stretches overactive muscle groups and prevents asymmetries while asleep (Goldsmith 2000, Pountney et al. 2001, Hankinson and Morton 2002). Usually slight abduction of the hips, a symmetrical pelvis and a straight back are the primary considerations. Some families and some children cannot tolerate the idea of such postural control, but many children sleep comfortably (Goldsmith 2000) and there is mounting evidence for their beneficial effect for the profoundly disabled child *for whom prevention of deformity may need to be the primary physical management aim*. Night thermoplastic orthoses, controlling the ankle and foot posture (AFO) or maintaining knee extension (KO), are frequently used but getting a correct fit, particularly for a splint controlling both the knee and the ankle/foot (KAFO) can be difficult and often they act more on the knee than the ankle. Using an AFO on one leg with a KO on the other, changing sides alternate nights, is often a better method and more acceptable to the child. Anything other than a soft and light orthosis is difficult to use on the arm as it can fall on to the child's face with sudden movement when asleep.

Muscle strengthening

In the recent past, strengthening muscles which were also spastic was not encouraged. It was considered that this might increase the spasticity (or at least the power of the spasticity). In the 1930s Phelps had advocated strengthening (Slominski 1984), as had Eirene Collis, who founded the first CP treatment unit in England in 1942, but it fell out of use with the advent of the more neurologically based treatments and somehow got lost. However, spastic muscles are also weak muscles and there is no good reason for thinking that strengthening the muscle will increase the disability. Over the last 10 years or so this omission has been rectified (Darrah et al. 1997, Wiley and Damiano 1998, Schindl et al. 2000, Dodd et al. 2002) and muscle strengthening is once again part of many treatment programmes. Many of these children have a crouched-leg gait and their hip and knee extensors, although ineffective, are working much harder than normal and tire quickly. Increased strength can improve their dynamic posture (Damiano et al. 1995). Anything

which can help a muscle take part in activities nearer normal use is an advantage.

The hip, hip/pelvis and pelvis/spine

Hip

For the hip to develop properly the head of the femur (the ball at the top of the thigh bone) needs to be firmly located in the acetabulum (the socket in the pelvis) during the first few years of life (Figure 25.13c) and it locates better when the thigh is *abducted*. Therefore an important part of the treatment is based on preventing continual hip adduction. This can be done by manual handling of the young child, padding (things like wide nappies), stretching the adductor muscles, lying and seating systems or orthoses (Bower 1990) and some adapted standing frames (but most frames, although probably beneficial, do not allow enough abduction). For some children adductor muscle tightening and hip subluxation are probably inevitable and then the adductor muscles will need to be treated either by preventing them working (for example, with botulinum toxin) or surgery (usually to lengthen the muscle/tendon), followed by maintaining the improved position with an abduction splint of some sort.

Even if an X-ray much earlier had shown there was no problem, it is suggested that it should be repeated at around 30 months. To allow one X-ray to be compared with another, the child should be in the same position each time (and it is often the carer who ensures this happens).

Hip/pelvis

The most serious problems arise when the deformity at the hips is asymmetric because this tips and rotates the pelvis and transmits the asymmetry to the spine. For example, when sitting the pelvis is thrust forward on the least adducted side so that the trunk is not facing forwards but to one side (Figure 25.2b). One method of correcting this position in sitting is to control the pelvis by thrusting back on the forward side with a pad on the knee (Figure 25.18); this is only possible if that hip is not dislocated (Scrutton 1978, Pountney et al. 2001).

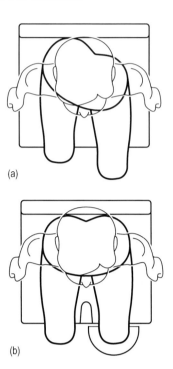

(a)

(b)

Figure 25.18 • The effect of windswept hips upon sitting. (a) The child's natural way to sit. (b) How this may be corrected by thrusting back on the forward knee to rotate the pelvis back into a symmetrical seating position.

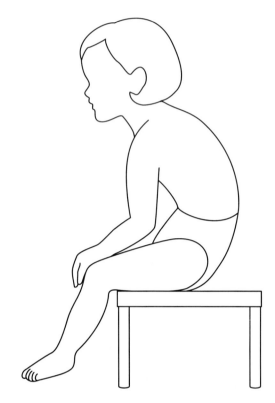

Figure 25.19 • Effect of an incorrectly positioned pelvis upon sitting and spinal posture. Sitting in a chair requires hip flexion and if that is not possible then the spine has to compensate and the neck must hyperextend to allow the child to look ahead.

Pelvis/spine

Although pelvic and spinal posture may need controlling in lying, the major problems arise when the child sits. If the *sole* treatment aim were to prevent deformity, then many of the children with profound disability would *never* be sat up: their control of spinal posture is simply not up to the task. But there is more to life than that and, for social and mobility reasons, sitting is part of life, although it brings problems. Whether there is limited range of flexion or only spasm, if the hips are not sufficiently flexed then the pelvis will be in a position nearer to lying than sitting and the spine will have to bend forwards massively if the child's back is to be forced into the vertical (Figure 25.19); alternatively the backrest will have to slope back. A flexed spine means that the neck has to be overextended or children will look at their knees all the time. Both the flexed spine

and the extended neck will lead to tightening of these shortened muscles as time passes.

Without consistent correction all too often the spine of severely affected children can side-flex and rotate, over time creating a scoliosis. Once even mild scoliosis has started a spine cannot be sufficiently supported by a chair to prevent increasing deformity. A close-fitting supportive trunk orthosis can be fitted but few curves can be contained satisfactorily in this way during rapid growth. Surgery to correct and fix a scoliotic spine is a lengthy and difficult procedure in CP and is made more difficult because many of those with the worst spines have involuntary movements as well as hypertonia. But it can be very successful and transform the child's comfort and ease of daily care. This is one area in these children's management where there is unanimous agreement: prevention of scoliosis (and so also prevention of hip dislocation) is essential wherever possible. Modified lying or seating positions or orthotics may be needed to prevent and correct this habitual asymmetry (Robson 1968, Fulford and Brown 1976, Letts et al. 1984, Bower 1990, Pountney et al. 2001, Hankinson and Morton 2002).

Carers should respect gravity. It never stops, never gives up. Never give it an opportunity to dictate habitual posture, because gradually and inevitably it will create deformity.

Deformity and walking

Any postural or fixed deformity of the legs can affect how children walk, perhaps so that it is no more than a mild cosmetic problem. More severe deformity can cause children to walk more slowly and fatigue easily, or be so severe that with growth and weight gain they gradually go off their feet altogether. Preventing deformity is our initial aim, but once children *can* walk they *will* walk, and to stop them simply because they walk in a way which will produce deformity would be wrong: they have social and independent lives to develop. Most children with CP who can walk will do it less than perfectly. Often we can help them walk better by correcting how the foot hits the ground with an orthosis or by surgery to lengthen a tendon across the ankle, knee or hip because, apart from other advantages, the better they can walk, the less likely they are to develop deformity. The treatment decision may be aided by gait analysis.

Gait analysis

Over the last 20 years or so computer analysis of data has rapidly advanced and it has become possible to collect and usefully analyse vast amounts of data from televising a child walking. From this a computer can model in three dimensions how children walk and indicate how they might walk better if certain things were changed, either by the use of orthotics or by surgical correction. Quite as importantly, it allows walking before and after treatment to be compared.

Short bones

Differences in arm lengths are usually greater than in the legs (Holt 1961) and no physiotherapy or medical treatment can correct this. As already mentioned, leg length affecting gait can usually be compensated by a shoe raise. Surgical correction is possible but is *very seldom* considered necessary for CP as (unlike some other disorders) leg length differences are usually quite small.

Rotated bones

If the thigh or shin bone is twisted (so that the knee or the foot turns in), no amount of twisting, stretching or exercise will correct it. Attempting correction by vigorous twisting can harm joints. If essential, rotational deformity can be corrected surgically and occasionally this can improve walking considerably.

Hemiplegia

Nearly all children with hemiplegic CP walk and do so at a near-normal age; but they frequently do so with a postural or fixed equinus deformity combined with some varus or valgus of the foot. Walking with one leg in tiptoe is difficult. It increases the effective length of the leg on one side, which makes it difficult to clear the ground when swinging through and gives a poor base when it is the supporting leg. Consequently it is common to use an AFO to keep the ankle/foot in a more normal position. The angle the ankle is set by the AFO varies with the child's problem; but it will be aiming to get the knee and the hip to adopt more normal movements in walking. Frequently the Achilles tendon behind the ankle becomes too tight and it needs to be surgically lengthened. It is not an onerous operation for the child, has a high success rate and can transform walking; but often an AFO will still be worn afterwards as the dorsiflexor muscles (which pull the foot up) do not function well enough to do this alone. If a child with spastic hemiplegia walks for several years with equinus and a semiflexed knee and hip, the knee and hip flexors can become short and (more often at the knee) these muscles need lengthening. The key to preventing this is to establish the best foot ankle posture as early as possible (see Scrutton 2000).

Diplegia

Most of the children with bilateral CP who walk have a spastic or dystonic disorder and, as far as walking is concerned, they can be seen as having hemiplegia on both sides. Having both sides involved makes balance and walking much more difficult and allows postural tendencies full reign, particularly a crouch gait.

Typically the child stands and walks with the feet in equinus, the knees and hips semiflexed, but with the hips also adducted and internally rotated (Figure 25.20). This does not make for

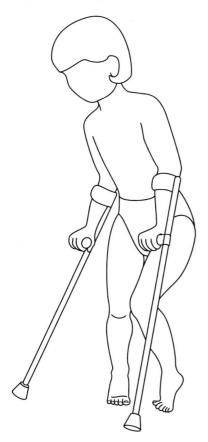

Figure 25.20 • A typical standing and walking posture of a child with spastic diplegia. The semiflexed hips and knees are liable to flex more as the child grows and the equinus position of the feet/ankles gives a poor base. Walking like this is very hard work.

efficient walking and there is a marked tendency for some children to sink gradually into greater flexion. These children may be encouraged to wear orthoses at night to maintain knee extension. However, unlike hemiplegia, lengthening of the heel cord for children with diplegia is not always straightforward. Lengthening on one side is successful, but on both sides it causes some children to have difficulty extending the hips and knees. Gravity is the great enemy of diplegia.

Flexion of the hips and knees and hip adduction can be a problem, and all too often knee flexors and hip adductors require surgical lengthening. Correcting deformity does not automatically lead to better gait and judicious and timely decisions are needed if the gait is to be improved significantly. It is here that many surgeons consider that gait analysis has most to offer. Readers interested in gait analysis and its use with CP might refer to James Gage's book (2004), listed in the Further Reading section.

An early well-established and efficient gait can usually be maintained through to adult life. It is those who can only just walk, with a cosmetically worrying semiflexed unstable gait, who may have difficulty maintaining it through their teens: the two great enemies of maintaining walking are increasing deformity and weight gain.

Conclusion

The aim of this chapter has been to explain how growth, posture and gravity can combine to increase these children's disability and how health workers try to prevent the development of deformity and to encourage the role of carers. At times the treatment needed can be relatively uncomfortable and intrusive to the child's and the family's life: equipment, stretches, orthoses, serial casting and surgery. But we would not recommend them if they were not better than the alternatives: deformity, loss of function and perhaps discomfort throughout life. There are those who decry what they call our *medical model* of managing CP, preferring their *social model*; but I think of the social implications of hip dislocation, scoliosis and the other soft-tissue problems and wonder how their preferred model might prevent or manage these problems.

CP is a health problem and, however great the social implications may be (and they are great for the child and the family), the *health problems* require *health care solutions*.

References

Booth CM, Cortina-Borja MJF, Theologis TN. Collagen accumulation in muscles of children with cerebral palsy and correlation with severity of spasticity. Dev Med Child Neurol 2001; 43:314–320.

Bower E. Hip abduction and spinal orthosis in cerebral palsy (an alternative to the use of special seating, lying and standing frames). Physiotherapy 1990; 76:658–659.

Cooperman DR, Bartucci E, Dietricke E et al. Hip dislocation in spastic cerebral palsy: long term consequences. J Pediatr Orthoped 1987; 7:268–276.

Cornall C. Splinting and contractures. Synapse 1992; April: 50–54.

Cosgrove AP, Corry IS, Graham HK. Botulinum toxin in the management of the lower limb in cerebral palsy. Dev Med Child Neurol 2004; 36:386–396.

Damiano DL, Kelly LE, Vaughn CL. Effects of quadriceps femoris muscle strengthening on crouch gait in children with spastic diplegia. Phys Ther 1995; 75:658–667.

Darrah J, Fan JSW, Chen LC et al. Review of the effects of progressive resisted muscle strengthening in children with cerebral palsy: a clinical consensus exercise. Pediatr Phys Ther 1997; 9:12–17.

Dodd KJ, Taylor NF, Damiano DL. A systematic review of the effectiveness of strength-training programs for people with cerebral palsy. Arch Phys Med Rehabil 2002; 83:1157–1164.

Frank C, Akeson WH, Woo S et al. Physiology and the therapeutic value of passive joint motion. Clin Orthop Rel Res 1984; 185:113–125.

Fulford GE, Brown JK. Position as a cause of deformity in children with cerebral palsy. Dev Med Child Neurol 1976; 18:305–314.

Glanzman AM, Kim H, Swaminathan K et al. Efficacy of botulinum toxin A, serial casting, and combined treatment for spastic equinus: a retrospective analysis. Dev Med Child Neurol 2004; 46:807–811.

Goldsmith S. Postural care at night within the community. Physiotherapy 2000; 86:528–534.

Hankinson J, Morton RE. Use of a lying hip abduction system in children with bilateral cerebral palsy: a pilot study. Dev Med Child Neurol 2002; 44:177–180.

Holt KS. Growth disturbances. In: Hemiplegic cerebral palsy in children and adults. Little Club Clinics in Developmental Medicine no. 4. MacKeith Press, London, 1961, pp. 39–53.

Kalen V, Bleck EE. Prevention of spastic paraplegic dislocation of the hip. Dev Med Child Neurol 1985; 27:17–24.

Letts M, Shapiro L, Mulder K et al. The windblown hip syndrome in total body cerebral palsy. J Pediatr Orthoped 1984; 4:55–62.

O'Dwyer NJ, Nielson PD, Nash J. Mechanisms of muscle growth related to muscle contracture in cerebral palsy. Dev Med Child Neurol 1989; 31:543–552.

Paterson JMH. Cerebral palsy. In: Banta JV, Scrutton D (eds) Hip disorders in childhood. Clinics in Developmental Medicine No. 160. MacKeith Press, London, 2003, pp. 163–179.

Phillips WE, Audet M. Use of serial casting in the management of knee joint contractures in an adolescent with cerebral palsy. Phys Ther 1990; 70:521–523.

Pountney T, Mandy A, Green E et al. Management of hip dislocation with postural management. Child Care Health Dev 2001; 28:179–185.

Robson P. Persisting head turning in the early months: some effects in the early years. Dev Med Child Neurol 1968; 10:82–92.

Schindl MR, Forstner C, Kern H et al. Treadmill training with partial body weight support in non-ambulatory patients with cerebral palsy. Arch Phys Med Rehabil 2000; 81:301–306.

Scrutton DR. Developmental deformity and the profoundly retarded child. In: Apley J (ed.) Care of the handicapped child. Clinics in Developmental Medicine no. 67. MacKeith Press, London, 1978, pp. 83–91.

Scrutton D. Physical assessment and aims of treatment. In: Neville B, Goodman R (eds) Congenital hemiplegia. Clinics in Developmental Paediatrics no. 150. MacKeith Press, London, 2000, pp. 65–80.

Scrutton D, Baird G. Surveillance measures of the hips of children with bilateral cerebral palsy. Arch Dis Child 1997; 56:381–384.

Scrutton DR, Gilbertson M. Physiotherapy in paediatric practice. Butterworth-Heinemann, London, 1975.

Scrutton D, Baird G, Smeeton N. Hip dysplasia in bilateral cerebral palsy: incidence and natural history in children aged 18 months to 5 years. Dev Med Child Neurol 2001; 43:586–600.

Sharrard WJW. Paediatric orthopaedics and fractures. Blackwell Scientific, Oxford, 1979.

Slominski AH. Winthrop Phelps and the Children's Rehabilitation Institute. In: Scrutton D (ed) Management of the motor disorders of children with cerebral palsy. Clinics in Developmental Medicine no. 90. MacKeith Press, London, 1984, pp. 59–74.

Tardieu C, Lespargot A, Tabary C et al. For how long must the soleus muscle be stretched each day to prevent contracture? Dev Med Child Neurol 1988; 30:3–10.

Wiley ME, Damiano DL. Lower extremity strength profiles in spastic cerebral palsy. Dev Med Child Neurol 1998; 40:100–107.

Williams PE, Catanese T, Lucey EG et al. The importance of stretch and contractile activity in the prevention of connective tissue accumulation in muscle. J Anat 1988; 158:109–114.

Further reading

Damiano DL, Abel MF. Functional outcomes of strength training in spastic cerebral palsy. Arch Phys Med Rehabil 1998; 79:119–125.

Damiano DL, Dodd K, Taylor NF. Should we be testing and training muscle strength in cerebral palsy? Dev Med Child Neurol 2002; 44:68–72.

Gage JR. The treatment of gait problems in cerebral palsy. Clinics in Developmental Medicine no. 164/5. MacKeith Press, London, 2004.

Graham HK. Mechanisms of deformity. In: Scrutton D, Damiano D, Mayston M. (eds) Management of the motor disorders of children with cerebral palsy. Clinics in Developmental Medicine no. 161, 2nd edn. MacKeith Press, London, 2004, pp. 105–129.

Horstmann HM, Bleck EE. Orthopaedic management in cerebral palsy. Clinics in Developmental Medicine no. 173/4. MacKeith Press, London, 2007.

Morris C, Dias LS (eds) Paediatric orthotics. Clinics in Developmental Medicine no. 175. MacKeith Press, London, 2007.

Scrutton D, Damiano D, Mayston M (eds) Management of the movement disorders of children with cerebral palsy, 2nd edn. Clinics in Developmental Medicine no. 161. MacKeith Press, London, 2004.

Watt J, Sims D, Harckham F et al. A prospective study of inhibitive casting as an adjunct to physiotherapy for cerebral-palsied children. Dev Med Child Neurol 1986; 28:480–488.

Williams PE. Use of intermittent stretch in the prevention of serial sarcomere loss in immobilised muscle. Ann Rheum Dis 1990; 49:316–317.

Williams PE, Goldspink G. Connective tissue changes in immobilised muscle. J Anat 1984; 138:343–350.

Chapter Twenty Six

26

Orthoses and children with cerebral palsy

Christopher Morris

CHAPTER CONTENTS

Orthoses are items of individualized medical equipment worn over various parts of the body that are sometimes referred to as braces or splints. *Ortho* is the Greek word meaning 'to make straight' and in simple terms that is what orthoses do: they hold joints of the limbs or spine straight by applying forces to the body. Whilst remaining rather rudimentary in concept, contemporary orthoses are predominantly made from light-weight plastics such as polypropylene rather than traditional metal and leather materials. The science of studying the effect of forces generated by the body and created through the interaction of the body with the environment, and especially gravity, is called biomechanics. Children with cerebral palsy (CP) are prone to developing deformities of their limbs and spine because of unbalanced forces created by spastic and weak muscles and the effect of gravity. Additionally, the growing skeleton can compound these problems as muscles may struggle to lengthen in proportion to their adjacent long bones, causing loss of the range of movement at joints. Children may be limited in some activities due to their inability to coordinate their body posture and movement adequately. Orthoses can be used to alter body posture in an attempt to prevent deformities and may make some activities easier. However, orthoses may also be an encumbrance for children and make some activities such as crawling, toileting and dressing more difficult. Therefore, a careful assessment of the benefits of using orthoses versus any disadvantages is often necessary.

Terminology

There are a confusing number of ways used to name and describe orthoses. The simplest and most common method describes the parts of the body within the orthosis. These expressions are then frequently abbreviated as acronyms. Thus in the leg, ankle foot orthoses (AFOs) enclose the ankle and foot; knee ankle foot orthoses (KAFOs) additionally include the knee joint; and hip knee ankle foot orthoses (HKAFOs) extend above the hip. Similarly, for the trunk, thoracolumbar sacral orthoses (TLSOs) encase all parts of the spine except the neck but are often referred to as jackets. Wrist hand orthoses (WHOs) or elbow orthoses (EOs) are used for the arm. This apparently straightforward system is complicated by the need to distinguish between different designs of orthoses. The names of people or places where orthoses were first used or commercial product names are commonly used, as well as terms such as 'dynamic'.

Supply process

Orthotists are the clinically trained health professionals who specialize in designing, making and fitting orthoses. The decision about whether any orthosis should be prescribed for a child should be made by the team of health professionals involved in the child's physical management programme in consultation with the family. The team should consider prescribing an orthosis when a clear treatment goal is identified. Typical treatment goals for children with CP include preventing deformities, enabling sitting or standing activities or improving the efficiency and pattern of walking. Biomechanical objectives that may enable these goals to be achieved include limiting the range of movement at specific joints and improving overall stability. The need for orthotic prescription may vary according to the severity and extent of a child's CP and consideration of any associated problems.

Once the objectives are agreed the orthotist will design and fabricate an orthosis. This will involve taking appropriate measurements and sometimes a plaster cast model. All orthoses are constructed with parts that apply forces to the body, a structure to hold these together and straps to fasten the device to the child's body. The fit of the orthosis will be judged by the orthotist as adequate and families instructed on appropriate use and care of the orthosis. The effectiveness of the orthosis in achieving the intended biomechanical effect and overall treatment goal should be evaluated by the team at regular intervals. The effect of wear should also be reviewed every few months so that any necessary repairs can ensure the safe and appropriate function of the orthosis. The orthosis cannot work if it is not being used; therefore children with CP require a responsive orthotic service and need to

be provided with contact details should any problems occur. A reputable paediatric orthotic facility should be able to carry out straightforward repairs and adjustments on the day. Occasional rubbing of the skin is inevitable with such close-fitting devices and is usually easily resolved by the orthotist either by heating and reshaping the plastic or by the addition of appropriate padding. In general, children outgrow most orthoses somewhere between 10 and 18 months and a review of how the child benefits from the orthosis should precede replacement.

Many therapeutic interventions other than orthoses will be considered as part of the physical management regimen for a child. These treatments may be prescribed to supplement using an orthosis or perhaps make orthotic treatment redundant. Professionals adopting a family-centred approach to organizing individual physical management programmes are more likely to encourage compliance with the prescribed regimen. The health care team must therefore be well coordinated, work in partnership with the family, provide adequate information about the role of interventions and their expected outcomes, as well as generally supporting the family.

Lower-limb orthoses

One of the most common problems for children with CP is an equinus or tiptoe posture of the foot and ankle due to spasticity or tightness in the calf muscles (Figure 26.1), sometimes referred to as plantarflexion of the ankle. This often causes changes to the flexible structure of the ankle and foot, making the foot roll excessively inwards (valgus) or outwards (varus). Fixed deformities of the hind and midfoot can develop when the range of movement available at the ankle is reduced by either spasticity, or muscle shortening relative to the limb, or both. AFOs can be used to restrict ankle movement and prevent the foot from pointing downward. The corrective force applied under the forefoot is achieved in combination with forces applied to the back of the calf and through the strap over the instep (Figure 26.2). Therefore it is important that the strap is fastened securely and the orthotist will often make a mark on the

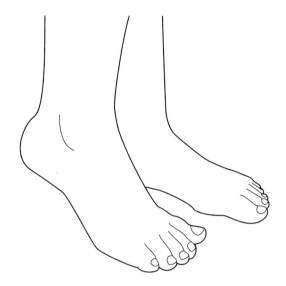

Figure 26.1 • Plantarflexion or equinus of the ankle.

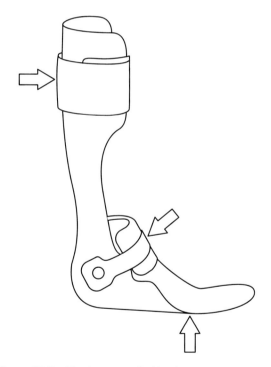

Figure 26.2 • The forces applied by the ankle foot orthosis to prevent plantarflexion.

strap to indicate the appropriate tension. Given the need for the foot to be correctly positioned in the orthosis, the knee should be well flexed when putting the orthosis on, as this renders the joints

of the foot and ankle more flexible. A sequence of steps to be undertaken when fitting an AFO is suggested in Figure 26.3.

Flexible foot and ankle deformities can be corrected during the casting process and the position maintained using a close-fitting AFO and corrective strapping. Fixed deformities must be accommodated in their best-corrected posture. Persistent ankle and knee deformities secondary to spasticity may benefit from intramuscular injections of botulinum A toxin to weaken spastic muscles, often combined with short periods of serial casting to increase the range of ankle movement, in order to facilitate ongoing management in orthoses. Children wearing AFOs usually manage these inside ordinary shop-bought shoes. As all the support for the leg is provided by the orthosis, the shoe does not need to include any special features other than being light-weight and provide a non-slip sole. However, if profound fixed ankle and foot deformities become established then fitting of ordinary shoes can become a problem and custom-made footwear may be necessary.

The issue of for how many hours AFOs should be worn is an issue of dosage of the medical intervention. The only available research suggests that ensuring calf muscles spend more than 6 hours in each 24-hour period in an elongated position may help to prevent them becoming shortened. If the orthosis also aims to improve the child's function then the orthosis must surely be worn during daily activities. However, some health professionals may recommend wearing an AFO at night either in addition to daytime wear or as an alternative if maintaining range of movement is the primary goal. Orthoses should only be used at night if their intrusion does not disrupt normal sleeping patterns, as time the child spends in an AFO whilst reading or watching television may be more easily negotiated and similarly beneficial. Supplementing the AFO with a stiffened fabric gaiter, to hold the knee extended and foot dorsiflexed simultaneously, will significantly intensify the stretching force on the calf muscle. The most common regimen for school-age children is for them to wear the orthosis during time spent at school and not at home. This allows the child a reasonable period of time where movements

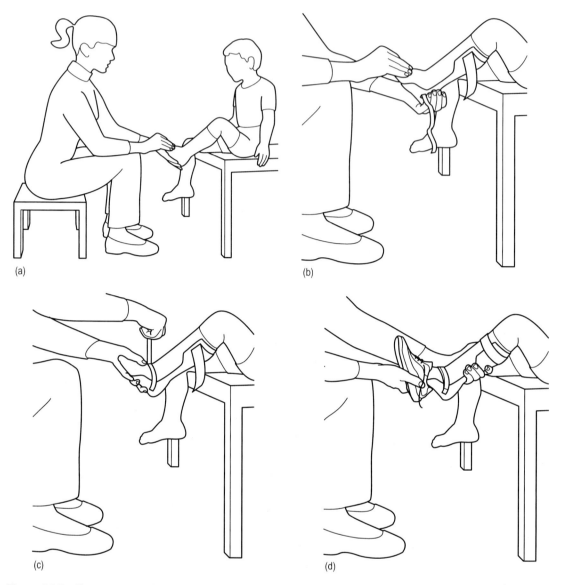

(a)

(b)

(c)

(d)

Figure 26.3 • The sequence of steps to be undertaken when fitting an ankle foot orthosis (AFO). (a) The child's foot posture is more easily corrected when the child is sitting in a relaxed position with the knee well flexed. (b) Keeping the foot corrected and the knee flexed, the AFO is introduced from behind. (c) Once the foot is within the AFO then the heel strap is securely fastened first. (d) Then the calf strap is fastened and an ordinary shoe is fitted over the AFO.

are unrestricted. It should be stressed that a programme for using AFOs in the school holidays should also be negotiated, as several weeks of not using the orthosis can allow loss of range of joint movement at the ankle and cause problems tolerating the AFO when school resumes.

Although it may seem counterintuitive to restrict movement at the ankle to improve function, recent reviews of the efficacy of orthoses for children with CP conclude that preventing plantarflexion improves the efficiency of gait. Using an AFO to prevent plantarflexion has been shown to improve stability in standing and walking, positioning of the foot and clearance of the swinging leg during gait, thereby reducing energy expenditure and increasing step length and walking speed. For children who are not walking, maintaining foot and ankle position will enable more comfortable posture in seating systems by allowing some of the weight of the lower limbs to be supported by footplates.

AFOs may be designed to prevent all movement (solid or rigid AFOs) or include hinges to allow partial movement. This may make climbing stairs and inclines slightly easier. However, the potential benefits of this flexibility are often negated by the disadvantage that children using hinged AFOs may flex their hips and knees excessively and sink into a crouched posture; particularly when there is tightness of the calf muscles or when the hip and knee muscles are also affected by spasticity. Occasionally the aim of the AFO is to assist in extending the knee during standing and walking, such as when children are prone to crouching, in which case the AFO must be very rigid at the ankle to prevent buckling. This is common after orthopaedic surgery to the leg when muscles may become temporarily weakened.

There is no evidence to support any 'tone-reducing' effect on gait from orthoses that incorporate specially moulded footplates. Therefore, the prescription of foot orthoses that provide no leverage to prevent plantarflexion would seem to offer little benefit in the goal to improve gait efficiency. However, foot orthoses may be beneficial for children whose gait deviations are an essential mechanism for achieving ambulation, or for children whose problem has resolved following surgery.

Some children walk with their feet pointing inward (in-toeing) and other children with the foot turned outwards. This is often a combination of foot posture and rotational deformities in the femur and tibia, the two long bones of the leg. It may be possible to gain some rotational control of the leg using an orthosis. Incorporating a flexible sprung cable as part of the HKAFO or winding elastic fabric straps around the limb attaching to AFOs from a waistband may improve in-toeing. However, this is one circumstance when the bulkiness of the orthosis may impede the child

rather than make walking easier. When the cause of internal hip rotation is due to fixed torsion in the femur, these problems are often not controlled using orthoses and children may require surgery to align the foot to the leg better. Pelvic rotation, when the child leads with the less impaired limb during walking, is part of the neurological problem and cannot be influenced by orthotic management.

Spinal orthoses

The spine is usually slightly curved in the lumbar and thoracic segments from front to back; any lateral curvature of the spine is referred to as scoliosis. Scoliosis is usually aggravated by the effect of gravity when children are artificially placed in sitting positions. Tightness of the hamstring muscles can also reduce the lumbar curve and tilt the pelvis backwards in sitting (sometimes called sacral sitting). When taking a mould for a spinal orthosis (TLSO), it is desirable to remove the deforming effect of gravity by laying the child supine on a bed or casting frame. Plastic spinal orthoses or TLSOs may reduce spinal curvature and improve sitting ability whilst the orthosis is worn. Children with poor levels of sitting ability may also demonstrate excessive forward trunk-leaning, or kyphosis, which spinal orthoses can prevent. A consensus on the length of time a spinal orthosis should be worn is not well established and current recommendations range from only whenever the child is upright to 23 out of 24 hours. Whatever the regimen, TLSOs are unlikely to prevent some spinal deformities progressing over time and surgery may be required to stabilize the child's spine internally when major scoliosis occurs.

Hip orthoses

Some children with CP are prone to problems with the development of their hip joints, and those children who do not walk are most vulnerable. The rounded top of the femur usually fits snugly into a socket in the pelvis. Children with CP may have an underdeveloped socket and the femur may be pulled away from its proper place due to spastic muscles, reduced movement and not bearing weight through the hip. Orthoses can be used to position the hip better and to stretch hip muscles. For non-ambulant children, the benefits of the TLSO in controlling the position of the centre of gravity and stabilizing the trunk as a single segment can be combined with hip abduction orthosis, providing a stable base in an HASO. HASOs offer an alternative to the wheelchair, allowing the child to sit in regular furniture, but do not replace the need for a wheelchair.

The commercially available Standing, Walking and Sitting Hip (SWASH) orthosis comprises a pelvic section and thigh cuffs linked to a posterior curved connecting bar. The hip hinge of the SWASH encourages a wider hip posture when the hip is flexed, helping with sitting stability. Although there is a slightly narrow hip posture when the hip is extended the SWASH orthosis may help to prevent the legs crossing (scissoring) during standing and walking. Despite the efficacy of hip orthoses to hold the legs apart, there is as yet limited evidence that they can alter the natural history of progressive hip migration, even in combination with botulinum A toxin to weaken spastic muscles. Surgical reconstruction of the hip joint may become necessary if the hip is painful or limiting activities of sitting or toileting. Orthoses may be used in the postoperative regimen to avoid the problems of immobilizing the child in total body casts. The most versatile design of orthosis for use in the postoperative period includes a hip hinge that allows incremental adjustment of hip movement that can be locked in the selected position.

Upper-limb orthoses

Children for whom control and coordination in the upper limb are affected may have impaired manual dexterity and reduced ranges of movement at the elbows, wrists or fingers. The principles of orthotic management are the same as for the lower limbs – to stretch spastic or tight muscles, sometimes in combination with botulinum A toxin injections and serial casting. Stiffened fabric gaiters can be used to hold the elbows extended for periods to maintain range of elbow movement. Wrist Hand Orthoses (WHOs) may be usefully employed to support the wrist in a more functional position. This may help the child to use both hands if only one is affected, as in hemiplegia, or to improve ease of using hand controls on wheelchairs or other forms of assistive technology. There has been some experimental research using fabric garments as gloves; however, this currently remains a fringe rather than mainstream treatment. If the orthosis is solely required to stretch the wrist, fingers and thumb, then dexterity will be impeded and it should only be worn during resting periods.

Conclusion

There have been few clinical trials to determine how effective orthoses are in achieving their goals, in part because of the confounding effects of other treatments. In the absence of compelling evidence, health professionals use a variety of different treatment approaches with different types or no orthoses. The advice given to families by different professionals may conflict at times, causing confusion. Although some therapists are rightly reluctant to restrict any of children's available movement, orthoses can enhance children's interaction with their environment and help them overcome activity limitations precisely by restricting unhelpful movements. At other times, the utility of orthoses must be balanced with the family's lifestyle and changing priorities and, although perhaps worth trying in the first instance, may not be worth pursuing if there is no demonstrable benefit.

Further reading

Journal of Prosthetics and Orthotics in 2002 freely available on http://www.oandp.org/jpo/Library/2002_04_150.asp.

Morris C, Dias I (eds). Paediatric orthotics. Clinics in Developmental Medicine no. 175. Mackeith Press, London, 2007.

Chapter Twenty Seven

27

Spasticity

Daniel S Roy • John F McLaughlin

CHAPTER CONTENTS

Spasticity is characterized by high muscle tone that increases in response to fast stretching of muscles. This muscle tightness results from interruption of brain and spinal cord control of movement, and is only one of several motor control problems that can occur as a result of brain malformation or injury. Spasticity is present in a number of medical conditions, and is considered a defining characteristic for approximately 85% of children with cerebral palsy (CP). Spasticity does not need to be treated in all children. Treatment of spasticity is considered when the increased muscle tightness results in pain, impaired function, positioning problems, or increased care difficulties. A variety of treatment options are currently available. No single treatment is appropriate for every individual. This chapter reviews treatment of spasticity with oral medications, intrathecal baclofen pump, selective dorsal rhizotomy (SDR) and botulinum toxin injections, and reviews orthopaedic interventions intended to address complications of spasticity.

Oral medications

Oral medications used to treat spasticity include baclofen, diazepam, tizanidine, dantrolene and gabapentin. Although oral medications are considered to be the least invasive means to treat spasticity, none of these medications corrects the underlying problem. As spasticity seems stronger when muscles grow larger, each can become ineffective over time, and each has potential side-effects that limit their use. Despite these limitations, for some children oral medications may be all that is ever required to treat their spasticity.

Baclofen is the medication most often prescribed to treat spasticity. Its chemical structure resembles gamma-aminobutyric acid (GABA), a chemical normally produced in the nervous system that inhibits the response of nerves to other signals. This interference with other nervous system signals reduces spasticity. Baclofen is absorbed rapidly from the gastrointestinal tract, and reaches a peak blood concentration within 2–3 hours. Approximately one-third of a dose remains bound to proteins in the blood and is not available for use by the body. Because baclofen is rapidly cleared from the body, repeat dosing approximately three times daily is required. To be effective, baclofen must reach the spinal cord. This medication does not cross well from the blood into the spinal fluid, and so relatively high oral dosages are required to treat spasticity. Increased dosages may also increase side-effects, most commonly sedation, constipation, problems swallowing and confusion. Occasionally baclofen is associated with an increased frequency of seizures in children who already have a seizure disorder. Side-effects may often be prevented or minimized by building up the dose slowly and usually decrease after several weeks of use. Dosages typically begin between 2.5 and 10 mg/day and are gradually increased to effect, with maintenance dosages of 20–90 mg/day required for effective treatment. Some patients' spasticity can be managed with this medication for years, whereas for others its effectiveness decreases over time. Baclofen must be discontinued gradually over 1–2 weeks to prevent withdrawal symptoms, including agitation and hallucinations.

Diazepam is commonly used to treat spasticity. Like baclofen, diazepam has its effect within the central nervous system. Diazepam is thought to work by increasing sensitivity to GABA. This increased sensitivity also produces side-effects, most notably sedation. Despite a markedly longer duration of action that would suggest the possibility of once-a-day dosing, by dividing the dose into multiple-times-per-day increments these side-effects can be minimized. Dosages are based upon the individual child's weight, with doses typically beginning at 0.5 mg and gradually increased every 3–7 days to a maximum dose of 20 mg/day. Most children obtain optimal effect with doses of 1–5 mg three times a day. Tolerance to diazepam is reported to occur in some children after a few months, requiring adjustment of the dosage. Additionally, some become dependent upon this medication at high doses and must be tapered off gradually. There is some evidence that baclofen and diazepam may have a synergistic effect, which means that small doses of both may work better than large doses of a single drug.

Tizanidine is a newer spasticity management medication, approved for use in adults in the USA in 1996. Like baclofen and diazepam, tizanidine works in the central nervous system but is thought to have its effects by regulating central nervous system chemicals that stimulate muscles. Unlike baclofen and diazepam, there is no published experience with its use in children. Its use is also limited by its side-effects, causing sedation in almost half of individuals, but also causing dizziness and dry mouth, and lowering blood pressure. Blood tests are periodically required to monitor liver function as this medication is cleared from the body by the liver, and severe liver injury has been reported with its use in a few cases. Dosage of tizanidine typically starts between 1 and 2 mg four times daily, and is increased as needed to doses of 2–6 mg four times daily.

Dantrolene works directly at the muscles to reduce resting muscle tone and relieve spasticity. Because of this direct method of action, dantrolene may reduce muscle strength, counteracting the benefits gained from the reduced spasticity, and many children experience no functional gain with its use. Like tizanidine, this medication can be harmful to the liver and requires periodic blood tests for monitoring of liver function. The risk of liver damage appears to be less in children than in adolescents or adults. No fatalities have been reported in individuals under the age of 20. Other more commonly reported side-effects of dantrolene include sedation, fatigue, vomiting and diarrhoea, although these side-effects typically decrease over time. Dantrolene is likely best reserved for children who do not respond to the other medications when the main intent is pain relief. Initial dosage of dantrolene is weight-based, and the dose is gradually increased every 4–7 days to a maximum maintenance dosage administered four times daily.

Gabapentin is a medication used primarily to treat seizures. It has been observed to decrease spasticity and does not appear to have many side-effects. A dose range of 50–400 mg two or three times a day is considered sufficient. More data are needed on the benefits and side-effects of all these medications.

Botulinum toxin

Botulinum toxin is rapidly becoming the 'go-to' intervention for spasticity that interferes with limb function. This toxin was identified in the 19th century as the cause of botulism. It is a bacterial protein that causes weakness or paralysis of muscle by permanently blocking chemical communication between nerves and muscles. Publications of the use of purified botulinum toxin A to treat spasticity began in 1993. Today botulinum toxin is used to improve dynamic contractures, to reduce pain and to improve both function and cosmetic problems. Botulinum toxin can be used at the same time that a child is receiving other treatments for spasticity. Botulinum toxin temporarily weakens the muscles into which it is injected. Challenges in deciding when to use botulinum toxin include the timing of the intervention, which muscles to target for injection and the optimum location and preparation dosage for injection.

It is generally agreed that botulinum toxin may benefit children with increased muscle stiffness, especially when specific functional benefit and focal goals are defined, such as improved range of motion to aid walking or hand use, increased ease of care or relief of pain. It is often a choice for treatment of either lower-extremity or upper-extremity problems in children ages 2 to 6, but only for focal upper-extremity problems in older children. Children with fixed contractures, bony deformity, unstable joints or widespread spasticity involving numerous muscles are less likely to benefit from this therapy. There is little clinical experience with the use of botulinum toxin in children under the age of 1 year, largely because of the difficulty in determining specific functional goals in this age population. The timing of botulinum toxin therapy remains a clinical decision based upon the child's symptoms, the physicians' and therapists' experience and parental desires.

While many different measures have been tried to determine which muscles to target for therapy, most physicians rely on clinical examination and experience to choose target muscles and then monitor the effectiveness of the intervention using objective measurements of functional improvement and parental report of beneficial effects and problems.

There are currently two commercially available botulinum toxin A preparations approved for use, Botox and Dysport, and one commercially available botulinum B preparation, Myobloc. Although these preparations have similar clinical effects, manufacturing differences result in very different dosage recommendations. Each preparation has a peak dose response, with dosages above this level resulting in minimal further effect. Maximum dosing is also limited by the desired response, as too large a dose also results in either local muscle weakness that impairs function or systemic side-effects. Some children eventually develop antibodies against the specific toxin being used, rendering further treatment with that toxin ineffective.

The procedure itself involves multiple intramuscular injections of small amounts of toxin. The precise location and injection dosage vary according to the size of the muscles and the severity of the spasticity. Immediate side-effects of the procedure are similar to those encountered with any intramuscular injection and include injection site pain, redness and swelling. Injection pain may be reduced by the use of topical anaesthetic cream, intravenous sedation or light general anaesthetic. Desired effects of the therapy are usually seen within 12–72 hours from injection and reach their peak in a few weeks. Effects of the blockade disappear within 3–6 months, due to either the formation of new nerve buds or recovery of the nerves. Side-effects are rarely reported with this therapy, and are usually caused by either too robust an effect at the locally injected muscle or systemic spread. Reported side-effects include frequent falls, generalized fatigue and, rarely, temporary urinary and faecal incontinence. For children with difficulties swallowing there is an additional concern of worsening aspiration due to either systemic spread or from direct injection of neck muscles. Sometimes botulinum toxin does not have a noticeable effect despite proper technique.

Intrathecal baclofen pump

Spasticity can be treated by continuously infusing baclofen directly to the spinal cord with an implanted pump. This is called continuous intrathecal baclofen. As noted previously, use of baclofen orally to treat spasticity is limited by side-effects resulting from the dosage of medication required to achieve effective levels of medication in the spinal nerves where baclofen has its effect. Intrathecal baclofen avoids these limitations by directly injecting the medication into the spinal fluid. The doses required are 50–100 times less than the oral doses and the effects on tone are considerably greater. Baclofen cannot be detected in the blood stream during continuous delivery of baclofen into the spinal fluid. Intrathecal baclofen is most often used in children with Gross Motor Function Classification System (GMFCS) IV or V (severe) CP who are experiencing pain and extreme stiffness. Children who have a floppy (hypotonic) trunk and poor head control despite severe spasticity in their limbs may not do well with this treatment.

Children are evaluated to determine whether they will respond appropriately to medication administered into the spinal fluid. They are given one or more injections of medication into their spinal fluid and monitored for response. If they respond as desired, they then undergo a 1-hour surgical procedure in which a hockey puck-sized pump containing medication is surgically implanted under the skin of the abdomen at approximately waist level. A tube is then placed under the skin, leading from the pump around the waist to the back, and the end is inserted between the bones of the spine into the space surrounding the spinal cord. Children must lie flat for up to 3 days following the surgery to minimize risks of spinal fluid leakage before slowly resuming their daily activities. Most children experience some degree of soreness requiring pain management, but the majority of children have minimal pain by the time of discharge.

When activated the pump administers a steady low dose of baclofen directly into the spinal fluid, typically at one one-hundredth of the typical oral dose, minimizing the potential for medication side-effects. The baclofen dose is then slowly increased in increments of 10–15% until an optimal dose rate is achieved. The pump most commonly used is calibrated using a special small computer maintained by the child's physician. Because the pump can be programmed, it is possible to customize dosages so that the amount of baclofen can be adjusted through the day to the child's needs. Depending upon the pump size and the individual child's dosing requirement, the pump contains enough medication to last 2–4 months. The pump is easily refilled in approximately 15 minutes using a refill kit that includes a special needle, syringe and guide to insert the needle into a refill port on the pump. The pump is battery-operated, with a battery life expectancy of approximately 5–7 years, after which the old pump must be surgically replaced. There is also a simpler pump that is powered by hydraulic pressure but does not have the flexible programming of the battery-operated pump.

Surgical risks such as bleeding and infection accompany placement of an intrathecal baclofen pump. Infection with placement of a pump typically requires the temporary removal of the device. The most common non-surgical complications are medication side-effects, including nausea, headache, dizziness, drowsiness and weakness. These are typically temporary and respond to supportive care. Dose-dependent side-effects respond to lowering of the dose rate. More severe, but rarely encountered, complications are reported in response to intrathecal baclofen overdose, and include breathing problems and reversible coma. As of this writing, although potentially life-threatening, all children reported to have intrathecal baclofen overdose recovered and returned to using their pumps. The pump is highly reliable but occasionally the tubing that carries baclofen to the spinal cord becomes dislodged or breaks, leading to a decrease of effect. Pumps can never be allowed to run dry. Sudden withdrawal of intrathecal baclofen can lead to rapid return of severe spasticity. When this happens, the muscle spasm can be so severe that the muscle tissue breaks down and releases harmful chemicals into the blood stream. Fatalities have occurred when a pump failure was not recognized or treated properly.

Selective dorsal rhizotomy

SDR is another intervention available to reduce spasticity and improve function. SDR interrupts spinal circuitry and is thought to decrease excitatory stimulation of motor nerves. SDR is a surgical procedure that is expected to result in permanent elimination of spasticity in the muscles receiving input from the nerve rootlets that are cut. SDR can only be done to decrease spasticity in the legs, not the arms. To think of SDR as a purely surgical procedure is misleading, however, as for maximum benefit a rigorous programme of intensive physical therapy is required following the surgery. The evaluation needed to make good decisions about the use of SDR requires a team of experienced health professionals, and includes the parents and child in the decision-making process.

Because of both the surgical nature of the procedure and its permanent effects, SDR is not a good choice for all children with CP. Typically children who benefit from SDR are between 3 and 10 years old, and have either spastic diplegia or quadriplegia of GMFCS III severity. SDR only works for spasticity so care must be taken to be sure that spasticity is really causing the problems. Orthopaedic conditions must also be evaluated, as severe scoliosis increases the risks and complexity of the surgery, and fixed contractures limit the potential benefits of this procedure. Severe visual impairment may also limit the functional benefits. The child and family must be able to participate effectively in the postoperative physical therapy programme. Each of these factors is evaluated prior to the procedure, as are the extent and distribution of the spasticity in order to guide the neurosurgeon in preparation for the procedure.

Performed under general anaesthesia, the procedure itself begins with an incision along the spinal column to expose the individual vertebrae that make up the backbone. The length of this first incision varies from 2 to 8 vertebral bodies depending upon the neurosurgeon's preferred technique. A portion of each of the backbone segments is opened to expose the nerves emerging from the spinal cord. Each exposed nerve is tagged and then tested by electrical stimulation to separate the sensory dorsal root from its paired motor ventral root. The surgeon then considers the preoperative examination to determine which

rootlets to cut – typically the dorsal roots from the first lumbar vertebra to the first sacral vertebra – with recommended rates ranging around 50% of the nerve root tissue.

For several days following the procedure children may experience pain and muscle spasms, and so are typically given potent high-dose pain medications directly into the wound through tubes placed during the operation. Some children also experience a temporary inability to urinate and require bladder catheterization following the procedure for a few days, whereas others experience a temporary tingling or numbness in the affected limb. All children must lie on their stomach for 3–4 days, and typically feel both weak and sleepy. The sutures are removed after approximately 10 days, after which the children can be moved in wheelchairs.

The postoperative physical therapy regime begins while the children are still at bedrest. Although most children can resume their preprocedure activities after only 1 month, their physical therapy continues for several months. Specific physical therapy programmes vary widely, ranging from several weeks of inpatient therapy programmes to several hours per week of outpatient therapy programmes. These therapy programmes all focus on muscle strengthening and gait training, and are supplemented by parent-assisted stretching and strengthening activities.

Although spasticity is almost immediately reduced and permanently so in most children receiving SDR, functional abilities improve more gradually over the first 6–9 months following the procedure. It is important to note that functional abilities do not always improve, and that there are significant side-effects to this procedure besides risks associated with any surgical procedure. Temporary changes in sensation are often reported. Less frequent side-effects include loss of bladder function, excessive weakness and perceptions of difficulty with balance. Additionally, other movement problems may be unmasked following reduction of spasticity, limiting functional improvements postoperatively. Even when SDR effectively reverses functional difficulties resulting from spasticity, it does not eliminate the potential need for future orthopaedic surgeries, as this procedure does not halt the progression of hip and back problems. In some rare individuals the procedure may actually worsen these problems, although there is insufficient information in the medical literature to document accurately the incidence of these problems in either treated or untreated children with CP. The long-term consequences of SDR during the adult life of a child with CP are unknown.

Orthopaedic interventions

Despite the best physical therapy, orthotics and medications, spasticity combined with skeletal growth can result in the formation of joint contractures or dislocation. In typically developing children, bone length in the arms and legs doubles in the first 4 years of life, and doubles again between age 4 and adulthood. During growth in children with spasticity, the tendons attaching the muscles to the bones become too short, limiting the range of motion in the affected joint. Over time the abnormal stresses caused by these contractures change the shape of the affected bones, eventually resulting in a fixed deformity. The goals of orthopaedic surgery are identical to those of spasticity management; relief of pain, and preservation and improvement of function. All musculoskeletal surgeries result in temporary loss of function due to weakness and immobilization, requiring postoperative therapies to regain full function.

The true art of orthopaedic surgery is not in the performance of the technical procedure, but rather in determining the best time and sequence for surgical intervention. The decision on whether surgical treatment is needed begins, like all medical decisions, with evaluation of the child. The observations of physical therapists, parents and children themselves are important since the physician usually only sees the child for a brief period of time. The evaluation typically consists of a review of the child's medical history and physical examination. Findings on this portion of the evaluation guide the physician's decision on whether to obtain X-rays. Videotapes of the front and side views of the child that can be replayed at normal and slow speeds help the physician define

the problem and determine the most appropriate intervention. Computerized gait analysis that simultaneously records video, electrical activity of muscles, the force of walking and energy use is in use in some centres. This type of gait analysis is not universally available, and probably is only necessary for more complicated situations. Gait analysis is a tool that provides additional information to help guide physician or surgeon decisions. There is debate as to whether this technology adds enough information to justify the time and expense involved. A paediatric orthopaedic surgeon with special interest and experience in treating CP will usually see a child more than once and listen carefully to parents and other health professionals who know the child before recommending surgery unless there is an urgent problem. Frequently there will be a need to deal with other health problems such as seizures, respiratory problems and nutritional status to assure that the child will tolerate anaesthesia, heal quickly, and be in a condition to take advantage of the changes that happen because of the surgery itself.

The muscles of the hips are among the largest and strongest in a child. Hip spasticity can lead to hip dislocation, one of the earliest possible musculoskeletal problems resulting from spasticity that requires orthopaedic surgical correction. Other problems commonly appear and include shortening of the tendons (contractures), displacement of the bones of the hands and feet (deformities) and inappropriate twisting of the bones (torsion) Procedures designed to address these problems include tendon lengthening, tendon transfer, tendon release, cutting of the bones (osteotomy) and joint fusion (arthrodesis). It must be emphasized that orthopaedic procedures do not correct the underlying neurological problems. All have potential for common intraoperative complications, including bleeding, infection and complications of anaesthesia. Surgical procedures are typically delayed as long as possible, and then multiple procedures are performed at the same time to reduce the risks of surgery.

The least complicated of these procedures is tendon lengthening. In this procedure the surgeon exposes the affected tendon, divides the tendon lengthwise and finally sews the two halves back together to create a single longer tendon. This procedure typically requires approximately 30 minutes per tendon to complete. Following the procedure the muscle is immobilized in a position that keeps the muscle stretched to prevent shortening of the muscle and tendon during healing which improves range of motion. The muscle needs to adapt to the new length and may be weak at first. A complication specific to this procedure is weakening of the tendon.

Tendon transfer procedures are usually performed to correct deformities of the wrists, knees and ankles. This procedure involves the disconnection of a tendon from its bony insertion and then reconnection of that tendon at a new site. Although typically requiring only 45 minutes per tendon to complete, this procedure is more complex due to differences in muscle strength and the sequence in which muscles typically contract. Following the surgery, families should anticipate several weeks of casting or bracing. Retraining to take advantage of the new tendon position may require months of practice.

Tendon release is perhaps the simplest of the orthopaedic interventions, and involves the cutting of the tendon that attaches a spastic muscle to the bone. This procedure is primarily indicated for children who have maximized their functional potential and do not require use of the affected muscle.

More involved procedures are required when prolonged spasticity results in bony deformity or instability. Osteotomy is usually performed on the hip, pelvis, foot and/or ankle. This involves cutting and reattaching the affected bone to place it in proper alignment, which may improve joint function, increase useful range of motion, provide easier fit for braces or wheelchairs and improve appearance. Once correctly positioned the bone is reconnected with a metal plate and screws which maintain the new position until bone healing is complete, usually 9–12 months later. This procedure typically requires an hour or more in surgery, and usually requires postoperative casting and bracing. Once the patient has healed, the metal plate and screws can be removed through the original incision. The hardware removal is usually performed as an outpatient procedure, with

children able to resume their regular activities within 2 days.

Joint fusion or arthrodesis is usually reserved for children who would not benefit from one or more of the procedures previously described, yet who have unstable joints or deformities that cannot be braced. As the name suggests, this procedure permanently attaches bones to one another. It is commonly used to correct ankle, thumb, wrist and spine deformities. Metal devices used in fusion procedures are usually left in place permanently.

Scoliosis, or curvature of the spine, deserves special mention. This problem is not often apparent in young children but the stage is set for its development early in life by the abnormal neurological control of movement that is the hallmark of CP. Scoliosis usually becomes apparent in early adolescence and may become rapidly worse during the main adolescent growth spurt. This growth spurt, which is ultimately under the control of brain regulation of hormone production, may occur earlier or later than usual in children with CP. Scoliosis usually occurs in children whose CP affects the selective motor control and balance of the trunk. Most such children have GMFCS class IV or V CP. At present, there is no known method of preventing scoliosis. Families and health professionals often feel guilty that they did not provide enough treatment, but there is no evidence that any current treatment will prevent scoliosis. Medicines, custom positioning systems for wheelchairs, dorsal rhizotomy and intensive physical therapy are all helpful, but do not prevent scoliosis. Custom body jackets may help maintain a comfortable body position in which the child can use both hands, but may impair respiratory effort and cause skin breakdown. Surgical repair is complex but highly effective if done by a skilled surgeon who has lots of experience and a highly effective team including anaesthesiology, postoperative nursing, physical therapists, nutritionists and doctors to look after medical problems and pain management. Scoliosis repair is never an emergency and deserves careful planning that includes the 6–12 months of recovery during which the child and family may need extra supports to assure a successful outcome. There are some children who have been through many complications from severe CP who do not benefit from yet another highly stressful surgical procedure. Families are usually the ones who know best about how the stresses of CP and the other health problems associated with it affect the quality of life of their child.

Useful websites

American Academy for Cerebral Palsy and Developmental Medicine: http://www.aacpdm.org.

CanChild Centre for Child Disability Research: http://www.fhs.mcmaster.ca/canchild/.

Information from the National Library of Medicine: http://www.medlineplus.gov.

KidsHealth, Nemours Foundation: http://www.kidshealth.org/parent/medical/brain/cerebral_palsy.htmMedlinePlusHealth.

National Institute for Neurological Disorders and Stroke: http://www.ninds.nih.gov/disorders/spasticity/spasticity.htm.

Scope: Major British charity serving people with CP: http://www.scope.org.uk.

United Cerebral Palsy: Major US charity serving people with CP: http://www.ucp.org/.

WeMove Worldwide Education and Awareness for Movement Disorders: http://www.wemove.org/spa/.

28

Complementary and alternative medicine in cerebral palsy

Mark Bower

Nowhere is there a more consensus view about complementary and alternative medicine (CAM) than among practitioners who work in areas of treatment for patients with cancer or cerebral palsy (CP). Parents confronted with a diagnosis of CP may feel a void at a vulnerable stage in their own and their child's life – a void that may be readily filled with complementary treatments, alternative therapies and quackery.

Patients and their carers are introduced to an area of medicine where conventional therapies have limited success. It is scarcely surprising that they seek complementary and alternative treatments. There is good reason for thinking that the unmet emotional needs of patients and their carers are responsible for the increasing use of unconventional treatments.

This makes it doubly important that all should understand what CAM is and the reasons why medical practitioners have serious reservations about many of the treatments put forward.

What is complementary and alternative medicine?

The Cochrane Collaboration, founded in 1993 and named after the British epidemiologist, Archie Cochrane, is an international not-for-profit independent organization that aims to publish accurate and proven information about the effects of health care interventions. It produces evidence-based reviews by examining the facts from clinical trials and other studies of therapies. According to the Cochrane project, CAM is a 'broad domain of healing resources that encompasses all health systems, modalities, and practices and their accompanying theories and beliefs, other than those intrinsic to the politically dominant health system of a particular society or culture in a given historical period'. Thus, although orthodox conventional medicine is politically dominant, CAM practises outside this system and is for the most part isolated from the universities and hospitals where health care is taught and delivered. As some CAM disciplines, for example acupuncture, become increasingly incorporated into conventional medicine they lose their 'alternative' status. Indeed, it is this cooperation between health systems that led to the introduction of the term 'complementary medicine' rather than 'alternative medicine'. Although frequently used interchangeably, the two terms imply these differences: complementary therapies are used in conjunction with conventional treatments whereas alternative therapies are used in place of conventional medicine.

What CAMs are used in cerebral palsy?

The National Centre for Complementary and Alternative Medicine (NCCAM) is a branch of the National Institutes of Health (NIH) in the USA and undertakes large surveys of CAM usage. They classify CAMs into five groups: (1) biologically based therapies; (2) energy therapies; (3) manipulative and body-based practices; (4) mind–body therapies; and (5) whole medical systems.

Biologically based therapies

These use naturally occurring substances such as herbs, special diets and vitamins (in doses outside those used in conventional medicine). It should be remembered that many conventional drugs originated from natural sources, for example, Botox used in children with CP to relieve spasticity, was derived from the bacterium *Clostridium botulinum* that causes a severe form of food poisoning known as botulism. An example of biologically based alternative therapy that has been used in CP is amino acid therapy. Based on the theories of Professor Khokhlov, amino acid therapy is a prime example of pseudoscience, using the language and authority of science but without recognizing its methods or providing a plausible biological mechanism. No published studies have tried to evaluate whether there are any benefits or side-effects from this therapy.

Energy therapies

These approaches use energy fields such as magnetic fields or biofields (energy fields that advocates believe surround and penetrate the human body). One example of a biotherapy is hyperbaric oxygen therapy (HBOT) which was thought to increase oxygenation of the brain in children with CP. It involves breathing 100% oxygen in a hyperbaric chamber similar to a diving bell that is pressurized at up to three times greater than atmospheric pressure. A session typically lasts 1–2 hours although the length, frequency and total number of sessions have not been standardized. The first status of HBOT was as an alternative therapy based on anecdotal evidence; thereafter an initial pilot study was encouraging (Montgomery et al. 1999) and HBOT became thought of as a complementary therapy. As a consequence two sizeable and well-controlled randomized trials were undertaken to evaluate the role of HBOT in children with CP. However both found that there was no benefit from HBOT (Collet et al. 2001, Hardy et al. 2002) and this is also the conclusion of a systematic review of the evidence sponsored by the US Department of Health (McDonagh et al. 2003). Moreover, it should not be assumed that because HBOT does no good that it also does no harm. Ear, breathing and neurological side-effects have all been described with HBOT (Nuthall et al. 2000, Collet et al. 2001).

Therapeutic (subthreshold) electrical stimulation (TES) involves giving small electrical shocks to the skin overlying selected muscles, usually those that work opposite muscles affected by spasticity. TES is often delivered when the child is asleep and aims to strengthen the stimulated antagonist muscles in an attempt to balance out the spasticity. TES was studied in a randomized cross-over study in Norway to measure whether it improved leg function in CP children with spastic diplegia. The study showed no benefit from TES in any objective, measurable index of muscle strength or walking capacity (Sommerfelt et al. 2001). Despite this, almost all of the parents reported that TES helped their children and it is this subjective but unreal effect that is a common finding in CAM users and that may relate to the increased attention and input that result in emotional gains ('At least we're doing something'; 'I'll try anything for my child').

Manipulative and body-based practices

These treatments are based on manipulation or movement of body parts and are widely used physical therapies for children with CP. Many of the conventional therapies prescribed for CP are physical treatments and are closely related to the complementary exercise-related treatments such as aquatic exercises (hydrotherapy), martial arts training, t'ai chi and hippotherapy (therapeutic horse riding). Most of these are enjoyable pastimes that encourage muscle strength and coordination and, although they may not have all been formally evaluated, many are advocated by conventional medicine and evaluated scientifically (McGibbon et al. 1998, Benda et al. 2003).

However another more suspect alternative therapy approach is Adeli suit therapy, based on the Adeli suit, first used by Russian cosmonauts in the early 1970s to prevent muscle atrophy in space. The straightjacket-like suit is laced up with cords to adjust the pressure exerted on different muscle groups during exercise. Patented by Professor Siemionowa and quite widely used, there have been no published, scientifically credible attempts to evaluate the suit or to assess its safety in children with CP.

Mind–body therapies

These therapies include a number of techniques designed to enhance the mind's ability to affect bodily function and symptoms. Conductive education (CE) is a programme of developmental learning (physical, social, emotional and academic) for children with motor disorders designed to improve motor skills and increase independence for many aspects of common living. CE was developed in the 1940s by Dr Andreas Petö in Hungary and has now been widely established in a number of centres in Europe and increasingly further afield. A careful meta-analysis of CE for children with CP has been undertaken for the American Academy for Cerebral

Palsy and Developmental Medicine (AACPDM), including all published studies. In all there were 20 statistically significant outcome measures, 10 favouring the CE groups and 10 the control groups (Darrah et al. 2004). The report concludes that the present literature provides no conclusive evidence to support (or refute) the use of CE. Despite this lack of any supporting evidence families and friends of children with CP dig deep into their pockets to afford this expensive unproven treatment.

Whole medical systems

These complete systems of theory and practice of alternative medicine often hark back to earlier approaches to medicine that predate conventional Western medicine. One example is the traditional Chinese practice of acupuncture.

Acupuncture

Acupuncture originated over 2000 years ago in China. It was used by William Osler, the most celebrated Canadian-born physician who was both Chief of Staff at Johns Hopkins University and subsequently Regius Professor of Medicine at Oxford University at the start of the 20th century. The recent resurgence in popularity of acupuncture dates from President Nixon's visit to China in the 1970s. The stimulation of acupuncture points by fine needles is intended to control the qi energy circulating between organs along channels or meridians. The 12 main meridians correspond to 12 major functions or 'organs' of the body and acupuncture points are located along these meridians. The analgesic actions of acupuncture may be explained by a conventional physiological model and acupuncture is known to release endogenous opioids. There is convincing evidence supporting the value of acupuncture in the management of both nausea and acute pain. The evidence base for the use of acupuncture in chronic pain is less secure and current evidence suggests that it is unlikely to be of benefit for obesity, smoking cessation and tinnitus. For most other conditions the available evidence is insufficient to guide clinical decisions.

Acupuncture appears to be a relatively safe treatment in the hands of suitably qualified practitioners, with serious adverse events being extremely rare. Despite these limitations it has been estimated that one million acupuncture treatments are given on the National Health Service (NHS) in England each year, at an estimated cost of £26 million, equivalent to all other complementary therapies combined. A further two million acupuncture treatments are given in the private sector annually.

Acupuncture has been widely used in the care of children with CP, with many anecdotal reports of benefits. However a recent randomized controlled trial of tongue acupuncture has been undertaken in 33 children with CP in Hong Kong and the results have been published in a peer-reviewed medical journal of high repute (impact factor 3). This trial evaluated the effects of acupuncture or no acupuncture as measured by the Gross Motor Function Measure (GMFM) and the Paediatric Evaluation of Disability Inventory (PEDI) – two validated scales widely used in conventional medicine. There was a statistically significant improvement in motor function seen following a short course of acupuncture (Sun et al. 2004). This type of evaluation of an alternative therapy by conventional trial methodology leads to the acceptance of new approaches by conventional medicine, so that acupuncture becomes a complementary treatment accepted within the overall management of children with CP rather than an alternative therapy whose value is unknown, or a quack treatment that is harmful.

Who uses CAM?

Every year around 20% of the population in the UK use CAM and this is interpreted as a measure of disillusionment with conventional medicine. In contrast, the prevalence of use in the USA is 40% and in Germany is > 60%. There is a prolonged history in Germany of CAM use and indeed Samuel Hahnemann (1755–1843), who first described homeopathy, was a German physician. The pantheon of complementary and alternative therapies includes alternative therapies with recognized professional bodies (e.g. acupuncture, chiropractic, herbal medicine, homoeopathy

and osteopathy), complementary therapies (e.g. Alexander technique, aromatherapy, Bach and other flower extracts, body work therapies including massage, counselling stress therapy, hypnotherapy, meditation, reflexology, shiatsu, healing, Maharishi ayurvedic medicine, nutritional medicine and yoga) and alternative therapies that lack professional organization but have established and traditional systems of health care (e.g. anthroposophical medicine, ayurvedic medicine, Chinese herbal medicine, Eastern medicine (Tibb), naturopathy and traditional Chinese medicine) and finally there are other 'new-age' alternative disciplines (e.g. crystal therapy, dowsing, iridology, kinesiology and radionics). Surveys suggest that about 2 in 3 children with CP have used CAM (Hurvitz et al. 2003, Sanders et al. 2003) mostly in addition to, rather than as replacement for, conventional treatments.

The worst form of CAM – quackery

The word 'quack' is supposedly derived from quacksalver, a 17th-century variant spelling of quicksilver or mercury which was used in certain remedies which the public came to recognize as harmful. Pseudoscience uses the language and authority of science without recognizing its methods. It produces claims that cannot be proven or refuted and often poses as the victim ('scientists are suppressing the truth'). A quack may reasonably be defined as a pseudoscientist who is selling something, and a charlatan as a cynical pseudoscientist who knows he or she is deceiving the public. It is a sorry monument to human greed and stupidity that more money is spent on health frauds every year than on medical research.

Quacks are convincing because they tell people what they want to hear. Moreover it is almost impossible for the CP quack to fail. When a patient deteriorates, the CP quack resorts to lines such as, 'If only you had come to me sooner'. However professionals should appreciate that quacks can teach us a great deal whilst we retain an honest and informed practice of medicine. Their popularity is attributed to their patience and ability to listen carefully and show both interest and affection. As well as this, quacks encourage patients to take an active role in their health care, thus empowering them.

The internet appears to have made CP quackery even easier. Although much health information on the web is evidence-based and of high quality, the open access has also been abused. Entrepreneurs have recognized the value of the web as a free-for-all market and have used it to promote fraudulent CP treatments. A Google search with the terms 'cerebral palsy cure' yields 575 000 hits in 0.07 seconds, despite the fact that to date there is no cure for CP and that no CAM therapies have been scientifically demonstrated to improve brain function for the control of muscle spasticity, or improvement in motor coordination.

Worries about using CAM

Many doctors remain concerned about the use of CAM. These concerns may be based on a number of factors, including that patients may be seen by unqualified practitioners, may risk delayed or missed diagnosis, may decline or stop conventional therapies, may waste money on ineffective therapies and may experience dangerous adverse effects from treatment. Moreover, the scientific academic training in medicine leads many doctors to question the value of these therapies where a plausible mechanism of action is not available. At present practitioners of CAM in the UK are free to practise as they wish without clear regulation. Greater cooperation and respect between conventional doctors and complementary therapists might help to improve patient care.

Advice to parents, carers and health care professionals about CAM

So, how should parents and carers of children with CP react to people who suggest CAM treatments? Almost all of these suggestions will be benevolent in origin, from grandparents or other relatives, friends and the parents of other children with CP. As I have described, the CAMs most frequently proposed for children with CP either have not been shown to work or have been found to be detrimental to the child's health. Moreover, they are often very expensive and in health systems such as the NHS or insurance-based health schemes, CAMs are rarely funded for children with CP. Despite these caveats, parents may be put under great pressure by those advocating CAMs. Seeking the advice of traditional medical professionals may seem like a cop-out, as it is often dissatisfaction with these professionals and the results of their approaches that encourages parents to seek CAM. Parents and carers need to consider critically the evidence in favour and the expense of any suggested CAMs and may seek the advice of independent evidence evaluators such as the Cochrane project. Similarly, mainstream health care professionals need to react sympathetically to parents/carers following an alternative therapy regimen. After all, we need to recognize that it is the failure of conventional medicine that encourages parents and carers of children with CP to seek CAMs. Parents of children with pneumonia rarely seek CAM, as the traditional medical treatment with antibiotics is so successful. If only this were true of our therapies for children with CP.

References

Benda W, McGibbon NH, Grant KL. Improvements in muscle symmetry in children with cerebral palsy after equine-assisted therapy (hippotherapy). J Altern Complement Med 2003; 9:817–825.

Collet JP, Vanasse M, Marois P et al. Hyperbaric oxygen for children with cerebral palsy: a randomised multicentre trial. HBO-CP Research Group. Lancet 2001; 357:582–586.

Darrah J, Watkins B, Chen L et al. Conductive education intervention for children with cerebral palsy: an

AACPDM evidence report. Dev Med Child Neurol 2004; 46:187–203.

Hardy P, Collet JP, Goldberg J et al. Neuropsychological effects of hyperbaric oxygen therapy in cerebral palsy. Dev Med Child Neurol 2002; 44:436–446.

Hurvitz EA, Leonard C, Ayyangar R et al. Complementary and alternative medicine use in families of children with cerebral palsy. Dev Med Child Neurol 2003; 45:364–370.

McDonagh M, Carson S, Ash J et al. Hyperbaric oxygen therapy for brain injury, cerebral palsy, and stroke. Evid Rep Technol Assess (Summ) 2003; 85:1–6.

McGibbon NH, Andrade CK, Widener G et al. Effect of an equine-movement therapy program on gait, energy expenditure, and motor function in children with spastic cerebral palsy: a pilot study. Dev Med Child Neurol 1998; 40:754–762.

Montgomery D, Goldberg J, Amar M et al. Effects of hyperbaric oxygen therapy on children with spastic diplegic cerebral palsy: a pilot project. Undersea Hyperb Med 1999; 26:235–242.

Nuthall G, Seear M, Lepawsky M et al. Hyperbaric oxygen therapy for cerebral palsy: two complications of treatment. Pediatrics 2000; 106:E80.

Sanders H, Davis MF, Duncan B et al. Use of complementary and alternative medical therapies among children with special health care needs in southern Arizona. Pediatrics 2003; 111:584–587.

Sommerfelt K, Markestad T, Berg K et al. Therapeutic electrical stimulation in cerebral palsy: a randomized, controlled, crossover trial. Dev Med Child Neurol 2001; 43:609–613.

Sun JG, Ko CH, Wong V et al. Randomised control trial of tongue acupuncture versus sham acupuncture in improving functional outcome in cerebral palsy. J Neurol Neurosurg Psychiatry 2004; 75:1054–1057.

Appendix 1
An overview of the first five stages of sensorimotor development in a child with typical movement

The purpose of this overview is to illustrate that, when helping a child with cerebral palsy (CP) towards functional independence skills it is useful to have an understanding of the sensorimotor development underlying such skills.

Given such an understanding of the development of a child as a basis, it is easier to appreciate the differences between the child with typical movement and that of the child with CP, enabling one to realize how atypical postures and movements interfere with future achievement. Although there are many stages in the sensorimotor development of the child during the period covered in this book, such as getting up to sitting, moving from sitting to standing and from standing to walking, only the early stages of development are described to point out how the gross motor movements in supine, prone and sitting underlie the fine movements of the hands and overlap with the development of vision, hearing and speech.

The posture of a child during the first few months is predominantly one of flexion. At this early stage the head is rarely in the midline, the child has no active head control other than the ability to turn the head sideways to breathe when placed on the tummy. The arms are usually bent and apart. The mass movements are abrupt and follow no set pattern. The child reacts to light and loud sounds by blinking or by a Moro reaction: neither stimulus has real meaning to the child.

Stage 1

The first significant stage in motor development is that of midline orientation and the start of head control.

Both of these activities make it possible for the child to begin to make contact with the environment, first with the eyes and later exploring with the hands.

Rolling

The first time that the child starts to move from one position to another is usually by rolling to either side from the back. To begin with the child will often hold the hands together while rolling. The movement of rolling starts with the turning of the head which causes the body to follow; later the child self-initiates the entire movement.

Vision and the beginning of eye–hand regard

Gradually the child starts to select what is seen. The child is able to follow the mother with the eyes as she moves around the cot and also to follow a simple dangling toy 150–300 mm (6–12 inches) above the face through a half-circle from side to side. The child begins to turn to the sound of a voice and smiles when the mother speaks to her child. The child is already learning to smile when wanting to be picked up and to know that crying will get attention.

Figure A.1 illustrates the child at stage 1 in supine.

Figure A.2 illustrates the child at stage 1 in prone.

Figure A.3 illustrates the child at stage 1 in sitting.

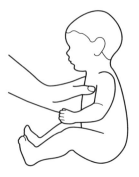

Figure A.3 • At this stage the child must be supported when sitting. The child holds the head erect but only for a few seconds. The back is straight, except for the lumbar region. The body has to be supported in sitting long after head control is established in this position. The arms and legs are bent and abducted, feet dorsiflexed.

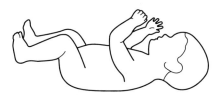

Figure A.1 • At this stage the child prefers to lie on the back. The head is now usually in the midline. The child brings the hands together over the chest and looks at them. This combination of touch and vision is the first step in self-exploration. The child takes the hands to the mouth, at first accidentally, then purposefully, to suck, later touching and exploring the lips, cheeks and tongue with the fingers. The eyes start to coordinate and the child becomes preoccupied with the mother's face, but at first only at a distance of 150 mm (6 inches).

Stage 2

The next important stage in motor development is the beginning of extension/abduction of the limbs, overlapping with flexion/abduction in conjunction with the extension of the whole body. The child practises this extension in all positions but at the same time is able to undertake activities in flexion.

Vision and the beginning of eye–hand coordination

The child can, as it were, now 'grasp' an object with the eyes but is still unable to reach out and grasp it with the hands. The child displays excitement and demonstrates wanting something by kicking with both legs and waving both arms, opening and closing the fingers while doing so. At first this is done with the arms bent and near the body but gradually progresses to opening and closing the hands while both following and reaching out for an object, although being still unable to grasp or manipulate at this stage. It is worth noting that this is the time when one sees the child making a deliberate attempt to move the arms towards an object with the intention of trying to get it.

The child can follow an object if it is moved slowly from left to right in front of the face.

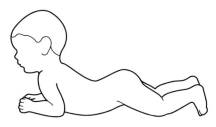

Figure A.2 • Head control starts to develop first when the child lies on the tummy. The top of the spine extends sufficiently to enable the child to get the shoulders and arms forwards. Weight is taken on the forearms, which helps to raise the upper part of the body. The hands remain loosely closed. The pelvis, which was previously up in the air when lying on the tummy, is now flat on the support. The hips and legs are bent and apart, feet dorsiflexed.

If a rattle is placed in the child's hand it will be grasped with a strong grip using the inner side of the hands and fingers. The child can look at it for a second but will then often wave the arms about in an uncoordinated fashion and maybe hit him- or herself and complain loudly. The child cannot at this stage let go. Rattles vary in shape and sound and are a good way of encouraging development of the eyes and ears at this stage.

Hearing and speech

The child responds momentarily to loud sounds, vocalizing while moving and answering back in a way to sounds made by others. In conjunction with a variation in pitch the child's repertoire enlarges; for example, sounds of anger appear. The child blows raspberries, syllables come into the babbling and the child starts to make the sounds 'm', 'mm', and 'ddd'.

Figures A.4 and A.5 illustrate the child in supine at stage 2.

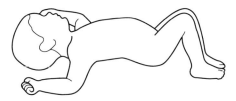

Figure A.4 • The child practises extension while lying on the back. The shoulders are retracted, arms bent, hands loosely closed. The feet are flat on the floor and the bottom lifted slightly off the support. Soon the child will push backwards; thus the child is able to lift the head forward despite the shoulder retraction.

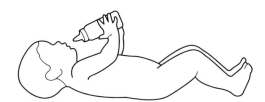

Figure A.5 • Although supine tends to be a position of extension, the child can bring the arms forwards to have a bottle placed into the hands. Hand regard and taking them to the mouth are practised at this stage.

Figures A.6 and A.7 illustrate the child in prone at stage 2.

Figure A.8 illustrates the child in sitting at stage 2.

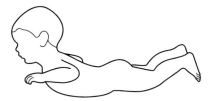

Figure A.6 • High lifting of the head helps extension of the body, including the lumbar spine. The child lifts the arms either bent and off the support as shown, or off the support and extended sideways, 'swimming' on the tummy. The legs are lifted, extended and apart, but the feet remain dorsiflexed.

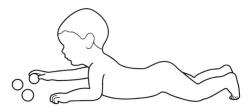

Figure A.7 • At this stage the child can also take weight on the forearms and reach out to touch a toy. The feet are dorsiflexed and toes bent, pressing against the floor. Later the child will use this position of the feet when starting to creep.

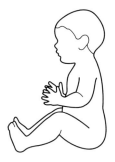

Figure A.8 • The child's head is now steady, the body straighter, including for the first time extension of the lumbar spine. The arms are bent, abducted and retracted at the shoulders or forward as shown. The legs are bent and apart, feet dorsiflexed. At this stage of development it is often difficult to bend the child's hips for sitting. The child enjoys pushing back and still needs support to sit.

Stage 3

The child has progressed from being a flexed individual to being an extended individual and now has good head control. The child has now reached an important stage in development when a greater variety of motor postures appear. This is the stage of stronger extension abduction of the limbs. Whereas previously movements of the limbs were taking place predominantly at the shoulders and hips, an increase in active movements is now seen at the elbows and knees. The development of the arms is in advance of the legs.

Rolling

The child can now roll over from the tummy on to the back, a movement that includes rotation and active extension of the whole body, essential later on when standing and walking.

Vision and manipulation

As head control is now good the child can follow objects with the eyes in all directions. The child is also able to fix the gaze on small objects. Whereas earlier when seeing an image of him- or herself in a mirror the child was puzzled, the child is now aware that it is an image, recognizes it and will reach forward and pat the image. Self-exploration continues as the child becomes increasingly aware of the feet.

Object exploration begins as the child now has the ability to look, reach, touch and clutch an object with a whole hand. Manipulation is still very crude and for this reason everything is quickly taken to the mouth. The mouth plays an important role in providing information such as taste, shape and consistency.

The child still does not have fine movements of the fingers, flapping and scooping with the hands, needing to open the whole hand widely before grasping but succeeding in this fashion to pick up for example a 25-mm (1-inch) wooden cube. The grasp is called a *palmar* one, that is, with a whole hand. Movements at the wrist are becoming noticeably more refined. The child can hold and transfer two cubes of 25 mm, but if one is dropped no notice is taken. The child will accept large objects with both hands, look at them and immediately take them to the mouth. Wooden spoons, bricks and plastic cups are much preferred at this stage to soft toys.

Hearing and speech

The child now immediately turns to sounds except for those which come from directly over the head, which tend to confuse. The child responds when spoken to by laughing, chuckling and squealing, vocalizing with variations in a tuneful way. The continuous sounds made are forerunners of future speech; the babbling is repetitive, using syllables such as 'ppp' and 'sss'.

Figure A.9 illustrates the child in supine at stage 3.

Figure A.10 illustrates the child in prone at stage 3.

Figure A.11 illustrates the child in sitting at stage 3.

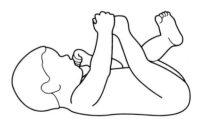

Figure A.9 • At this stage the child starts making movements for a desired result. The child reaches out with the arms when mother approaches to pick the child up. As the child reaches out with the hands the hips may be bent but the legs straight, a position used later when getting up from sitting or sitting with legs out in front. Reaching out coincides with the ability to grasp. The child now finds the feet for the first time and is able to integrate the ability to see, feel and grasp by holding on to the feet, becoming aware of how they look both still and moving. The feet are taken to the mouth in further exploration.

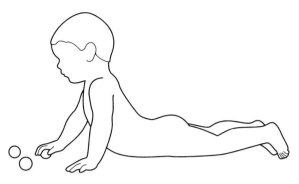

Figure A.10 • When on the tummy the child not only raises the head high with a straight upper back but, whereas a few weeks earlier weight was taken on a closed hand, the hand is now open. Resulting from the mobility of the arms when using them for support, the child is soon able to take weight on one arm and reach for toys with the other, forwards and later backwards.

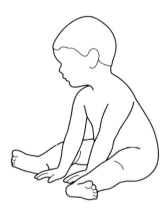

Figure A.11 • The child now sits with the legs apart and straight out in front, the feet dorsiflexed. There is still no sitting balance and a tendency to throw oneself backwards when sitting. Resulting from the lack of sitting balance and sideways support, the child often falls sideways. The child begins to use the hands for support at this stage, but only in front.

Stage 4

The child now reaches the stage in development when *the ability to rotate becomes well coordinated*. Whereas rotation was previously present when the child rolled, when the child reached across for an object while lying on the back and when lying on the tummy supporting on one arm while reaching back with the other, now, with arm support developing both sideways and forwards, *spontaneous rotation, trunk control and sitting balance appear.*

Rolling

The child now rolls from the back to the tummy in a well-coordinated manner whereas previously the child was rather disorganized.

Vision and manipulation

As already pointed out, a child's ability to reach and grasp objects is dependent on balance and the ability to look at what is being done. It is therefore not surprising to find that at this stage the child makes exaggerated movements of the whole body, often overbalancing in attempts to reach out for a toy. During the following months these exaggerated movements gradually diminish.

The ability to manipulate improves rapidly at this stage and grasp becomes more refined; the child can now hold one object in each hand and transfer from hand to hand and bang two cubes together. The child begins to take objects out of a container and tries unsuccessfully to pick up small objects. The child starts to drop large objects on to the floor – a basic movement for future release – but once the object has been dropped shows no further interest.

Speech

The child uses sounds to express anger and hunger and 'nnn' sounds to express dislikes and imitates dialogue using chains of sounds with intonation.

Figure A.12 illustrates the child at stage 4 beginning to move from sitting to prone.

Figure A.13 illustrates the child at stage 4 sitting.

Figure A.14 illustrates the child at stage 4 in crawling position.

Figure A.15 illustrates the child at stage 4 sitting and reaching for a toy backwards and upwards with rotation.

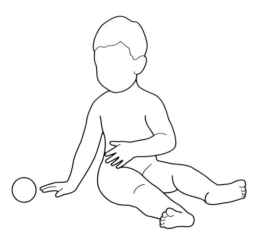

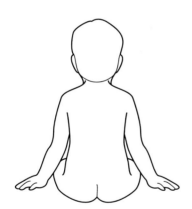

Figure A.12 • The child now uses the ability to support on one hand to push up to sitting at the same time as rotating the body. The child pivots on the tummy, also pushing backwards, with the legs remaining rather inactive – another example of the arms still being in advance of the legs in development. Later the child will creep forward, the legs participating strongly in the movement, especially the feet.

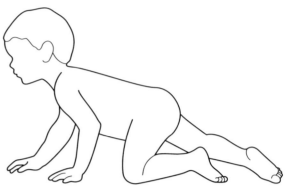

Figure A.14 • Movement is important at this time. The child only plays on the tummy for short periods, now preferring to get on all fours where the child rocks in preparation for crawling. Crawling requires both balance and reciprocal movements of the legs.

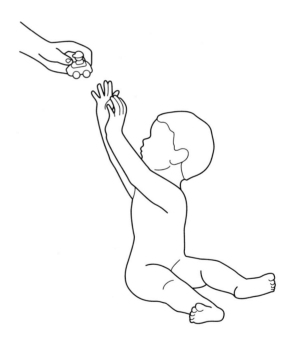

Figure A.13 • At first unsupported sitting is of short duration, probably no longer than a minute. The child will then lean forward to support him- or herself. Gradually with the development of trunk control and sitting balance the child learns to support sideways. Arm support is first with a loosely closed hand and later the hand opens in preparation for weight-bearing.

Figure A.15 • Backward protective extension of the arms is now starting. Balance in sitting is good and the hands are no longer required for support. As shown, the child can turn to look and grasp a toy with rotation of the trunk or alternatively pivot in sitting.

Stage 5

The final developmental stage to be dealt with is the acquisition of balance and beginning of moving in and out of positions requiring balance.

Most activities at this time start from the sitting position. Moving round is an important function for the child at this stage. It is an opportunity to explore the environment and the child's relationship to the environment.

Supine

On the rare occasions when the child does lie on the back this is now done with the legs straight and slightly apart.

Eye–hand development

At this time isolated movements of the fingers are developing, enabling the child to explore objects with the fingertips and poking them with the index finger. The thumb and index finger now play an important part in manipulation. Small objects are picked up and inspected. One needs to note however, that at this stage, although manipulation has reached a more constant phase, release of an object is still difficult. The child attempts to release by pressing an object against a surface. Play is now more purposeful and the child becomes engrossed for longer periods at a time. The child is also becoming aware of the permanence of objects and when dropping a toy will look to see where it has gone.

Speech

The child vocalizes deliberately as a means of communication and understands 'no' and 'bye-bye' and enjoys copying adults, for example, when they cough.

I hope that the first five stages of sensorimotor development described above will help parents and carers to understand the role of gross movement development in relation to the development of eye–hand dexterity, hearing and speech development. This in turn may help parents and carers to appreciate some of the difficulties that may occur in children with CP when this development of gross motor movement is atypical and/or absent.

Appendix 2
A typical child's gross motor development

Age	Lying	Sitting	Standing
0–6 months	Supine; holds head up and pushes up on hands Rolls from prone to supine	Sits with support Sits leaning forwards on hands	Can be stood on feet with support
6–12 months	Rolls from supine to prone Crawls	Sits independently Sits and turns and reaches Saving reaction in sitting	Pulls to stand
12–24 months		Moves in and out of sitting position Rights self if tilted in sitting	Walks independently
2–4 years			Kicks a ball Jumps

Appendix 3
Validated measures of motor development and function which can be used for children with cerebral palsy (listed alphabetically)

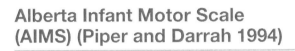

Alberta Infant Motor Scale (AIMS) (Piper and Darrah 1994)

Age range: birth–18 months
Time to administer: 10–20 minutes
Appraises: by observation and analysis of the spontaneous movements of a child in prone and supine lying, sitting and standing

Obtainable from: Saunders Elsevier, UK

Bayley Scales of Infant and Toddler Development (3rd edn) (Bayley 2005)

Age range: 1–42 months
Time to administer: 30–90 minutes
Appraises: by observation and administration of 'the mental scale', 'the motor scale' and 'the behaviour rating scale'

Obtainable from: Harcourt, UK

Gross Motor Function Measure (GMFM 66 and 88) (Russell et al. 2002)

Age range: birth–16 years
Time to administer: 30–60 minutes
Appraises: by observation of motor abilities in:

1. Lying and rolling
2. Sitting
3. Crawling and kneeling
4. Standing
5. Walking, running and jumping

Obtainable from: MacKeith Press, UK

Movement ABC-2 test (Henderson and Sugden 2007)

Age range: 3–6 years
Time to administer: 20–40 minutes
Appraises: by observation of:

1. Manual dexterity
2. Ball skills
3. Static and dynamic balance

Obtainable from: Harcourt, UK

Paediatric Evaluation of Disability Inventory (PEDI) (Haley et al. 1992)

Age range: 6 months–7 years
Time to administer: 45–60 minutes
Appraises: by interview/report of:

1. Self-care, mobility and social function
2. Care-giver assistance
3. Modifications
   (a) Environmental
   (b) Equipment

Obtainable from: Harcourt, UK

Peabody Developmental Motor Scale (2nd edn) (Folio and Fewell 2000)

Age range: birth–6 years
Time to administer: 45–60 minutes
Appraises: by observation of:

1. Gross motor quotient (large-muscle systems)
   (a) Reflexes (birth–11 months)
   (b) Stationary body control
   (c) Locomotion
   (d) Object manipulation (throw, catch and kick)
2. Fine motor quotient (small-muscle systems)
   (a) Grasping
   (b) Visual motor integration

Obtainable from: Harcourt, UK

WeeFIM (Msall et al. 1994)

Age range: all persons with a 'mental age' below 7 years
Time to administer: 30 minutes
Appraises: by observation of:

1. Motor abilities in self-care, sphincter control, transfers and locomotion
2. Cognitive abilities in communication and social cognition

Obtainable from: The Centre for Functional Assessment Research, Uniform Data System for Medical Rehabilitation, 232 Parker Hall, Sunny South Campus 3435 Main Street, Buffalo NY 141214-3007, USA

References

Bayley N. Bayley Scales of Infant and Toddler Development, 3rd edition. Harcourt Assessment, TX, 2005.

Folio MR, Fewell RR. Peabody Developmental Motor Scale, 2nd edition. Therapy Skill Builders, TX, 2000.

Haley SM, Coster WJ, Ludlow LH et al. Paediatric Evaluation of Disability Inventory (PEDI). New England Medical Center Hospitals, Boston, 1992.

Henderson SE, Sugden DA. Movement Assessment Battery for Children, 2nd edition (Movement ABC-2). Harcourt Assessment, TX, 2007.

Msall ME, DiGaudio K, Duffy LC et al. WeeFIM. Normative sample of an instrument for tracking functional independence in children. Clinical Pediatrics 1994; 33: 431–438.

Piper M, Darrah J. Alberta Infant Motor Scale Score Sheets (AIMS). Saunders, Philadelphia, 1994.

Russell DJ, Rosenbaum PL, Avery LM, Lane M. Gross Motor Function Measure (GMFM 66 and 88). MacKeith Press, Cambridge, 2002.

Appendix 4
Using the Gross Motor Function Classification System (GMFCS) for intervention planning in children 0–5 years
(cognitive, behaviour and sensory characteristics may further influence all of these suggestions)

Level	Abilities	Ideas for intervention
Age 1–2 years		
I	Sits with both hands free for use Moves in and out of sitting Crawls. Pulls to stand Walks holding on to furniture 18 months–2 years: walks independently	Opportunities may be needed to encourage the improvement of speed, balance and coordination in all activities
II	Maintains floor sitting but may need support from hands Creeps on stomach or crawls on hands and knees May pull to stand and take steps holding on to furniture	Opportunities to encourage independence in sitting plus the use of hands, crawling and transfers
III	Maintains floor sitting with support at lower back Rolls. Creeps forward on stomach	Provide a suitable chair Opportunities to encourage moving about on the floor, sitting independently using the hands and pulling up to standing from sitting
IV	Able to control head position Requires trunk support for floor sitting Rolls prone to sitting but has difficulty with supine to prone	Provide a suitable chair Provide a suitable bathing aid Opportunities to encourage rolling
V	No antigravity head or trunk control in prone or sitting Needs adult assistance to roll	Provide a suitable chair Provide a suitable bathing aid Opportunities to encourage head control
Age 2–4 years		
I	Walks independently	Opportunities to encourage climbing stairs

II	Floor sits but may have difficulty with balance when using hands Moves in and out of sitting Pulls to stand on stable surface Crawls with reciprocal movements Cruises holding on to furniture Walks with mobility device	Provide mobility device Opportunities to encourage independence in all upright activities (standing and walking)
III	Maintains floor sitting, often in 'W' position Creeps or crawls on hands and knees May pull to stand and cruise short distances May walk with mobility device but needs help to steer and turn	Provide mobility device Opportunities to encourage pull-up to standing, cruising, transfer and walking with device Assess for a self-propelled wheelchair for outdoor use and bathing aid
IV	Floor sits if placed in position using hands for support Rolls and creeps on stomach Crawls without reciprocal movements	Provide wheelchair for inside and outside use Provide a standing frame Opportunities to encourage use of hands in supported sitting and floor mobility Assess for powered electric wheelchair, stair lift and hoist
V	No independent mobility	Provide a wheelchair for inside and outside use Assess for possible use of electric-powered wheelchair, stairlift and hoist

Age 4–6 years

I	Walks in community, climbs stairs	
II	Chair sits with both hands free for use Moves from floor sitting to standing and from chair sitting to standing but may require a stable surface to push and pull up on arms Walks independently inside and outside on level surfaces Climbs stairs using one rail	Mobility device should no longer be needed Provide stair rail Opportunities to encourage walking on uneven surfaces, inclines, in crowds and in wide open spaces
III	Sits on a regular chair but may need pelvic/trunk support Walks with a mobility device May need adult assistance on stairs or two rails May be transported outside	Provide two stair rails Opportunities to encourage moving on and off a regular chair and wheelchair, stepping up and down a kerb or steps Train in outside use of self-propelled wheelchair
IV	Sits on chair with adaptations for trunk control Needs help to move in and out of sitting May walk very short distances with help from an adult or very supportive device	Train in use of powered electric wheelchair or self-propelled wheelchair as appropriate inside and outside Opportunities to encourage transfers
V	No change	Train in use of electric-powered wheelchair if appropriate

Appendix 5
Glossary of some of the terms used by therapists
(most terms are described as used in the chapters)

Abduction	The movement of the limbs away from the midline of the body
Active movements	Purposeful, spontaneous movements undertaken by the child
Adduction	The movement of the limbs towards the midline of the body
Agnosia	An inability to recognize the relevance of sensory stimuli, that is, the significance of objects seen, sounds heard and/or textures felt. A perceptual deficit
Aphasia	An impairment or loss of language
Associated reactions	An increase in muscle tone resulting from the effort required to undertake a task. Sometimes actual movements of other parts of the body occur, for example, movements in the unaffected hand when using the affected hand in a child with hemiplegia
Astereognosis	The inability to appreciate size, shape, form or texture
Asymmetrical	One side of the body differs from the other
Asymmetrical tonic neck reflex	The limbs on the side to which the face is turned extend and on the other side the limbs flex
Ataxia	Unsteadiness. This may apply to the limbs or trunk. Movements are poorly timed, graded and directed
Athetosis	Unpredictable fluctuating muscle tone and impairment of postural control causing involuntary movements. Static postural control is absent and automatic reactions are exaggerated
Atrophy	The wasting of muscles
Audiometry	The process of measuring the activity of hearing
Audiotory	This relates to the ability to hear
Automatic reactions	See Equilibrium, Protective reactions/saving reactions and Righting reactions
Balance	Maintaining equilibrium
Bilateral	Relating to both sides
Bite reflex	A reflex that causes the child to close the mouth tightly when touched on the lips, tongue or gums
Body awareness	A knowledge of one's body, in terms of both the idea of one's body's different parts and their relation to each another

Body image	An appreciation of one's body parts. Body image plays a significant role in the development of motor and perceptual skills
Cerebral palsy	A disorder of movement and posture resulting from a non-progressive defect of the brain occurring in earliest childhood
Clonus	Shaking movements of hypertonic (spastic) muscles after the muscles have been suddenly stretched
Cognitive	Involving a learning rather than a physical process
Colour perception	The recognition and differentiation of hues and intensity of colour
Concentration	Taking interest in and trying to understand a task
Concept of space	An understanding of the body acting as a point of reference in relation to objects in the environment, for example up/down, under/over, in front/behind
Conductive loss	A hearing loss due to blockage or infection
Contracture	Permanently tight soft tissues (muscles, tendons etc.)
Contralateral	Refers to the opposite side, usually referring to extremities
Coordination	Control of the action of the muscles of the body working together in different areas
Cyanosis	Blue discoloration due to circulation of imperfectly oxygenated blood
Deformities	Body or limbs fixed in abnormal positions
Developmental scales	These indicate the mean ages at which different skills in various areas of development are achieved, but there is a wide variation
Diplegia	A descriptive term used to describe the motor involvement when the lower limbs are more affected than the upper limbs
Dorsiflexion	Lifting the foot up towards the lower leg
Dysarthria	Difficulty in articulation due to an impairment of nerve muscular control. Speech is slow, sluggish and monotonous
Dyslexia	Difficulty in reading due to an inherent inability to understand or reproduce written symbols
Dyspraxia	Difficulty in planning movements and putting them into the necessary sequence
Equilibrium	State of balance
Equinus	Walking on the toes due to a shortening of the calf muscles/soft tissues
Eversion	Turning-out of the foot so that the sole of the foot faces outwards – a valgus position
Extension	Straightening of any body parts
Eye–motor coordination	Ability to coordinate vision with motor activities
Fine motor skills	Hand and finger movements such as grasp and release, handwriting and using a pair of scissors
Finger grasp	Grasping between thumb and one or more fingers
Flexion	Bending of any body parts
Fluctuating tone	Combination of high and low muscle tone
Form perception	The ability to see a pattern of parts making a whole

Function	The ability to deal with tasks of daily living such as eating and toileting
Gestures	Movements used to communicate
Gravity	The pull of gravity cannot be seen but affects all one's movements from birth onwards
Gross motor skills	Movements and position of the head, trunk and limbs such as sitting, crawling and walking
Handling	Holding and moving a child
Head control	The ability to control the movements of the head
Hemiplegia	A descriptive term which is used to describe the motor involvement when one side of the body is affected
Hypertonus	Increased tension in a muscle (high tone/spasticity)
Hypotonia	Decreased tension in a muscle (low tone/floppiness)
Intelligence	Cognitive/learning ability enabling the child to understand the world, including information about the environment
Inversion	Turning-in of the foot so that the sole of the foot faces inwards – a varus position
Involuntary movements	Uncontrolled movements
Kinaesthetic	The ability to perceive movement
Kyphosis	Rounded upper spine
Language	1. Inner language is used for thinking and talking to oneself
	2. Receptive language is an understanding of what is said to one
	3. Expressive language is the ability to communicate one's ideas to others using words, gestures and written symbols appropriately
Laterally	The sides, for example, of the body
Locomotion	Means of propulsion, to move through space
Muscle tone	The state of tension in muscles at rest and when one moves, regulated under normal circumstances subconsciously in such a way that the tension is sufficiently high to withstand the pull of gravity, that is to keep one upright, but that it is never too strong to interfere with one's movements
Nystagmus	Continual oscillation of the eyeballs
Otitis media	Glue ear
Palmar grasp	An object grasped between the palm and two or more fingers
Passive	That which is done to the child without help or cooperation from the child
Pathological	Abnormal
Pelvic tilt	1. Anterior tilt, extension of the lumbar spine (hollow back)
	2. Posterior tilt, flexion of the lumbar spine (rounded back)
Perceptual behaviours	The process of organizing and interpreting the sensations an individual receives from both internal and external stimuli, for example auditory, tactile, vestibular and kinaesthetic stimuli
Perseveration	The unnecessary repetition of movement and/or speech

Phonation	The ability to utter vocal sounds
Pincer grasp	The use of thumb and index finger to grasp small objects
Plantar flexion	Pointing of the foot downwards
Plantar surface	The sole of the foot
Postural stability	An antigravity mechanism, essential if one is to move and balance in a smooth, controlled, coordinated manner from one position to another
Postural tone	The potential a muscle has for action. The degree of muscle tension at a particular point in time constantly alters in response to movements and changes in posture
Posture	The positioning and alignment of the body and the position from which a movement takes place
Primitive movements	Early movements
Pronation	Turning-in of the forearm with the palm of the hand facing downwards
Prone	Lying on the tummy
Proprioception	Information from the muscles, joints and vestibular systems providing one with information about one's body position and movement
Protective reactions/saving reactions	Automatic reactions which protect the head and body following loss of balance, for example throwing out the arms and hands to protect the face when falling
Protraction	Pulling forward of part of the body, for example the shoulders
Quadriplegia	A descriptive term which is used to describe the motor involvement when all four limbs are affected
Reciprocal movements	Alternate movements of the arms and/or legs
Reflexes	Postures and movements beyond a child's voluntary control
Retardation	Slowing down of physical and/or mental development
Retraction	Drawing back of part of the body, for example the shoulders
Righting reactions	Automatic reactions which enable one to maintain the normal position of the head in space and in relation to the trunk, for example when the body moves, the face remains vertical, the mouth horizontal
Rigidity	Very stiff posture
Rotation	Usually refers to movement taking place between the shoulder and pelvic girdles but can also refer to movement of the head or limbs
Scoliosis	Curvature of the spine (usually a long C curve in children with cerebral palsy)
Sensorimotor integration	Movements of the limbs send stimuli (messages) to the brain to modify the strength, speed and frequency of the limb movements
Side flexion	Bending of the body/trunk sideways
Skilled activity	A programme of action directed towards the attainment of a specified task
Spasticity (hypertonus)	The muscles in a varying state of cocontraction (stiffness)
Speech	The process of producing sounds and combining these with words

Stereognosis	The ability to recognize shape, size and/or weight of objects
Stereotype	Unchanging
Subluxation	Partial dislocation of a joint, usually the hip
Supination	Turning-out of the forearm, so that the palm of the hand faces upwards
Supine	Lying on the back
Symmetry	Equality between the body parts, usually between the two sides
Trunk	The body as distinct from the limbs
Unilateral	Relating to one side
Valgus	A pronated position of the feet (flat feet)
Varus	A supinated position of the feet
Vestibular apparatus	This is found in the inner ear, influencing equilibrium/balance, posture and special orientation
Visual memory	The ability to retain and reproduce objects seen
Visual organization	The ability to scan and sequence with the eyes
Voluntary movements	Movements undertaken with intention
Weight shift	The ability to shift one's weight against gravity, allowing an adjustment in the trunk so that movements of the limbs can take place, for example walking
Windswept hip	When lying the pelvis is usually elevated and rotated (retracted) on one side with the hip adducted and inwardly rotated on that side. When sitting one leg appears shorter than the other

Index

A

Ability
  assessment of, 2–3
  learning, assessment of, 75–76
Acceptance
  of CP, 57–58, 86
  of help, 60
  social, 60
Accidents, epilepsy association, 53
Activity centres, 314
Acupuncture, 377–378
Adeli suit therapy, 377
Adjustment to CP, 58–59
Admission to hospital, *See* Hospital, admissions
Aids/adaptations, *See* Equipment; *individual functions/*
    purposes (e.g. bathing)
Air travel, 299
Alberta Infant Motor Scale (AIMS), 391
Alternative therapies, *See* Complementary and alternative
    medicine (CAM)
Anaesthesia, general, in epilepsy, 53
Anal sphincters, 182
Ankle
  deformities, 362
  examination, 343
  plantar flexion, *See* Equinus
  problems, 25–26, 362, 363
Ankle foot orthoses (AFOs), 353, 355, 361, 362–365
  aims and benefits, 365
  duration of use, 363–364
  fitting, process, 363, 364
Antiepileptic drugs
  cognitive and behavioural effects, 50
  commonly used, 51–52
  discontinuation, 50
  monitoring, 50
  in status epilepticus, 46–47
  treatment targets, 49, 50
  when to start treatment, 49
  See also Epilepsy
Appointments, hospital, 7–8
Approval, of behaviour/actions, 65–66
Arm
  examination, 311
    See also Upper-limb
  length differences, 357
Arthrodesis, 373
Aspiration, 22
  milk/food, 151
Assessment
  of ability, 2–3
  hand function, 251–252
  hospital, 7–8, 10–11
  learning ability, 75–76
  risk, moving and lifting, 167–168
  seating, 285–286
  speech, 234, 235–236
  swallow safety, 159
  upper-limb function, 251–252
Ataxia, 17, 103
Ataxic cerebral palsy, 17, 103
Athetoid cerebral palsy, 17, 103
  abnormal postures, 114–115, 121
  bouncing, 134
  bridging movement, 110
  bunny hopping movement, 112
  carrying child with, 170–171
  creeping movement, 110, 111
  dressing, 204, 205, 208
  handling recommendations, 121–125, 128–129, 131
  pulling up to sitting, 133